T0293661

Antibiotic Drug Discovery and Development

Antibiotic Drug Discovery and Development

Edited by Trish Grantham

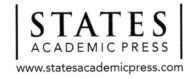

www.statesacademicpress.com

States Academic Press,
109 South 5th Street,
Brooklyn, NY 11249, USA

Visit us on the World Wide Web at:
www.statesacademicpress.com

ISBN: 978-1-63989-770-4

Cataloging-in-Publication Data

Antibiotic drug discovery and development / edited by Trish Grantham.
    p. cm.
Includes bibliographical references and index.
ISBN 978-1-63989-770-4
1. Antibiotics. 2. Drug interactions. 3. Drugs--Physiological effect.
4. Pharmaceutical chemistry. I. Grantham, Trish.
RM267 .A58 2023
615.792 2--dc23

Table of Contents

Preface

Antibiotic drugs or antibacterial drugs are a group of substances that combat disease-causing bacteria. Antibiotic drug discovery refers to a process through which new antibiotic drugs are identified. Antibiotic drugs can be discovered using different models such as computational, experimental, translational, and clinical models. The process of discovering new medications based on knowledge of biological targets is known as drug design. After a lead compound has been identified through the drug discovery process, the process to bring a new pharmaceutical drug to the market begins. This process is called drug development. There are three major steps involved in the process of drug discovery and development. The first step includes carrying out preclinical research using cell-based and animal models. The second step involves carrying out clinical trials on humans. The last step involves obtaining approval from the required regulatory authority for marketing the drugs. This book is a compilation of recent developments in antibiotic drug discovery and development. A number of latest researches have been included to keep the readers up-to-date with the latest advancements in this field.

This book is the end result of constructive efforts and intensive research done by experts in this field. The aim of this book is to enlighten the readers with recent information in this area of research. The information provided in this profound book would serve as a valuable reference to students and researchers in this field.

At the end, I would like to thank all the authors for devoting their precious time and providing their valuable contribution to this book. I would also like to express my gratitude to my fellow colleagues who encouraged me throughout the process.

Editor

Reprogramming of the Antibacterial Drug Vancomycin Results in Potent Antiviral Agents Devoid of Antibacterial Activity

Zsolt Szűcs [1,2], Lieve Naesens [3], Annelies Stevaert [3], Eszter Ostorházi [4], Gyula Batta [5], Pál Herczegh [1] and Anikó Borbás [1,*]

[1] Department of Pharmaceutical Chemistry, University of Debrecen, Egyetem tér 1, H-4032 Debrecen, Hungary; szucs.zsolt@pharm.unideb.hu (Z.S.); herczegh.pal@pharm.unideb.hu (P.H.)
[2] Doctoral School of Pharmaceutical Sciences, University of Debrecen, Egyetem tér 1, H-4032 Debrecen, Hungary
[3] Rega Institute for Medical Research, KU Leuven, B-3000 Leuven; Belgium; lieve.naesens@kuleuven.be (L.N.); annelies.stevaert@kuleuven.be (A.S.)
[4] Department of Medical Microbiology, Semmelweis University, Nagyvárad tér 4, H-1089 Budapest, Hungary; ostorhazi.eszter@med.semmelweis-univ.hu
[5] Department of Organic Chemistry, University of Debrecen, H-4032 Debrecen, Hungary; batta@unideb.hu
* Correspondence: borbas.aniko@pharm.unideb.hu

Abstract: Influenza A and B viruses are a global threat to human health and increasing resistance to the existing antiviral drugs necessitates new concepts to expand the therapeutic options. Glycopeptide derivatives have emerged as a promising new class of antiviral agents. To avoid potential antibiotic resistance, these antiviral glycopeptides are preferably devoid of antibiotic activity. We prepared six vancomycin aglycone hexapeptide derivatives with the aim of obtaining compounds having anti-influenza virus but no antibacterial activity. Two of them exerted strong and selective inhibition of influenza A and B virus replication, while antibacterial activity was successfully eliminated by removing the critical N-terminal moiety. In addition, these two molecules offered protection against several other viruses, such as herpes simplex virus, yellow fever virus, Zika virus, and human coronavirus, classifying these glycopeptides as broad antiviral molecules with a favorable therapeutic index.

Keywords: glycopeptide antibiotic; vancomycin aglycone hexapeptide; antiviral; influenza virus; human coronavirus

1. Introduction

Seasonal infections by influenza A and B viruses are each year responsible for significant morbidity and mortality [1]. Besides, zoonotic influenza A viruses occasionally enter the human population to cause serious pandemics with a high number of fatalities [2]. Antiviral drugs are essential for influenza treatment and prevention, including in the context of pandemic preparedness. At the moment, four drug classes are available: The M2 ion channel blockers and neuraminidase inhibitors, approved in all countries [3], and two polymerase inhibitors, recently approved in a few countries [4,5]. For each of these drugs, emergence of resistant mutants is possible; this is particularly problematic when the mutant viruses are fit and human-to-human transmissible [6–9]. Hence, additional drug classes with a distinct mechanism of action remain essential [10–12].

Several recent investigations demonstrated that some antibiotics from bacterial origin display interesting antiviral properties [13] representing a unique example of drug repurposing [14].

Glycopeptide antibiotics like teicoplanin, dalbavancin, oritavancin, and telavancin were shown to inhibit Ebola pseudovirus infection [15] and prevent the host cell entry process of Ebola virus, Middle East respiratory syndrome coronavirus (MERS-CoV) and severe acute respiratory syndrome coronavirus (SARS-CoV) [16]. Moreover, semisynthetic hydrophobic derivatives of vancomycin and teicoplanin antibiotics were reported to inhibit HIV [17,18], SARS-CoV [19], HCV [20], and flaviviruses [21]. The anti-influenza virus potential of lipophilic derivatives of glycopeptide antibiotics was first discovered by our group. We reported a class of molecules with various lipophilic modifications at the N-terminal part of the peptide core of ristocetin, showing robust inhibition of influenza virus replication in cell culture [22]. Mechanistic studies with the lead compound demonstrated interference with virus uptake by endocytosis [23]. Encouraged by the favorable selectivity of this compound, we prepared a series of ristocetin and teicoplanin analogues in a systematic manner, to gain further insight in the structure-activity relationship [24–29].

Recently, we prepared a series of teicoplanin pseudoaglycone (TC) derivatives by coupling one or two lipophilic side chains to the N-terminus of the glycopeptide core, using triazole, sulfonamide or maleimide linking elements [30]. Some of the modifications yielded remarkably effective inhibitors of influenza A and B viruses with low cytotoxicity. Besides the potent antiviral effect, most analogues proved to be also active against Gram-positive bacteria including vancomycin resistant enterococci. Due to the global threat of antibiotic resistance, the antibacterial activity in this case represents a drawback that could hinder application of these types of derivatives as antiviral agents. The undesirable antibacterial activity of antiviral glycopeptides has been suggested by others as well. Several glycopeptide analogues have been synthesized and evaluated against retroviruses [17,18]. As the antibacterial activity of these derivatives was a concern, the same researchers prepared and evaluated aminodecyl and adamantyl functionalized compounds with partially destroyed peptide cores [31]. These degradation products lacking antibacterial activity typically displayed more-or-less weaker antiviral properties than the intact analogues. Similarly, in the present work we decided to overcome the issue of intrinsic antibacterial activity by using a degraded glycopeptide aglycone, but also exploiting the results of our study on antiviral TC derivatives [30] at the same time.

The first step in the synthetic plan was to select three TC derivatives with optimal antiviral activity combined with low cytotoxicity from our former antiviral study. As for the elimination of the antibacterial activity, obtaining a degradation product with no antibacterial activity from teicoplanin antibiotics is a very difficult task. Even after destroying one or more amide bonds of the peptide core (which are key in binding to the target bacterial cell-wall precursors) some activity still persists [32,33]. The complete elimination of the antibacterial activity requires the concurrent removal of amino acids 1 and 3, which is rather laborious [34]. As such, the simple postliminary degradation of the selected TC derivatives was considered implausible. On the other hand, in the case of vancomycin or its aglycone, the N-terminal N-methyl-D-leucine moiety can be easily removed by Edman-degradation [35,36] yielding hexapeptide derivatives that are inactive against bacteria, likely due to their inability to bind to the target cell-wall precursors terminating in D-Ala-D-Ala. Since we previously determined, that the antiviral activity of TC derivatives is primarily influenced by the structure of the side chains [30], we envisioned that we could reprogram vancomycin to create selective antiviral agents free of antibacterial activity by incorporating the appropriate lipophilic moieties of the former teicoplanins into vancomycin aglycone hexapeptide.

2. Results and Discussion

2.1. Chemistry

We synthesized a total of six derivatives by preparing two variants for the three selected side chains. These two variations consist of modifying the vancomycin aglycone hexapeptide in either the N- or C-terminal position. In this way, we wanted to learn whether the side chain attachment site influences the antiviral activity.

To synthesize the first variant, we used literature procedures to prepare vancomycin aglycone (1) and its hexapeptide derivative (2) by the Edman degradation (Scheme 1) [35,36]. Then, by the copper-catalyzed diazotransfer reaction, the N-terminal azido derivative (3) was successfully prepared in analogy to our previous work [24,30].

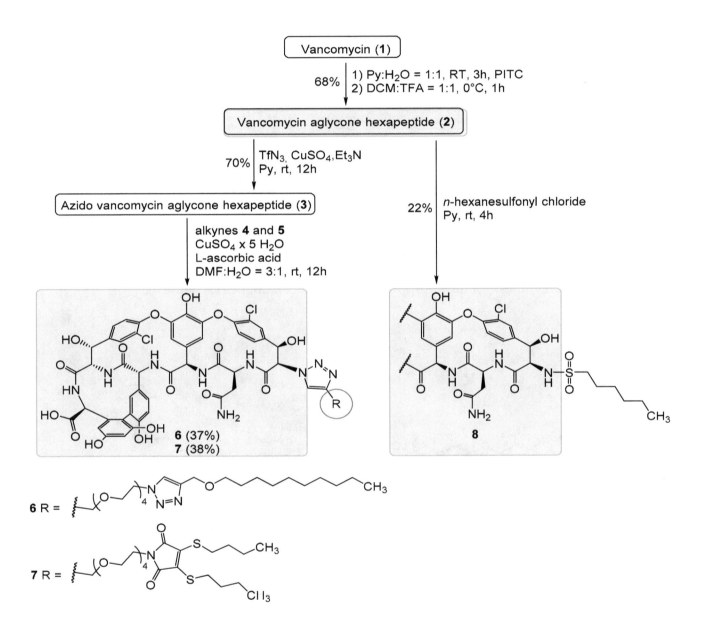

Scheme 1. Synthesis and structures of vancomycin aglycone hexapeptide derivatives 6–8 modified on the N-terminus. See Scheme 2 for the structures of alkynes 4 and 5.

The subsequent copper-catalyzed azide-alkyne click reaction using alkyne compound 4 (Scheme 2) yielded triazole derivative 6. The second compound modified on the N-terminus (7) was prepared by the same method using the already described maleimide derivative 5 [30] as the alkyne compound in the final step. The third derivative (8) in this group was synthesized using derivative 2 and hexanesulfonyl chloride by sulfonamide formation, similar to what we previously published for teicoplanin congeners [30].

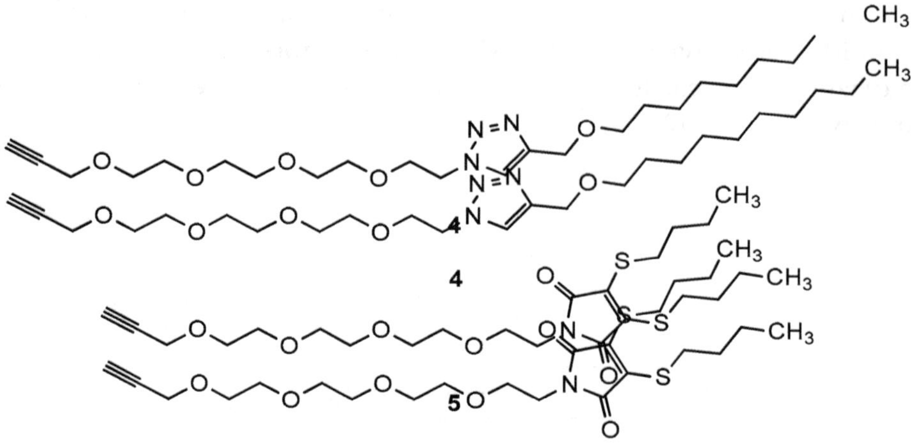

Scheme 2. Structures of previously prepared alkynes **4** and **5** used for the synthesis of derivatives **6** and **7**.

As for the *C*-terminal modifications, we decided to prepare two derivatives carrying a 1,2,3-triazole ring, since this moiety often generates bioactive analogues [37]. In order to minimize the structural difference between the side chain in the *N*-versus *C*-terminal position, we used 2-azidoethylamine as a small linker for the synthesis of the appropriate *C*-terminal analogues (Scheme 3).

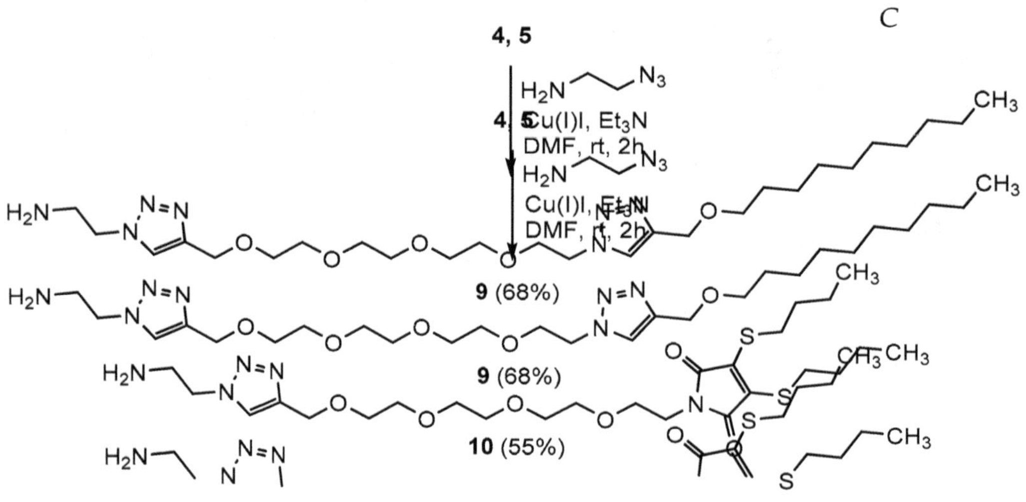

Scheme 3. Synthesis of amines **9-10** for the *C*-terminal modifications.

After preparation of the amines, the reaction of compound **2** with amine **9** using the PyBOP reagent gave amide derivative **11** (Scheme 4). Using the same conditions, the reaction between compound **2** and maleimide **10** as the alkyne compound yielded compound **12**. In the case of the *C*-terminal sulfonamide derivative **13** we also used the similar, small linker moiety. In this approach, an amine functionalized sulfonamide was first synthesized from *n*-hexanesulfonyl chloride and ethylenediamine, then the peptide coupling reaction between this compound and compound **2** using PyBOP yielded compound **13**.

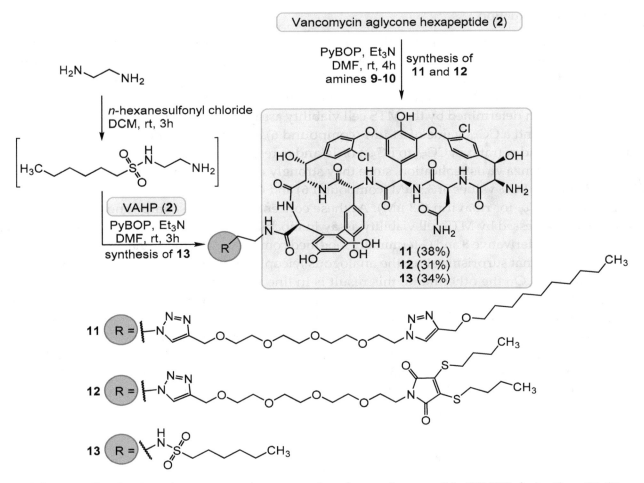

Scheme 4. Synthesis and structures of vancomycin aglycone hexapeptide (VAHP) derivatives **11–13** modified on the C-terminus.

2.2. Biology

2.2.1. Antibacterial Evaluation

Antibacterial tests were carried out by the broth microdilution method on a panel of eight Gram-positive bacterial strains, using vancomycin and teicoplanin as reference compounds. Neither of the new compounds exhibited significant activity against any bacterium, proving successful elimination of antibacterial activity, as anticipated (Table 1).

Table 1. Antibacterial evaluation of the new vancomycin aglycone hexapeptide derivatives.

Bacteria	In Vitro MIC in µg/mL							
	TEI	VAN	6	7	8	11	12	13
B. subtilis ATCC 6633	0.5	0.5	32	32	32	32	256	256
S. aureus MSSA ATCC 29213	0.5	0.5	128	256	256	256	256	256
S. aureus MRSA ATCC 33591	0.5	0.5	128	256	256	256	256	256
S. epidermidis ATCC 35984	4	2	32	32	32	256	128	128
S. epidermidis mecA	16	4	32	32	64	256	256	128
E. faecalis ATCC 29212	1	1	32	32	32	128	128	64
E. faecalis 15,376 VanA	256	256	128	256	256	256	256	256
E. faecalis ATCC 51,299 VanB	0.5	128	128	256	128	256	256	128

TEI: teicoplanin, VAN: vancomycin.

2.2.2. Antiviral Evaluation

With regard to antiviral activity, the two N-terminal triazole derivatives **6** and **7** displayed robust activity against the three influenza A or B viruses tested. Upon microscopic inspection, no virus-induced cytopathic effect (CPE) was observed in virus-infected cells treated with 6.25 µM of compound **6** or compound **7** (Figure 1A). The quantitative antiviral efficacy (EC$_{50}$) and cytotoxicity (CC$_{50}$) values, both determined by the MTS cell viability assay, are summarized in Table 2. With EC$_{50}$ values of ~3 µM and a CC$_{50}$ value of 41 µM (compound **6**) and 18 µM (compound **7**), the molecules had a selectivity index (ratio of CC$_{50}$ to EC$_{50}$) of 14 and 6, respectively. Both molecules exhibited clear inhibition of influenza virus replication, since they strongly reduced the virus yield in the supernatant (Figure 1B), giving EC$_{99}$ values of 3.5 µM (compound **6**) and 4.6 µM (compound **7**), which is 5- to 6-fold lower than the EC$_{99}$ for ribavirin (23 µM). At these concentrations, the compounds were devoid of cytotoxicity, as assessed by MTS cell viability assay in mock-infected cells (Figure 1C). The N-terminal n-hexanesulfonyl derivative **8** and C-terminally modified compound **11** proved inactive. For compound **8**, this was somewhat surprising since the analogous teicoplanin pseudoaglycone derivative showed high activity [30]. On the other hand, this result is in line with our previous findings on ristocetin and teicoplanin aglycone derivatives, indicating that even minor structural differences in the peptide core can lead to significantly different anti-influenza virus activity [27]. The C-terminally modified compounds **12** and **13** were only slightly active against one or both influenza A virus strains. Compared to compounds **6** and **7**, compound **13** displayed an 8-fold higher antiviral EC$_{50}$ value by MTS assay (Table 2); its lower potency was also evident in the virus yield reduction assay (Figure 1B). This points to the importance of the modification site, since the C-terminally modified compounds were clearly inferior to the N-terminal analogues.

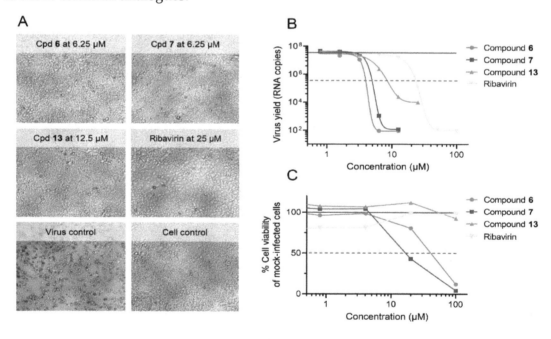

Figure 1. Anti-influenza virus activity of compounds **6**, **7**, and **13**, in MDCK cells at day 3 p.i. with A/PR/8/34 virus. (**A**) Representative images showing complete inhibition of viral cytopathic effect (CPE) at compound concentrations devoid of any cytotoxicity. (**B**) Reduction in virus yield, as determined by RT-qPCR for viral RNA in the supernatant (lower limit of detection: 10$^{1.6}$ copies). Curve fitting by GraphPad Prism, on two data points from one experiment performed in duplicate. Full grey line: Virus yield for untreated virus control; red dashed line: 100-fold reduction in virus yield. (**C**) Compound cytotoxicity in mock-infected cells, determined by MTS cell viability assay (mean data from three experiments). Full grey line: 100% viability in the cell control receiving no compound; red dashed line: 50% cell viability.

Table 2. Anti-influenza virus activity and cytotoxicity in MDCK [1] cells.

Compound	CC_{50} [2] (μM)	Antiviral EC_{50} [3] (μM)		
		Influenza A/H1N1	Influenza A/H3N2	Influenza B
6	41	4.1	1.4	3.2
7	18	3.6	2.0	3.2
8	100	>100	>100	>100
11	$\geq$20	>100	>100	>100
12	100	12	>100	>100
13	>100	34	14	>100
Ribavirin	>100	7.0	6.4	7.2
Zanamivir	>100	0.4	9.0	4.5

[1] Madin Darby canine kidney cells. Virus strains: A/H1N1: A/Ned/378/05; A/H3N2: A/Victoria/361/11; and B/Ned/537/05. [2] 50% Cytotoxic concentration based on the formazan-based MTS cell viability assay. [3] 50% Effective concentration, i.e., concentration producing 50% inhibition of virus-induced cytopathic effect, as determined by the MTS cell viability assay.

Encouraged by the promising anti-influenza virus activity of compounds **6** and **7**, we tested the two compounds against a range of DNA- and RNA-viruses evaluated in human embryonic lung (HEL) fibroblast, HeLa or Vero cells. For each virus, appropriate reference compounds were included. Protection against virus-induced cytopathicity as well as compound cytotoxicity were determined by the MTS cell viability assay. As shown in Table 3, the two compounds exhibited broad protection against a large variety of viruses, including herpesvirus types 1 and 2 and vaccinia virus. They retained full effectivity against a thymidine kinase deficient form of HSV-1, which was 61-fold (acyclovir) and 89-fold (ganciclovir) resistant to antiherpetic drugs.

Moreover, the compounds proved effective against two emerging pathogens for which no therapy is currently approved, i.e., coronavirus (inhibited by compounds **6** and **7**) and Zika virus (inhibited by compound **7**). At a non-toxic concentration of 25 μM of compound **6**, no coronavirus 229E-induced cytopathicity could be observed microscopically (Figure 2A), which agrees with an EC_{50} value of 11 μM as determined by MTS cell viability assay (Table 3).

In addition, treatment of infected cells with 25 μM of compound **6** resulted in a 1000-fold reduction of the viral RNA copy number in the supernatant, yielding an EC_{99} value of 20 μM for reduction of virus yield (Figure 2B). Hence, we established, by virus yield assays, that compound **6** suppresses the replication of influenza virus and coronavirus, and for the other viruses, activity was indicated by the protection against viral CPE. This broad activity against distinct viruses fits with our hypothesis that these molecules may act by disrupting the viral endocytosis process, similarly to what we reported for a glycopeptide active against influenza virus [23] and what was described for Ebola virus and MERS and SARS coronaviruses [15,16]. This should become clear from mechanistic work ongoing in our laboratory.

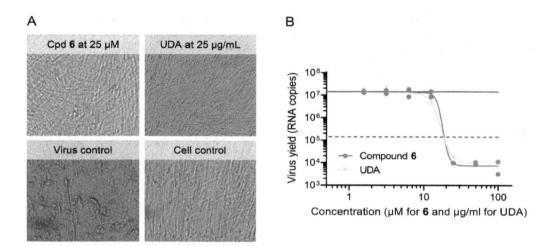

Figure 2. Activity of compound **6** in human embryonic lung (HEL) cells infected with human coronavirus 229E. (**A**) Representative images showing complete inhibition of viral CPE at non-toxic compound concentrations (reference compound: UDA lectin). (**B**) Reduction in virus yield, as determined by RT-qPCR for viral RNA in the supernatant at day 4 p.i. (lower limit of detection: 10^2 copies). Curve fitting by GraphPad Prism, on two data points from one experiment performed in duplicate. Full grey line: virus yield for untreated virus control; red dashed line: 100-fold reduction in virus yield.

Table 3. Evaluation of compounds **6** and **7** against a broad range of DNA- and RNA-viruses [1].

Compound	CC_{50} [2] (µM)			Antiviral EC_{50} [3] (µM) - cell line [4]							
	HEL	HeLa	Vero	HEL					HeLa	Vero	
				HSV-1	HSV-2	HSV-1/TK⁻	Vaccinia Virus	Human Coronavirus 229E	RSV	Yellow Fever Virus	Zika Virus
6	>100	>100	>100	20	7.8	7.4	7.2	11	7.7	>100	>100
7	>100	>100	>100	43	6.5	11	32	32	60	55	14
Cidofovir	>250	>250	>250	2.4	1.0	5.8	37	-	-	-	-
Aciclovir	>250	>250	>250	2.4	0.05	146	>250	-	-	-	-
Ganciclovir	>100	>100	>100	0.1	0.03	8.9	>100	-	-	-	-
UDA [5]	>100	>100	>100	-	-	-	-	1.8	-	-	-
Ribavirin	>250	>250	>250	-	-	-	-	-	5.0	119	-
Mycophenolic acid	>100	>100	>100	-	-	-	-	-	-	0.7	0.8

[1] Viruses: herpes simplex virus type 1 (HSV-1) or type 2 (HSV-2); a thymidine-kinase deficient (TK⁻) mutant of HSV-1; vaccinia virus; human coronavirus 229E; respiratory syncytial virus (RSV); yellow fever virus and Zika virus. [2] 50% Cytotoxic concentration, assessed in mock-infected cells by the MTS cell viability assay. [3] 50% Effective concentration offering 50% protection against virus-induced CPE, as determined by the MTS assay. [4] Cell lines: HEL, human embryonic lung fibroblast cells; HeLa, human cervix carcinoma cells; Vero, African Green monkey kidney cells. [5] UDA: Urtica dioica agglutinin lectin; for this compound, concentrations are expressed in µg/mL.

3. Materials and Methods

3.1. Chemistry

Vancomycin hydrochloride was a gift from TEVA Pharmaceutical Industries Ltd. (Debrecen, Hungary). Vancomycin aglycone hexapeptide, trifluoromethanesulfonyl azide, compounds **4** and **5** were prepared as described elsewhere [24,30]. TLC was performed on Kieselgel 60 F_{254} (Merck) with detection either by immersing into ammonium molybdate-sulfuric acid solution followed by heating or by using Pauly's reagent for detection. Flash column chromatography was performed using Silica gel 60 (Merck 0.040-0.063 mm) and Silica gel 60 silanized (0.063–0.200 mm). The ^{1}H NMR (500MHz, 400 MHz) ^{13}C NMR (125 MHz, 100 MHz) and 2D NMR spectra were recorded with a Bruker DRX-400 and Bruker Avance II 500 spectrometers at 300K. Chemical shifts are referenced to Me_4Si and to the solvent residual signals. MALDI-TOF MS analysis of the compounds was carried out in the positive reflectron mode using a BIFLEX III mass spectrometer (Bruker, Bremen, Germany) equipped with delayed-ion extraction. 2,5-Dihydroxybenzoic acid (DHB) was used as matrix and CF_3COONa as cationizing agent in DMF. Elemental analysis (C, H, N, S) was performed on an Elementar Vario MicroCube instrument.

Synthesis

Synthesis of azido vancomycin aglycone hexapeptide (3): 350 mg (0.34 mmol) vancomycin aglycone hexapeptide (2) was obtained from 750 mg (0.5 mmol) vancomycin hydrochloride (1) by Edman degradation as described in the literature [35,36]. Sodium azide (65 mg, 1.0 mmol) was added to dry pyridine (1.5 mL) cooled to 0–5 °C. Tf_2O (0.8 mmol, 134 µL) was added dropwise over the course of about 30 min. The reaction mixture was stirred for another 2 h at 0–5 °C. Then, 350 mg (0.34 mmol) of 2 was dissolved in 15 mL pyridine, then 95 µL (2.0 equiv., 0.68 mmol) Et_3N was added followed by the solution (1.5 mL) of the freshly prepared trifluoromethanesulfonyl azide, and finally 800 µL of a 10 mg/mL $CuSO_4 \cdot 5H_2O$ solution. The solution was stirred at room temperature overnight, then the solvents were evaporated. The crude product was dissolved in dilute NH_4OH, then the pH was set to 1-2 with 1N HCl, the resulting cloudy mixture was extracted with n-BuOH three times, the butanolic phase was washed with water, then evaporated and purified by flash column chromatography using step gradient elution (MeCN:H_2O = 100:0→97:3→94:6→92:8). The title compound was obtained in 250 mg yield (70%) as an off-white powder. NMR: see Table S1 in supporting information. MALDI-MS m/z calcd. for $C_{46}H_{37}Cl_2N_9O_{16}$ + Na^+ [M + Na]$^+$: 1064.16. Found: 1064.129.

Synthesis of compound 6: 132 mg (0.127 mmol) of 2 was dissolved in 2.0 mL of DMF:H_2O 3:1 mixture. Next, 72 mg (1.25 equiv., 0.16 mmol) of alkyne 4 was added, followed by 6 mg $CuSO_4 \cdot 5H_2O$. The reaction mixture was stirred at room temperature for 12 h. By this time TLC (cellulose, n-PrOH: cc. NH_4OH = 6:4) indicated good conversion. The solvents were evaporated until a syrupy residue was obtained. Ether was added, and the product was filtered off after precipitation and washed with additional ether to remove the excess alkyne. Purification was carried out by C_{18} reverse phase column chromatography (H_2O:MeCN = 70:30→60:40→55:45) followed by gel chromatography using Sephadex LH-20 in MeOH. The title compound was obtained as a white powder in 69 mg yield (37%). NMR: see Table S2 in supporting information. Elemental analysis: see Table S8 in supporting information. MALDI-MS m/z calcd. for $C_{70}H_{80}Cl_2N_{12}O_{21}$ + Na^+ [M + Na]$^+$: 1517.48. Found: 1517.68.

Synthesis of compound 7: 93 mg (0.09 mmol) of compound 3 was dissolved in 2.0 mL of DMF:H_2O 3:1 mixture. 54 mg (1.25 equiv., 0.111 mmol) of alkyne 5 was added followed 5 mg $CuSO_4 \times 5H_2O$. After 12 h stirring at room temperature, TLC indicated good conversion. The reaction mixture was worked up and purified by C_{18} reverse phase column chromatography as described above. The title compound was obtained as a yellow powder in 52 mg yield (38%). NMR: see Table S3 in supporting information. Elemental analysis: see Table S8 in supporting information. MALDI-MS m/z calcd. for $C_{69}H_{74}Cl_2N_{10}O_{22}S_2$ + Na^+ [M + Na]$^+$: 1551.369. Found: 1551.367.

Synthesis of compound 8: 78 mg (0.077 mmol) of 2 was dissolved in 3 mL dry pyridine and 0.5 mL dry DMF, then 19 µL (1.5 equiv., 0.115 mmol) of n-hexanesulfonyl chloride was added. After stirring 3 h at room temperature, ethyl acetate and ether was added, the resulting precipitate was filtered and washed with ether. The crude product was purified by flash column chromatography using Toluene: MeOH = 7:3→6:4 as eluent, followed by gel chromatography using Sephadex LH-20 with MeOH: H_2O = 6:4 as eluent. The yield was 20 mg (22%). NMR: see Table S4 in supporting information. Elemental analysis: see Table S8 in supporting information. MALDI-MS m/z calcd. for $C_{52}H_{51}Cl_2N_7O_{18}S$ + Na^+ [M + Na]$^+$: 1186.228. Found: 1186.276.

Synthesis of 2-(4-(13-(4-((decyloxy)methyl)-1H-1,2,3-triazol-1-yl)-2,5,8,11-tetraoxatridecyl)-1H-1,2,3-triazol-1-yl)ethanamine (9): 207 mg of 4 [24,30] (0.46 mmol) and 39 mg (0.46 mmol) of 2-azidoethylamine were dissolved in 2 mL dry DMF under argon. 70 µL (1.08 equiv., 0.5 mmol) Et_3N was added, then 17 mg (20 mol%, 0.09 mmol) Cu(I)I. The reaction mixture was stirred at room temperature for an hour. After evaporation of the solvents, the crude product was purified by flash column chromatography using DCM: MeOH = 95:5 (+0.1% v/v NH_4OH) as eluent. The title compound was obtained as an off white solid in 68% yield (171 mg).

^{1}H NMR (400 MHz, CDCl$_3$) δ 7.73 (s, 2H, 2 x triazole CH), 4.69 (s, 2H, NCH_2), 4.61 (s, 2H, NCH_2), 4.53 (t, J = 5.1 Hz, 2H), 4.41 (s, 2H), 3.87 (t, J = 5.0 Hz, 2H), 3.76–3.55 (m, 14H, 7 × CH_2), 3.51 (t, J = 6.7 Hz, 2H), 1.59 (p, J = 6.9 Hz, 2H), 1.35–1.21 (m, 14H, 7 × CH_2), 0.88 (t, J = 6.8 Hz, 3H). ^{13}C NMR (101 MHz, CDCl$_3$) δ 123.71 (2C, 2 x triazole CH), 70.95, 70.62, 70.56, 69.86, 69.58, 64.81, 64.35 (10C 10 × CH_2), 50.30 (N–CH_2), 31.97, 29.76, 29.67, 29.65, 29.57, 29.39, 26.21, 22.75 (8C, 8 × CH_2), 14.20 (CH_3). MALDI-MS m/z calcd. for C$_{26}$H$_{49}$N$_7$O$_5$ + Na [M + Na]$^+$: 562.37. Found: 562.37.

Synthesis of 1-(1-(1-(2-aminoethyl)-1H-1,2,3-triazol-4-yl)-2,5,8,11-tetraoxatridecan-13-yl)-3,4-bis(butylthio)-1H-pyrrole-2,5-dione (**10**): 208 mg (0.43 mmol) of compound **5 [30]** and 44 mg (1.2 equiv., 0.52 mmol) of azidoethylamine were dissolved in 2 mL dry DMF under argon. 66 μL (1.1 equiv., 0.47 mmol) Et$_3$N was added followed by 16 mg (20 mol%) Cu(I)I. The reaction mixture was stirred for 2 h at room temperature. After evaporation the crude product was purified by flash column chromatography using DCM: MeOH = 100:0→93:7 (+0.1% v/v NH$_4$OH) as eluent. The yield was 154 mg (55%), yellow syrup.

^{1}H NMR (400 MHz, CDCl$_3$) δ 7.77 (s, 1H), 4.69 (s, 2H, OCH_2), 4.44 (t, J = 5.9 Hz, 2H, N–CH_2), 3.73–3.57 (m, 16H, 8 x CH_2), 3.28 (t, J = 7.4 Hz, 4H, 2 x SCH_2), 3.21 (t, J = 5.9 Hz, 2H), 1.99 (s, 2H, NH_2), 1.63 (p, J = 7.4 Hz, 4H), 1.45 (h, J = 7.5 Hz, 4H), 0.93 (t, J = 7.3 Hz, 6H). ^{13}C NMR (101 MHz, CDCl$_3$) δ 166.42 (2C, 2 × C=O), 144.81 (triazole C$_q$), 135.61 (2C, 2 × S-C$_q$), 123.27 (triazole CH), 70.30, 69.80, 69.54, 67.75, 64.47 (8C, 8 x OCH_2), 53.01 (N-CH_2), 41.79, 37.64 (2 x CH_2), 32.32, 31.36, 21.48 (6C, 6 × CH_2), 13.43 (2C, 2 × CH_3). MALDI-MS m/z calcd. for C$_{25}$H$_{43}$N$_5$O$_6$S$_2$ + Na$^+$ [M + Na]$^+$: 596.25. Found: 596.238.

Synthesis of compound **11**: Vancomycin aglycone hexapeptide **2** (90 mg, 0.089 mmol) was dissolved in 1.0 mL dry DMF. 95 mg (2.0 equiv., 0.177 mmol) of compound **9** was added followed by 25 μL (2.0 equiv., 0.177 mmol) Et$_3$N and 55 mg (1.2 equiv., 0.107 mmol) of PyBOP. The reaction mixture was stirred for 2 h at room temperature, after which TLC (n-PrOH:NH$_4$OH = 7:3, cellulose) indicated complete conversion. The product was precipitated by the addition of 100 mL of cold EtOAc:Et$_2$O = 1:1 mixture, filtered off and washed thoroughly with diethyl ether. The crude product was purified by gel column chromatography using Sephadex LH-20 in MeCN:H$_2$O = 8:2 mixture, followed by flash column chromatography in MeCN:H$_2$O = 9:1 mixture. The product was obtained as a white powder in 52 mg yield (38%). NMR: see Table S5 in supporting information. Elemental analysis: see Table S8 in supporting information. MALDI-MS m/z calcd. for C$_{72}$H$_{86}$Cl$_2$N$_{14}$O$_{20}$ + Na$^+$ [M + Na]$^+$: 1559.54. Found: 1559.76.

Synthesis of compound **12**: Vancomycin aglycone hexapeptide **2** (90 mg, 0.089 mmol) was dissolved in 1.0 mL dry DMF, then 101 mg (2.0 equiv., 0.177 mmol) of compound **10** was added followed by 25 μL (2.0 equiv., 0.177 mmol) of Et$_3$N and 55 mg (1.2 equiv., 0.107 mmol) of PyBOP. The reaction was stirred for 2 h at room temperature, after which TLC (n-PrOH:NH$_4$OH = 7:3, cellulose) indicated complete conversion. The product was worked up and purified as described for compound **12**. The title compound was obtained as a yellow powder in 44 mg yield (31%). NMR: see supporting information. NMR: see Table S6 in supporting information. Elemental analysis: see Table S8 in supporting information. MALDI-MS m/z calcd. for C$_{71}$H$_{80}$Cl$_2$N$_{12}$O$_{21}$S$_2$ + Na$^+$ [M + Na]$^+$: 1593.43. Found: 1593.44.

Synthesis of compound **13**: Step 1: 837 μL (12.5 mmol) ethylenediamine was dissolved in 5 mL dry DCM and stirred at room temperature, while 115 mg (0.63 mmol) n-hexanesulfonyl chloride in 0.5 mL dry DCM was added via syringe over the course of about 30 min. The reaction mixture was stirred for 4 h, after which it was thoroughly evaporated. The crude product was purified by flash column chromatography using hexanes: acetone = 6:4 (+0.2% v/v Et$_3$N) as eluent. 95 mg of N-(2-aminoethyl)hexane-1-sulfonamide was obtained as a slightly yellow syrup with acceptable purity (based on ^{1}H and ^{13}C NMR spectra), which was suitable for the amide coupling in Step 2: Vancomycin aglycone hexapeptide **2** (90 mg, 0.089 mmol) was dissolved in 1.0 mL of dry DMF:DMSO mixture. 25 μL Et$_3$N (~2 equiv., 0.18 mmol) was added followed by 70 mg N-(2-aminoethyl)hexane-1-sulfonamide (~4 equiv., 0.34 mmol) obtained in step 1, followed by 54 mg (1.15 equiv., 0.103 mmol) PyBOP. The reaction was stirred at room temperature for 3 h, then the product was precipitated by the addition of ethyl acetate, filtered out and washed with diethyl ether. The product was purified by flash column chromatography using step gradient elution (toluene: MeOH = 7:3→1:1) then by gel column chromatography (Sephadex LH-20, acetone:H_2O = 1:1). The title compound was obtained as an off-white powder in 36 mg yield (34%). NMR: see Table S7 in supporting information. Elemental analysis: see Table S8 in supporting information. MALDI-MS m/z calcd. for $C_{54}H_{57}Cl_2N_9O_{17}S$ + Na^+ $[M + Na]^+$: 1228.29. Found: 1228.27.

3.2. Antiviral Procedures

3.2.1. Anti-Influenza Virus Activity

For antiviral testing, 25 mM compound stocks were prepared in 100% DMSO and stored at 4 °C. The compounds were fully soluble under these conditions. In the antiviral tests, the highest concentration tested was 100 μM, corresponding to a non-toxic DMSO content of 0.4%.

The virus strains (A/H1N1: A/Ned/378/05 and A/PR/8/34; A/H3N2: A/Victoria/361/11; and B/Ned/537/05) were propagated in embryonated hen eggs. The antiviral procedure was published elsewhere [38,39]. Madin-Darby canine kidney (MDCK) cells were seeded at 7500 cells per well into 96-well plates, using infection medium (UltraMDCK medium (Lonza) with 225 mg/L sodium bicarbonate, 2 mM L-glutamine, and 2 μg/mL N-tosyl-L-phenylalanine chloromethyl ketone (TPCK)-treated trypsin). One day later, virus (MOI: 0.001) was added together with 1:5 serial compound dilutions, to reach a total volume of 200 μL per well. Besides the test compounds, two references were included, i.e., zanamivir and ribavirin (positive controls) plus a condition receiving medium instead of compound (negative control). In parallel, the compound dilutions were also added to a mock-infected plate (in which medium was added instead of virus), to determine compound cytotoxicity. Each plate contained two wells in which all reagents yet no cells were added, to serve as blanks in the MTS calculations. After three days incubation at 35 °C, viral CPE was first monitored by microscopy. Then, the supernatants were replaced by MTS reagent (CellTiter 96® AQ$_{ueous}$ MTS Reagent from Promega) diluted 1:10 in PBS, and 4 h later, absorbance at 490 nm was measured in a plate reader. From all OD values, the blank OD was subtracted. The % protection against virus was defined as: $[(OD_{Cpd})virus-(OD_{Contr})virus]/[(OD_{Contr})mock-(OD_{Contr})virus] \times 100$, where (OD_{Cpd})virus is the OD for a given concentration of the compound in virus-infected cells; (OD_{Contr})virus is the OD for the untreated virus control; and (OD_{Contr})mock is the OD for the untreated mock-infected control. The % cytotoxicity was defined as: $[1-(OD_{Cpd})mock/[(OD_{Contr})mock] \times 100$, where (OD_{Cpd})mock is the OD for a given concentration of the compound in mock-infected wells. The values for EC_{50} (50% antivirally effective concentration) and CC_{50} (50% cytotoxic concentration) were calculated by interpolation based on semi-log dose response.

To monitor the inhibitory effect of the compounds on virus replication, MDCK cells were seeded, infected (with A/PR/8/34 virus; MOI: 0.001) and treated with 1:2 serial compound dilutions. The plate contained three virus controls (receiving no compound) and two cell controls (receiving no virus and no compound). At day 3 p.i., supernatants were collected and frozen at −80 °C, to quantify the virus yield by one-step qRT-PCR analysis of viral copy number [40]. Two μl supernatant was mixed with 10 μL resuspension buffer and 1 μl lysis reagent (CellsDirect One-Step RT-qPCR kit; Invitrogen) and heated during 10 min at 75 °C. Next, 10 μL lysate was transferred to a qPCR plate containing the qRT-PCR enzymes and buffer (CellsDirect One-Step RT-qPCR kit; Invitrogen), and influenza virus M1-specific primers and probe [40]. The program consisted of: 15 min at 50 °C; 2 min at 95 °C; and 45 cycles of 15 s at 95 °C followed by 90 s at 60 °C. Absolute quantification of vRNA copies was performed by including an M1-plasmid standard. The EC_{99} values were calculated by interpolation and defined as the compound concentration causing 100-fold reduction in vRNA copy number, as compared to the virus control receiving no compound. It was ascertained that the cell controls showed no detectable qPCR signal.

3.2.2. Other Antiviral Procedures

The viruses were propagated and evaluated in the following cell lines: Human embryonic lung (HEL) fibroblast cells, used for human coronavirus 229E [41], herpes simplex virus type 1 (HSV-1 strain KOS, including a thymidine kinase deficient HSV-1/TK⁻ mutant), herpes simplex virus type 2 (HSV-2, strain G) and vaccinia virus (strain Lederle); human cervixcarcinoma HeLa cells, used for respiratory syncytial virus (RSV, strain Long), and African Green Monkey kidney Vero cells, used for yellow fever virus (vaccine strain 17D) and Zika virus (strain MR766). The medium used for virus infection was Dulbecco's Modified Eagle's Medium supplemented with 2% fetal calf serum. To prepare virus stocks, confluent cell cultures in 75-cm^2 flasks were infected with the virus and frozen after 3 to 5 days incubation at 37 °C (or 35 °C in case of human coronavirus 229E), when full-blown CPE was visible. After freeze-thawing and centrifugation, the clarified lysates were stored at −80 °C. For the antiviral experiments, the cells were grown in 96-well plates until confluent. Virus was added (MOI: 0.001) together with 1:5 serial dilutions of the compounds. For each virus, appropriate reference compounds were included. The compound dilutions were also added to a mock-infected plate, to determine compound cytotoxicity. When manifest CPE was reached, i.e., after 3 to 5 days incubation at 37 °C (or 35 °C in case of human coronavirus 229E), CPE and compound cytotoxicity were quantified by the MTS assay, and EC$_{50}$ and CC$_{50}$ values were calculated as explained above for influenza virus.

To assess inhibition of human coronavirus 229E replication, HEL cells were infected and treated with 1:2 serial compound dilutions. The plate contained three virus controls (receiving no compound) and two cell controls (receiving no virus and no compound). At day 4 p.i., supernatants were frozen at −80 °C to determine the virus yield by one-step RT-qPCR assay. Two microliters supernatant was mixed with 11 µl lysis mix containing lysis enhancer and resuspension buffer at a 1:10 ratio (CellsDirect One-Step RT-qPCR kit; Invitrogen), and heated for 10 min at 75 °C. Five microliters of lysate was transferred to a PCR plate containing 9.75 µl RT-qPCR mix (CellsDirect One-Step RT-qPCR) and 0.25 µl Superscript III RT/Platinum Taq enzyme, and coronavirus-229E N-gene specific primers and probe (forward primer 5′-TTAGAGAGCGTGTTGAAGGTG-3′; reverse primer 5′-GTTCTGAATTCTTGCGCCTAAC-3′; probe 5′-FAM-TCTGGGTTG-ZEN-CTGTTGATGGTGCTA-IBFQ-3′). The RT-qPCR program consisted of 15 min at 50 °C, 2 min at 95 °C, and 50 cycles of 15 s at 95 °C and 45 s at 60 °C. An N-gene plasmid standard was included for absolute quantification. Compound activity was expressed as the EC$_{99}$ value, i.e., the concentration causing 100-fold reduction in vRNA copy number, as compared to the virus control receiving no compound. It was ascertained that the cell controls showed no detectable qPCR signal.

4. Conclusions

Starting from vancomycin, we have successfully prepared two derivatives with strong activity against influenza virus. The modifications that we introduced were based on our previous work on the glycopeptide antibiotic teicoplanin. Interestingly, some of these modifications yielded compounds **6** and **7** having the same antiviral potency as the analogous teicoplanin pseudoaglycon derivatives [24,30] but lacking antibacterial activity. The short work described here validates that the glycopeptide scaffold is an underexplored entity to conceive new antivirals with a broad activity spectrum, that besides influenza virus includes emerging pathogens like coronavirus and Zika virus.

Supplementary Materials: Table S1: NMR data for Compound **3**, Table S2: NMR data for Compound **6**, Table S3: NMR data for Compound **7**, Table S4: NMR data for Compound **8**, Table S5: NMR data for Compound **11**, Table S6: NMR data for Compound **12**, Table S7: NMR data for Compound **13**, Table S8: Elemental analysis data (C, H, N, S) for vancomycin derivatives **6⁻8′ 11⁻13·**

Author Contributions: Conceptualization, Z.S. and A.B.; methodology, Z.S., G.B., E.O., A.S., and L.N.; investigation, S.Z., E.O., and A.S.; writing, Z.S., A.B., P.H., and L.N.; supervision, A.B., P.H., and L.N.; funding acquisition, A.B. and G.B. All authors have read and agreed to the published version of the manuscript.

Acknowledgments: We acknowledge kind assistance of L. Persoons and her team, and of Ria Van Berwaer and Julie Vandeput.

References

1. Coleman, B.L.; Fadel, S.A.; Fitzpatrick, T.; Thomas, S.M. Risk factors for serious outcomes associated with influenza illness in high- versus low- and middle-income countries: Systematic literature review and meta-analysis. *Influenza Other Respir. Viruses* **2018**, *12*, 22–29. [CrossRef] [PubMed]
2. Richard, M.; Fouchier, R.A.M. Influenza A virus transmission via respiratory aerosols or droplets as it relates to pandemic potential. *FEMS Microbiol. Rev.* **2016**, *40*, 68–85. [CrossRef] [PubMed]
3. Von Itzstein, M. The war against influenza: Discovery and development of sialidase inhibitors. *Nat. Rev. Drug Discov.* **2007**, *6*, 967–974. [CrossRef] [PubMed]
4. Noshi, T.; Kitano, M.; Taniguchi, K.; Yamamoto, A.; Omoto, S.; Baba, K.; Hashimoto, T.; Ishida, K.; Kushima, Y.; Hattori, K.; et al. In vitro characterization of baloxavir acid, a first-in-class cap-dependent endonuclease inhibitor of the influenza virus polymerase PA subunit. *Antivir. Res.* **2018**, *160*, 109–117. [CrossRef]
5. Furuta, Y.; Takahashi, K.; Shiraki, K.; Sakamoto, K.; Smee, D.F.; Barnard, D.L.; Gowen, B.B.; Julander, J.G.; Morrey, J.D. T-705 (favipiravir) and related compounds: Novel broad-spectrum inhibitors of RNA viral infections. *Antivir. Res.* **2009**, *82*, 95–102. [CrossRef]
6. Dong, G.; Peng, C.; Luo, J.; Wang, C.; Han, L.; Wu, B.; Ji, G.; He, H. Adamantane-resistant influenza A viruses in the world (1902–2013): Frequency and distribution of M2 gene mutations. *PLoS ONE* **2015**, *10*, e0119115. [CrossRef]
7. Samson, M.; Pizzorno, A.; Abed, Y.; Boivin, G. Influenza virus resistance to neuraminidase inhibitors. *Antivir. Res.* **2013**, *98*, 174–185. [CrossRef]
8. Moscona, A. Global transmission of oseltamivir-resistant influenza. *N. Engl. J. Med.* **2009**, *360*, 953–956. [CrossRef]
9. McKimm-Breschkin, J.L. Influenza neuraminidase inhibitors: Antiviral action and mechanisms of resistance. *Influenza Other Respir. Viruses* **2013**, *7*, 25–36. [CrossRef]
10. Vanderlinden, E.; Naesens, L. Emerging antiviral strategies to interfere with influenza virus entry. *Med. Res. Rev.* **2014**, *34*, 301–339. [CrossRef]
11. Naesens, L.; Stevaert, A.; Vanderlinden, E. Antiviral therapies on the horizon for influenza. *Curr. Opin. Pharmacol.* **2016**, *30*, 106–115. [CrossRef]
12. Yip, T.-F.; Selim, A.S.M.; Lian, I.; Lee, S.M.-Y. Advancements in host-based interventions for influenza treatment. *Front. Immunol.* **2018**, *9*, 1547. [CrossRef]
13. Colson, P.; Raoult, D. Fighting viruses with antibiotics: An overlooked path. *Int. J. Antimicrob. Agents* **2016**, *48*, 349–352. [CrossRef]
14. Pizzorno, A.; Padey, B.; Terrier, O.; Rosa-Calatrava, M. Drug repurposing approaches for the treatment of influenza viral infection: Reviving old drugs to fight against a long-lived enemy. *Front. Immunol.* **2019**, *10*, 531. [CrossRef]
15. Wang, Y.; Cui, R.; Li, G.; Gao, Q.; Yuan, S.; Altmeyer, R.; Zou, G. Teicoplanin inhibits Ebola pseudovirus infection in cell culture. *Antivir. Res.* **2016**, *125*, 1–7. [CrossRef]
16. Zhou, N.; Pan, T.; Zhang, J.; Li, Q.; Zhang, X.; Bai, C.; Huang, F.; Peng, T.; Zhang, J.; Liu, C.; et al. Glycopeptide antibiotics potently inhibit cathepsin L in the late endosome/lysosome and block the entry of Ebola virus, Middle East respiratory syndrome coronavirus (MERS-CoV), and severe acute respiratory syndrome coronavirus (SARS-CoV). *J. Biol. Chem.* **2016**, *291*, 9218–9232. [CrossRef]
17. Balzarini, J.; Pannecouque, C.; De Clercq, E.; Pavlov, A.Y.; Printsevskaya, S.S.; Miroshnikova, O.V.; Reznikova, M.I.; Preobrazhenskaya, M.N. Antiretroviral activity of semisynthetic derivatives of glycopeptide antibiotics. *J. Med. Chem.* **2003**, *46*, 2755–2764. [CrossRef]
18. Preobrazhenskaya, M.N.; Olsufyeva, E.N. Polycyclic peptide and glycopeptide antibiotics and their derivatives as inhibitors of HIV entry. *Antivir. Res.* **2006**, *71*, 227–236. [CrossRef]
19. Balzarini, J.; Keyaerts, E.; Vijgen, L.; Egberink, H.; De Clercq, E.; Van Ranst, M.; Printsevskaya, S.S.; Olsufyeva, E.N.; Solovieva, S.E.; Preobrazhenskaya, M.N. Inhibition of feline (FIPV) and human (SARS) coronavirus by semisynthetic derivatives of glycopeptide antibiotics. *Antivir. Res.* **2006**, *72*, 20–33. [CrossRef]
20. Obeid, S.; Printsevskaya, S.S.; Olsufyeva, E.N.; Dallmeier, K.; Durantel, D.; Zoulim, F.;

Preobrazhenskaya, M.N.; Neyts, J.; Paeshuyse, J. Inhibition of hepatitis C virus replication by semi-synthetic derivatives of glycopeptide antibiotics. *J. Antimicrob. Chemother.* **2011**, *66*, 1287–1294. [CrossRef]

21. De Burghgraeve, T.; Kaptein, S.J.; Ayala-Nunez, N.V.; Mondotte, J.A.; Pastorino, B.; Printsevskaya, S.S.; de Lamballerie, X.; Jacobs, M.; Preobrazhenskaya, M.; Gamarnik, A.V.; et al. An analogue of the antibiotic teicoplanin prevents Flavivirus entry in vitro. *PLoS ONE* **2012**, *7*, e37244. [CrossRef] [PubMed]

22. Naesens, L.; Vanderlinden, E.; Rőth, E.; Jekő, J.; Andrei, G.; Snoeck, R.; Pannecouque, C.; Illyés, E.; Batta, G.; Herczegh, P.; et al. Anti-influenza virus activity and structure–activity relationship of aglycoristocetin derivatives with cyclobutenedione carrying hydrophobic chains. *Antivir. Res.* **2009**, *82*, 89–94. [CrossRef]

23. Vanderlinden, E.; Vanstreels, E.; Boons, E.; ter Veer, W.; Huckriede, A.; Daelemans, D.; Van Lommel, A.; Roth, E.; Sztaricskai, F.; Herczegh, P.; et al. Intracytoplasmic trapping of influenza virus by a lipophilic derivative of aglycoristocetin. *J. Virol.* **2012**, *86*, 9416–9431. [CrossRef]

24. Pintér, G.; Batta, G.; Kéki, S.; Mándi, A.; Komáromi, I.; Takács-Novák, K.; Sztaricskai, F.; Rőth, E.; Ostorházi, E.; Rozgonyi, F.; et al. Diazo transfer-click reaction route to new, lipophilic teicoplanin and ristocetin aglycon derivatives with high antibacterial and anti-influenza virus activity: An aggregation and receptor binding study. *J. Med. Chem.* **2009**, *52*, 6053–6061. [CrossRef]

25. Sipos, A.; Máté, G.; Rőth, E.; Borbás, A.; Batta, G.; Bereczki, I.; Kéki, S.; Jóna, I.; Ostorházi, E.; Rozgonyi, F.; et al. Synthesis of fluorescent ristocetin aglycone derivatives with remarkable antibacterial and antiviral activities. *Eur. J. Med. Chem.* **2012**, *58*, 361–367. [CrossRef]

26. Sipos, A.; Török, Z.; Rőth, E.; Kiss-Szikszai, A.; Batta, G.; Bereczki, I.; Fejes, Z.; Borbás, A.; Ostorházi, E.; Rozgonyi, F.; et al. Synthesis of isoindole and benzoisoindole derivatives of teicoplanin pseudoaglycone with remarkable antibacterial and antiviral activities. *Bioorg. Med. Chem. Lett.* **2012**, *22*, 7092–7096. [CrossRef]

27. Bereczki, I.; Mándi, A.; Rőth, E.; Borbás, A.; Fizil, Á.; Komáromi, I.; Sipos, A.; Kurtán, T.; Batta, G.; Ostorházi, E.; et al. A few atoms make the difference: Synthetic, CD, NMR and computational studies on antiviral and antibacterial activities of glycopeptide antibiotic aglycone derivatives. *Eur. J. Med. Chem.* **2015**, *94*, 73–86. [CrossRef]

28. Bereczki, I.; Kicsák, M.; Dobray, L.; Borbás, A.; Batta, G.; Kéki, S.; Nikodém, É.N.; Ostorházi, E.; Rozgonyi, F.; Vanderlinden, E.; et al. Semisynthetic teicoplanin derivatives as new influenza virus binding inhibitors: Synthesis and antiviral studies. *Bioorg. Med. Chem. Lett.* **2014**, *24*, 3251–3254. [CrossRef]

29. Szűcs, Z.; Csávás, M.; Rőth, E.; Borbás, A.; Batta, G.; Perret, F.; Ostorházi, E.; Szatmári, R.; Vanderlinden, E.; Naesens, L.; et al. Synthesis and biological evaluation of lipophilic teicoplanin pseudoaglycone derivatives containing a substituted triazole function. *J. Antibiot.* **2017**, *70*, 152–157. [CrossRef]

30. Szűcs, Z.; Kelemen, V.; Thai, S.L.; Csávás, M.; Rőth, E.; Batta, G.; Stevaert, A.; Vanderlinden, E.; Naesens, L.; Herczegh, P.; et al. Structure-activity relationship studies of lipophilic teicoplanin pseudoaglycon derivatives as new anti-influenza virus agents. *Eur. J. Med. Chem.* **2018**, *157*, 1017–1030. [CrossRef]

31. Printsevskaya, S.S.; Solovieva, S.E.; Olsufyeva, E.N.; Mirchink, E.P.; Isakova, E.B.; De Clercq, E.; Balzarini, J.; Preobrazhenskaya, M.N. Structure-activity relationship studies of a series of antiviral and antibacterial aglycon derivatives of the glycopeptide antibiotics vancomycin, eremomycin, and dechloroeremomycin. *J. Med. Chem.* **2005**, *48*, 3885–3890. [CrossRef]

32. Malabarba, A.; Ciabatti, R.; Kettenring, J.; Ferrari, P.; Vékey, K.; Bellasio, E.; Denaro, M. Structural modifications of the active site in teicoplanin and related glycopeptides. 1. Reductive hydrolysis of the 1,2- and 2,3-peptide bonds. *J. Org. Chem.* **1996**, *61*, 2137–2150. [CrossRef]

33. Cavalleri, B.; Ferrari, P.; Malabarba, A.; Magni, A.; Pallanza, R.; Gallo, G.G. Teicoplanin, antibiotics from Actinoplanes teichomyceticus nov. sp. VIII. Opening of the polypeptide chain of teicoplanin aglycone under hydrolytic conditions. *J. Antibiot.* **1987**, *40*, 49–59. [CrossRef] [PubMed]

34. Malabarba, A.; Ciabatti, R.; Maggini, M.; Ferrari, P.; Colombo, L.; Denaro, M. Structural modifications of the active site in teicoplanin and related glycopeptides. 2. Deglucoteicoplanin-derived tetrapeptide. *J. Org. Chem.* **1996**, *61*, 2151–2157. [CrossRef]

35. Booth, P.M.; Stone, D.J.M.; Williams, D.H. The Edman degradation of vancomycin - Preparation of vancomycin hexapeptide. *J. Chem. Soc Chem Commun.* **1987**, *1987*, 1694–1695. [CrossRef]

36. Crane, C.M.; Boger, D.L. Synthesis and evaluation of vancomycin aglycon analogues that bear modifications in the N-terminal D-leucyl amino acid. *J. Med. Chem.* **2009**, *52*, 1471–1476. [CrossRef]

37. Agalave, S.G.; Maujan, S.R.; Pore, V.S. Click chemistry: 1,2,3-triazoles as pharmacophores. *Chem. Asian J.*

2011, *6*, 2696–2718. [CrossRef]

38. Cihan-Üstündag, G.; Zopun, M.; Vanderlinden, E.; Ozkirimli, E.; Persoons, L.; Capan, G.; Naesens, L. Superior inhibition of influenza virus hemagglutinin-mediated fusion by indole-substituted spirothiazolidinones. *Bioorg. Med. Chem.* **2020**, *28*, 115130. [CrossRef]

39. Vrijens, P.; Noppen, S.; Boogaerts, T.; Vanstreels, E.; Ronca, R.; Chiodelli, P.; Laporte, M.; Vanderlinden, E.; Liekens, S.; Stevaert, A.; et al. Influenza virus entry via the GM3 ganglioside-mediated platelet-derived growth factor receptor beta signalling pathway. *J. Gen. Virol.* **2019**, *100*, 583–601. [CrossRef]

40. Stevaert, A.; Dallocchio, R.; Dessi, A.; Pala, N.; Rogolino, D.; Sechi, M.; Naesens, L. Mutational analysis of the binding pockets of the diketo acid inhibitor L-742,001 in the influenza virus PA endonuclease. *J. Virol.* **2013**, *87*, 10524–10538. [CrossRef]

41. Apaydin, Ç.B.; Cesur, N.; Stevaert, A.; Naesens, L.; Cesur, Z. Synthesis and anti-coronavirus activity of a series of 1-thia-4-azaspiro [4.5]decan-3-one derivatives. *Arch. Pharm.* **2019**, *352*, e1800330. [CrossRef] [PubMed]

2

Design, Synthesis, and Antibacterial and Antifungal Activities of Novel Trifluoromethyl and Trifluoromethoxy Substituted Chalcone Derivatives

Surendra Babu Lagu [1,*](ID), Rajendra Prasad Yejella [1](ID), Richie R. Bhandare [2,*](ID) and Afzal B. Shaik [3,*](ID)

1   Department of Pharmaceutical Sciences, Pharmaceutical Chemistry Division, A.U. College of Pharmaceutical Sciences, Andhra University, Visakhapatnam 530003, Andhra Pradesh, India; dryrp_au@rediffmail.com

2   Department of Pharmaceutical Sciences, College of Pharmacy & Health Sciences, Ajman University, Ajman P.O. Box 346, UAE

3   Department of Pharmaceutical Chemistry, Vignan Pharmacy College, Vadlamudi 522213, Andhra Pradesh, India

*   Correspondence: ysbabu033@gmail.com (S.B.L.); r.bhandareh@ajman.ac.ae (R.R.B.); bashafoye@gmail.com (A.B.S.).

Abstract: Despite the availability of many drugs to treat infectious diseases, the problems like narrow antimicrobial spectrum, drug resistance, hypersensitivities and systemic toxicities are hampering their clinical utility. Based on the above facts, in the present study, we designed, synthesized and evaluated the antibacterial and antifungal activity of novel fluorinated compounds comprising of chalcones bearing trifluoromethyl (**A1–A10**) and trifluoromethoxy (**B1–B10**) substituents. The compounds were characterized by spectroscopic techniques and evaluated for their antimicrobial activity against four pathogenic Gram-positive (*Staphylococcus aureus* and *Bacillus subtilis*) and Gram-negative (*Escherichia coli* and *Bacillus subtilis*) bacterial and fungal (*Candida albicans* and *Aspergillus niger*) strains. In this study, the compounds with trifluoromethoxy group were more effective than those with trifluoromethyl group. Among the 20 fluorinated chalcones, compound **A3/B3** bearing an indole ring attached to the olefinic carbon have been proved to possess the most antimicrobial activity compared to the standard drugs without showing cytotoxicity on human normal liver cell line (L02). Further, the minimum inhibitory concentration (MIC) for **A3/B3** was determined by serial tube dilution method and showed potential activity. These results would provide promising access to future study about the development of novel agents against bacterial and fungal infections.

Keywords: fluorinated compounds; chalcones; trifluoromethyl; trifluoromethoxy; antibacterial activity; antifungal activity; minimum inhibitory concentration; cytotoxicity

1. Introduction

Infectious diseases in human beings are caused by microbes including bacteria, fungi, and viruses. These diseases are treated by employing a range of antimicrobials available in the market. The utility of antimicrobials in therapy is ever-increasing, which is leading to the most dangerous problem, antimicrobial resistance (AMR) [1,2]. Resistance to antimicrobial agents is a major threat to public health and is responsible for significant rise in morbidity, mortality, and hospitalization. Keeping this in view, World Health Organization (WHO) introduced a preamble *"no action today no cure tomorrow"* to counteract the trouble of AMR [3–5]. The limitations of current antimicrobial agents like AMR, untoward side-effects, lengthier treatment period, and improper therapeutic outcomes compel the development of more effective novel antimicrobial chemical entities that can be employed as drugs. Scientists are in a continuous search for novel antimicrobial agents employing different strategies. One common strategy followed by researchers is the design and synthesis of small molecules for testing them as prospective antimicrobial drug candidates. Small molecule drugs play a significant role in treating different types of diseases. In recent years, according to United States-Food and Drug Administration (US-FDA), the development of small molecules has reduced to some extent (74% in 2017 and 71% in 2018). However, in 2019, nearly 70% of the total of approved targeted drugs were small molecules [6,7]. Advantages of small molecules include better pharmacokinetic properties, oral bioavailability, delivery, and production cost [8]. Small molecules bring chemical diversity in less time and with ease compared to isolation, structural elucidation and biological testing of natural products. Additionally, screening of small molecule libraries derived through laboratory synthesis is widely employed in the pharmaceutical industry to identify lead molecules with potential drug-like properties [9].

Chalcones are bichromophoric natural open-chain flavonoid small molecules containing a reactive propenone linkage connected to two aromatic rings. The propenone moiety of these molecules is highly reactive and is not only responsible for the assorted biological activities of chalcone derivatives [10] but also for the preparation of different heterocyclic derivatives from the chalcones. Chalcone is a privileged scaffold of interest to organic and medicinal chemists because of its ease of synthesis and multiple biological activities. Chulin et al. have published a critical and comprehensive review on this privileged scaffold [11]. Chalcone derivatives containing fluorine and or other types of substituents were reported to possess excellent anticancer, antimicrobial, antioxidant, anti-inflammatory, analgesic, cancer chemopreventive, antibacterial, and antifungal activities [12–21]. Xu et al. have reviewed the structural features of different chalcone derivatives and their influence on the antibacterial properties [16]. There is a difference in the biological potency of different chalcones, which is majorly attributed to the type of aromatic ring as well as the nature of the substituents present thereof. Literature survey and results from our own studies proved that fluorinated chalcones possess remarkable antibacterial and antifungal properties (Figure 1) [22–30]. The potent antimicrobial properties of the chalcones may be due to extra lipophilicity created by the fluorine atoms. With few exceptions, most of the antimicrobial fluorinated chalcones reported typically possess one or more fluorine atoms on the two aryl rings of the chalcone scaffold but not either a trifluoromethyl or trifluoromethoxy group. For instance, out of the eight compounds displayed in Figure 1, only compound 7 possesses a trifluoromethyl group. Hence, in the present study we considered synthesizing and evaluating novel chalcones with trifluoromethyl and trifluoromethoxy groups as prospective antibacterial and antifungal agents.

Presence of one or more fluorine atoms can be seen in a range of drugs used for different disorders including the antibacterials: fluoroquinolones; antifungal: fluconazole; antivirals: efavirenz, trifluridine; anticancer agents: 5-fluorouracil, bicalutamide, leflunomide; antifungals: 5-flucytosine; antidepressants: fluoxetine, escitalopram; steroids: dexamethasone, triamcinolone, fludrocortisone; selective COX-II inhibitors: celecoxib; antiulcer: lansoprazole; antihyperlipidemic agents: atorvastatin, rosuvastatin, ezetimibe, and an antischizophrenic agent: risperidone (Figure 2). The presence of fluorine atoms in the medicinally active compounds have imparted some special properties, including increased binding interactions, potency, permeability, metabolic stability, decreased *pka*, clearance, alteration of the conformation, modified physical properties, and selective reactivities [31–35].

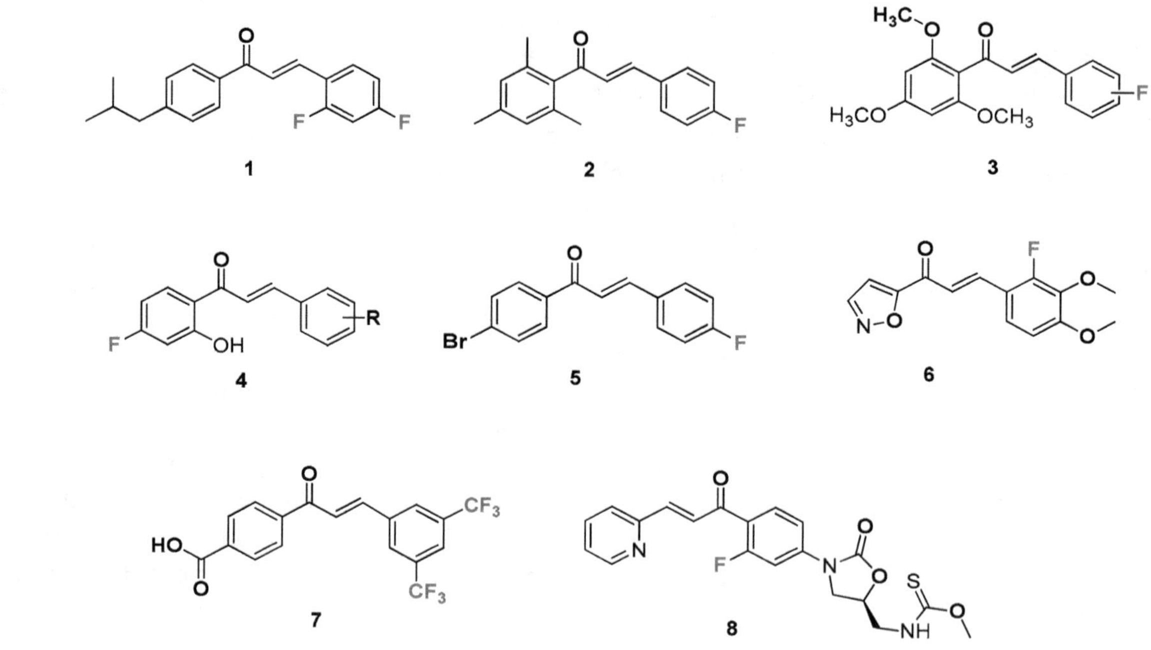

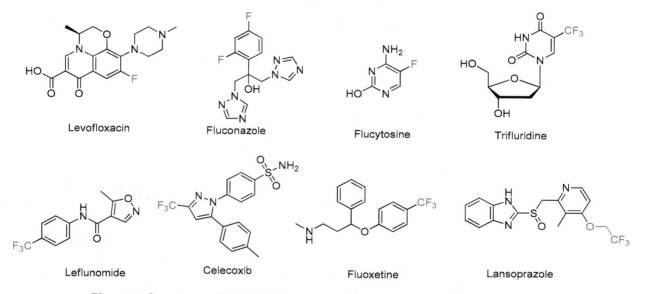

Figure 1. Structures of fluorinated chalcones with antibacterial and antifungal activities.

Levofloxacin   Fluconazole   Flucytosine   Trifluridine

Leflunomide   Celecoxib   Fluoxetine   Lansoprazole

Figure 2. Structures of selected drugs containing one or more fluorine atoms.

Motivated by the aforementioned facts, herein we have designed and prepared two series of novel chalcones substituted with trifluoromethyl (series-A) and trifluoromethoxy (series-B) groups (Figure 3) and evaluated further for their antibacterial and antifungal activities against selected clinically significant bacterial and fungal strains.

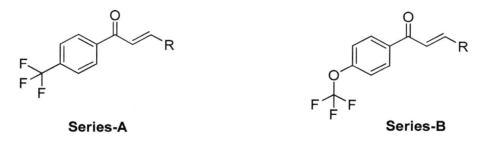

Series-A   **Series-B**

Figure 3. General structures of the designed target fluorinated chalcones.

2. Results and Discussion

2.1. Chemistry

The two series of chalcones were afforded by the Claisen–Schmidt condensation reaction of substituted aryl and unsubstituted heteroaryl aldehydes with two different types of ketones, i.e., 4'-trifluoromethyl acetophenone (series-A) and 4'-trifluoromethoxy acetophenone (series-B). The reaction time utilized for the formation of series-A chalcones was around 6–12 h, whereas for series-B chalcones, it was 12–15 h, and the yield of series-A chalcones was more than the latter. This may be due to the high electron-withdrawing nature of the trifluoromethyl substituent over the trifluoromethoxy group. The compounds were in yellow to orange color which may be due to the extensive conjugation of chalcone core and the additional electronic effects of the substituents on the ring-A and B.

All the compounds were characterized by elemental analysis, FT-IR and ^{1}H NMR, whereas the compounds **A3** and **B3**, were additionally characterized by ^{13}C NMR and mass spectral methods. The elemental analysis and spectroscopic data were consistent with the expected structures of the chalcones. All the compounds in their FT-IR spectrum showed two characteristic stretching absorption bands corresponding to the propenone linkage including C=O and C=C around the wave numbers 1656–1695 cm^{-1} and 1502–1514 cm^{-1} for the ten compounds in series-A and 1640–1656 cm^{-1} and 1502–1532 cm^{-1} for series-B compounds, respectively. The ^{1}H NMR spectra showed two diagnostic doublet signals corresponding to α- and β-protons resonating between the chemical shift values of 7.32–7.75 ppm and 7.76–8.04 ppm (series-A) and 7.51–7.65 ppm and 7.60–8.18 ppm (series-B). The coupling constant value, J, for these doublets ranged between 15 to 17 Hz, and such large coupling constant values indicate that the synthesized compounds have *trans* geometry at the olefinic bond of the propenone linkage.

The FT-IR spectrum of **A3** illustrated intense carbonyl band (C=O) of chalcones at 1695 cm^{-1} and strong stretching band at 1573 cm^{-1} accounting for vinyl (CH=CH) double bond. In addition, the other absorption bands were seen at wave numbers 3230 cm^{-1} (-NH in indole) and 1263 cm^{-1} (-CF$_3$). Two doublet peaks at 7.77 ppm and 8.13 ppm with the coupling constant value around 16 Hz in the ^{1}H NMR spectrum confirmed the formation of chalcone bridge of **A3** with trans geometry. The indole -NH proton showed a peak at 8.78 and the other nine aromatic protons showed two multiplets around 7.94–8.14 and 7.05–7.61, respectively. The ^{13}C NMR spectra of compound **A3** demonstrated three peaks at 189.93, 128.60, and 142.02 corresponding to the three carbons of the propenone moiety. The other ^{13}C peaks include 140.11 (C-1'), 128.60 (C-2' and 6'), 125.59 (C-3' and 5'), 137.30 (C-4'), 123.77 (C-4,'), 129.52 (C-6'), 112.06 (C-1"), 125.30 (C-2"), 130.30 (C-4"), 114.06 (C-5"), 120.71 (C-6"), 122.02 (C-7"), 117.44 (C-8"), 125.56 (C-9"). The mass spectrum of **A3** recorded in positive mode has given an [M + H]$^+$ peak at m/z 316.30. In the ^{19}F-NMR spectrum, **A3** showed signal at 63.27 ppm corresponding to -CF$_3$. The above spectral data confirmed the compound **A3** as (*E*)-3-(1"H-indol-3"-yl)-1-[4'-(trifluoromethyl)phenyl]prop-2-en-1-one.

The FT-IR spectrum of **B3** illustrated diagnostic intense carbonyl (C=O) and strong vinyl (CH=CH) absorption bands of chalcone linkage at wave numbers 1651 cm^{-1} and 1595 cm^{-1}, respectively. Additionally, the other absorption bands are seen at 3681 (-NH in indole), 1206 (-OCF$_3$), and 1248 (C-O-C). The ^{1}H NMR spectrum showed characteristic doublet signals at 7.53 ppm and 8.05 ppm with the coupling constant value (J) around 16 Hz. The larger coupling constant value represents the trans geometry of the chalcones. The other peaks seen are three singlets corresponding to the indole amine proton at chemical shift 8.78 and two multiplets around 7.38–8.02 and 7.05–7.66 corresponding to nine aromatic protons. The ^{13}C NMR spectra of compound **B3** showed three peaks corresponding to the three carbons of the propenone moiety at 189.97, 125.33, and 137.37, respectively. The peaks of other carbon atoms are seen at the following chemical shift values: 130.23 (C-1'), 130.71 (C-2' and 6'), 121.88 (C-3' and 5'), 139.61 (C-4'), 121.88 (C-4,'), 112.08 (C-1"), 123.63 (C-2"), 137.35 (C-4"), 114.41 (C-5"), 120.47 (C-6"), 122.69 (C-7"), 117.81 (C-8"), 123.63 (C-9"). The mass spectrum of **B3** recorded in positive mode showed $[M + H]^+$ peak at m/z 332.20. In the ^{19}F-NMR spectrum, **A3** showed signal at 63.27 ppm corresponding to -CF$_3$. The ^{19}F-NMR spectrum of **B3** showed signal at 58.64 ppm corresponding to -OCF$_3$. Based on the above spectral data, the compound **B3** was confirmed as (*E*)-3-(1"H-indol-3"-yl)-1-[4'-(trifluoromethoxy)phenyl]prop-2-en-1-one (Figure 4).

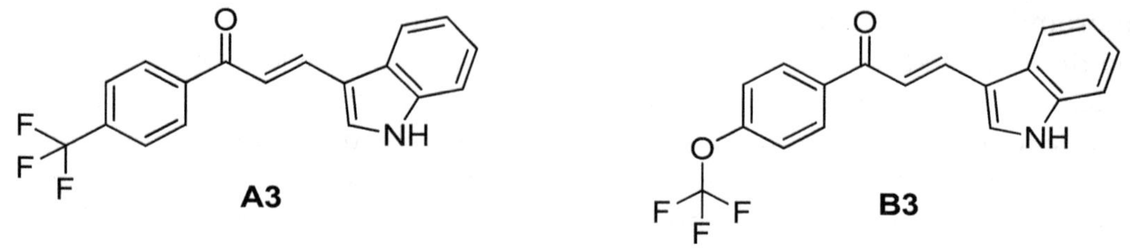

Figure 4. Structures of fluorinated chalcones **A3** and **B3**.

2.2. Biological Activities

2.2.1. Antibacterial and Antifungal Activities

All the 20 target compounds (**A1–A10** and **B1–B10**) were evaluated for their antibacterial and antifungal activities on selected pathogenic Gram-positive (*Staphylococcus aureus* and *Bacillus subtilis*) and Gram-negative (*Escherichia coli* and *Proteus vulgaris*) bacterial (Table 1) and fungal (*Candida albicans* and *Aspergillus niger*) strains (Table 2). The compounds were tested at 0.1% concentration. Benzyl penicillin was employed as standard drug against the bacterial isolates and fluconazole against the fungal strains. The compounds were partitioned into three different categories based on the type of ring-B portion of chalcones. Among the 20 target derivatives, **A2(B2)**, **A4(B4)**, **A5(B5)**, **A8(B8)**, and **A9(B9)** represents chalcones bearing a monosubstituted aryl ring, **A1(B1)** denotes compounds with a disubstituted aryl ring, and **A3(B3)**, **A6(B6)**, **A7(B7)**, and **A10(B10)** designate the compounds containing an unsubstituted heteroaromatic ring.

The compounds exhibited varying degrees of activity (Tables 1 and 2), i.e., some compounds were more active than the standard drugs, whereas some were moderately active and others were less active. When the results between the two series of compounds were compared, a greater number of the compounds belonging to series-B comprising of the -OCF$_3$ group exhibited more activity than the series-A compounds bearing -CF$_3$. However, against *Candida albicans*, five compounds belonging to series-A showed superior activity than series-B compounds. Out of the six microbial strains used in our study, the Gram-negative bacteria *Escherichia coli* and *Proteus vulgaris* were more vulnerable to both the series of chalcones than the Gram-positive bacterial species and fungal isolates. With few exceptions, the activity against Gram-positive bacterial and fungal strains is either intermediate or less.

Table 1. Antibacterial (zone of inhibition in mm) [a,b] of trifluoromethyl and trifluoromethoxy substituted chalcone derivatives (A1–A10 and B1–B10).

Series-A

Series-B

Series-A

Entry		Microorganisms			
Compound Code		S.aureus	B.subtilis	E.coli	P.vulgaris
A1		20.08 ± 0.02	21.16 ± 0.15	17.07 ± 0.02	20.02 ± 0.03
A2		18.13 ± 0.04	19.1 ± 0.26	13.11 ± 0.09	19.02 ± 0.02
A3		**25.05 ± 0.01**	**26.36 ± 0.32**	**20.03 ± 0.02**	**23.02 ± 0.02**
A4		20.06 ± 0.32	20.2 ± 0.17	16.04 ± 0.04	20.03 ± 0.03
A5		19.2 ± 0.81	20.13 ± 0.11	16.05 ± 0.04	20.06 ± 0.01
A6		18.10 ± 0.07	17.13 ± 0.15	15.18 ± 0.27	18.06 ± 0.01
A7		19.23 ± 0.04	18.66 ± 0.20	17.03 ± 0.02	19.20 ± 0.25
A8		15.23 ± 0.21	10.16 ± 0.20	15.05 ± 0.04	14.22 ± 0.22
A9		15.5 ± 0.16	17.13 ± 0.11	15.01 ± 0.02	12.09 ± 0.98
A10		12.1 ± 0.08	11.36 ± 0.05	13.03 ± 0.03	11.18 ± 0.07
Benzyl penicillin		24.06 ± 0.05	27.02 ± 0.02	14.05 ± 0.05	19.04 ± 0.03

Series-B

Entry		Microorganisms			
Compound Code		S.aureus	B.subtilis	E.coli	P.vulgaris
B1		21.06 ± 0.04	22.2 ± 0.11	18.05 ± 0.01	21.09 ± 0.12
B2		18.04 ± 0.03	20.46 ± 0.25	14.04 ± 0.00	20.03 ± 0.03
B3		**26.46 ± 0.04**	**29.43 ± 0.30**	**22.02 ± 0.02**	**21.02 ± 0.02**
B4		21.56 ± 0.04	20.18 ± 0.14	17.21 ± 0.20	20.04 ± 0.04
B5		23.53 ± 0.04	22.02 ± 0.02	17.20 ± 0.24	20.04 ± 0.03
B6		20.53 ± 0.04	19.61 ± 0.32	16.05 ± 0.03	17.04 ± 0.00
B7		21.36 ± 0.16	20.41 ± 0.33	15.05 ± 0.01	18.02 ± 0.01
B8		15.15 ± 0.05	16.3 ± 0.10	9.03 ± 0.01	12.05 ± 0.01
B9		16.3 ± 0.02	15.07 ± 0.04	8.06 ± 0.01	13.04 ± 0.52
B10		14.1 ± 0.04	15.21 ± 0.21	9.46 ± 0.25	10.05 ± 0.01
Benzyl penicillin		24.06 ± 0.05	27.02 ± 0.02	14.05 ± 0.05	19.04 ± 0.03

[a] Mean value ± SD (standard deviation from three experiments); [b] Bold value indicates best compounds.

Table 2. Antifungal activity (zone of inhibition in mm) [a] of trifluoromethyl and trifluoromethoxy substituted chalcone derivatives (A1–A10 and B1–B10).

Entry	Microorganisms		Entry	Microorganisms	
Compound Code	*C. albicans*	*A. niger*	Compound Code	*C. albicans*	*A.niger*
A1	18.03 ± 0.01	20.03 ± 0.02	B1	19.09 ± 0.01	21.04 ± 0.01
A2	15.05 ± 0.03	19.03 ± 0.03	B2	17.08 ± 0.01	20.05 ± 0.01
A3	20.05 ± 0.04	25.06 ± 0.01	B3	22.05 ± 0.03	26.07 ± 0.01
A4	17.07 ± 0.01	20.07 ± 0.01	B4	16.07 ± 0.01	20.05 ± 0.04
A5	17.05 ± 0.01	20.07 ± 0.01	B5	15.07 ± 0.01	20.02 ± 0.02
A6	10.08 ± 0.01	14.05 ± 0.04	B6	16.08 ± 0.01	15.04 ± 0.03
A7	11.07 ± 0.01	15.04 ± 0.04	B7	15.07 ± 0.01	17.08 ± 0.01
A8	11.03 ± 0.02	6.01 ± 0.01	B8	11.05 ± 2.32	12.05 ± 0.01
A9	12.05 ± 0.01	12.03 ± 0.02	B9	10.21 ± 0.24	11.05 ± 0.01
A10	13.04 ± 0.03	21.05 ± 0.03	B10	10.09 ± 0.01	12.05 ± 0.02
Fluconazole	19.05 ± 0.04	24.41 ± 0.52	Fluconazole	19.05 ± 0.04	24.41 ± 0.52

[a] Mean value ± SD (standard deviation from three experiments).

Among all the compounds, **A3** and **B3** containing an unsubstituted heteroaromatic 3-indolyl moiety showed more activity than the standard drugs against the tested bacterial and fungal species. This illustrates that the presence of a bicyclic heteroaromatic scaffold is a major contributing factor for the activity of chalcones bearing -CF$_3$ and -OCF$_3$ groups. Against *Staphylococcus aureus*, **A3** and **B3** showed a zone of inhibition (ZOI) of 25 and 26 mm, respectively. The activity of **B3** (ZOI = 29 mm) was more than benzyl penicillin (ZOI = 27 mm) against *Bacillus subtilis* but the activity of **A3** (ZOI = 26 mm) was less than the standard. **A3** and **B3** also exhibited more activity than benzyl penicillin against *Escherichia coli* (ZOI = 20 and 22 mm) and *Proteus vulgaris* with a ZOI of 23 and 21 mm, respectively. **A3** and **B3** showed a ZOI of 20 and 22 mm against *Candida albicans* and a ZOI of 25 and 26 mm, respectively, against *Aspergillus niger*. These ZOI values were more compared to the ZOI values obtained with standard fluconazole (19.05 and 24.41 mm).

Except **B3**, all the other compounds displayed intermediate-to-low activity against *Staphylococcus aureus*, *Bacillus subtilis*, *Candida albicans* and *Aspergillus niger* compared to the standard drugs. When the activities of other compounds against *Escherichia coli* were compared with the standard drugs, the compounds **A1(B1)**, **A4(B4)**, **A5(B5)**, **A6(B6)**, **A7(B7)**, **A8**, and **A9** were found to be more active. Further, among the above 12 compounds, **A1** and **A7** containing 2,3-dichlorophenyl and 2-furfuryl rings were next in potency to **A3** in series-A and **B1**, **B4**, and **B5** containing 2,3-dichlorophenyl, 2-nitrophenyl, and 3-nitrophenyl scaffolds after **B3** in series-B. The chalcones **A1(B1)**, **B2**, **A4(B4)**, and **A5(B5)** were more active than benzyl penicillin against *Proteus vulgaris*, and the compounds **A1** (2,3-dichlorophenyl), **A4** (2-nitrophenyl), **A5** (3-nitrophenyl), **B2** (3-chlorophenyl), **B4** (2-nitrophenyl), and **B5** (3-nitrophenyl) showed equal activity with a ZOI value of 20 mm, whereas the compound **B1** containing 2,3-dichlrophenyl moiety showed activity similar to **B3** (ZOI = 21 mm). These results suggest that presence of an electron-withdrawing group like chlorine or nitro at 2nd and 3rd positions of aryl ring are essential for the activity. The compounds **A2** and **A7** bearing 3-chlorophenyl and 2-furfuryl rings showed equal activity as benzyl penicillin (ZOI = 19 mm) against *Proteus vulgaris*, and **B1** exhibited equal potency as fluconazole against *Candida albicans* with a ZOI of 19 mm. All the other compounds including **A8(B8)** and **A9(B9)** containing 4-chlorophenyl and 4-nitrophenyl rings as well as **A6(B6)** and **A10(B10)** containing heteroaromatic 2-thienyl and 2-pyrrolyl rings, respectively, showed intermediate-to-poor activity relative to the standard drugs. Based on these results, we can summarize that either in series-A or B, the conditions of the ring B-portion of chalcones being either an aromatic ring with electron-withdrawing groups in the ortho and meta positions or a bicyclic heteroaromatic scaffold are essential to the promising antimicrobial activity of the fluorinated chalcones.

2.2.2. Determination of Minimum Inhibitory Concentration (MIC)

Minimum inhibitory concentration (MIC) is the lowest concentration of the antimicrobial agent that inhibits the visible growth of a microorganism after an overnight incubation. MICs are used to determine the resistance by the diagnostic labs mainly to confirm the resistance. However, frequently MIC is a research tool to determine the in vitro activity of novel natural and synthetic compounds. The two most potent compounds that emerged out of this study, i.e., **A3** and **B3** were further evaluated against all the six microbial strains by serial tube dilution to assess their minimum inhibitory concentration by serial tube dilution method (Table 3). Both the compounds showed MIC lower than the standard drugs benzyl penicillin and fluconazole against the tested bacterial and fungal strains and were in agreement with the zone of inhibition values. However, compound **A3** showed less activity against *Bacillus subtilis* (MIC = 101 µM) than benzyl penicillin (MIC = 95 µM). Both **A3** and **B3** exhibited nearly equal activity to that of fluconazole against the fungal strains and superior activity compared to benzyl penicillin. Compound **A3** (MIC = 51 µM) and **B3** (MIC = 48 µM) were 1.86- and 1.97-fold more active than benzyl penicillin (MIC = 95 µM) against *Staphylococcus aureus* and **B3** (MIC = 24 µM) was 3.95 times more active than benzyl penicillin against *Bacillus subtilis*. Against *Escherichia coli* and *Proteus vulgaris*, **A3** was 7.64 times more active than benzyl penicillin whereas **B3** was 7.95 and 3.97 times more active. These results show that the activity of **A3** containing a trifluoromethyl group favored the Gram-negative bacteria and **B3** with a trifluoromethoxy group favored Gram-positive bacteria. The obtained results were interesting and called for a synthesis and evaluation of other analogues to improve the potency.

Table 3. Minimum inhibitory concentration (MIC in µM) of compounds **A3** and **B3**.

Entry	Staphylococcus aureus	Bacillus subtilis	Escherichia coli	Proteus vulgaris	Candida albicans	Aspergillus niger
A3	51	101	25	25	50	25
B3	48	24	24	48	48	24
Benzyl Penicillin	95	95	191	191	-	-
Fluconazole	-	-	-	-	52	26

2.2.3. Cytotoxicity Studies

Compounds **A3** and **B3** were evaluated for their cytotoxicity study on normal human liver calls and were found to have an IC_{50} value greater than 50 µg/mL suggesting that the compounds were non-toxic against the tested normal human liver cell lines (Table 4).

Table 4. Cytotoxicity of compounds **A3** and **B3** against human normal liver cells (IC_{50}, µg/mL) [a].

S. No	Compounds	Human Normal Liver Cells (L02)
1	A3	>50
2	B3	>50

[a] Mean value from three experiments.

3. Materials and Methods

3.1. Chemicals and Instruments

All the chemicals used were of analytical grade and purchased from commercial sources. The organic solvents such as methanol, hexane, and ethyl acetate were of spectral grade and were used as such without further purification. Anhydrous methanol was obtained by fractional distillation and stored over type 4A° molecular sieves. Some of the solvents were purchased from local manufacturers and some from S.D. Fine Chem. Ltd., Mumbai, India. All the chemicals used in the synthesis were obtained from standard commercial sources. TLC chromatography was carried out on Merck grade precoated TLC silica gel 60 F_{254} plates (Merck KGaA, Darmstadt, Germany) and the spots were visualized under a UV lamp. 4'-trifluoromethylacetophenone and 4'-trifluoromethoxyacetophenone were obtained from Thermo Fisher Scientific-Alfa Aesar (Powai, Mumbai, India). Aldehydes were procured from Avra synthesis Pvt. Ltd. (Hyderabad, India). The melting points were determined in open capillaries, using a digital melting point apparatus (EZmelt, Stanford Research Systems) (expressed in °C) and are uncorrected. FT-IR spectra were scanned using Bruker OPUS 8.0 (BRUKER biospin International AG., Zug) and the ^{1}H- and ^{13}C-NMR spectra of the compound were recorded on a Bruker 400 Avance NMR spectrophotometer using Tetramethylsilane (TMS) as an internal standard (values are expressed in δ ppm). Mass spectra were recorded on SHIMADZU Lab Solution (ESI-MS) spectrometer at Indian Institute of Chemical Technology, Hyderabad, India (refer to the supplementary material).

3.2. Synthesis

General Procedure for Synthesis

The two series of chalcones were prepared (Scheme 1) by following Claisen–Schmidt condensation reaction [36]. Initially, 1 mmol of the ketone (4'-trifluromethyacetophenone/ 4'-trifluromethoxyacetophenone) was dissolved in 8 mL of ethanol. To the above solution, 1 mmol of the corresponding aldehyde was added and then 7.5 mL of 40% sodium hydroxide solution was added dropwise and stirred on a magnetic stirrer at room temperature for about 6–15 h. The progress and the completion of the reaction was monitored on precoated silica gel-G TLC plates and the spots on the plates were visualized using UV lamp and iodine vapors. After the completion of the reaction, the contents of the reaction mixture were transferred into a beaker containing crushed ice and then the mixture was neutralized with 50% hydrochloric acid, which resulted in the separation of the crude precipitate of the chalcone. The precipitate was filtered under vacuum, washed thoroughly with HPLC grade water, and dried in a desiccator. The dried crude mixture was further subjected to column chromatographic purification to obtain the pure product. Column chromatography was performed on 100–200-mesh silica gel as the stationary phase and a 1:15 ratio of hexane and ethyl acetate as mobile phase.

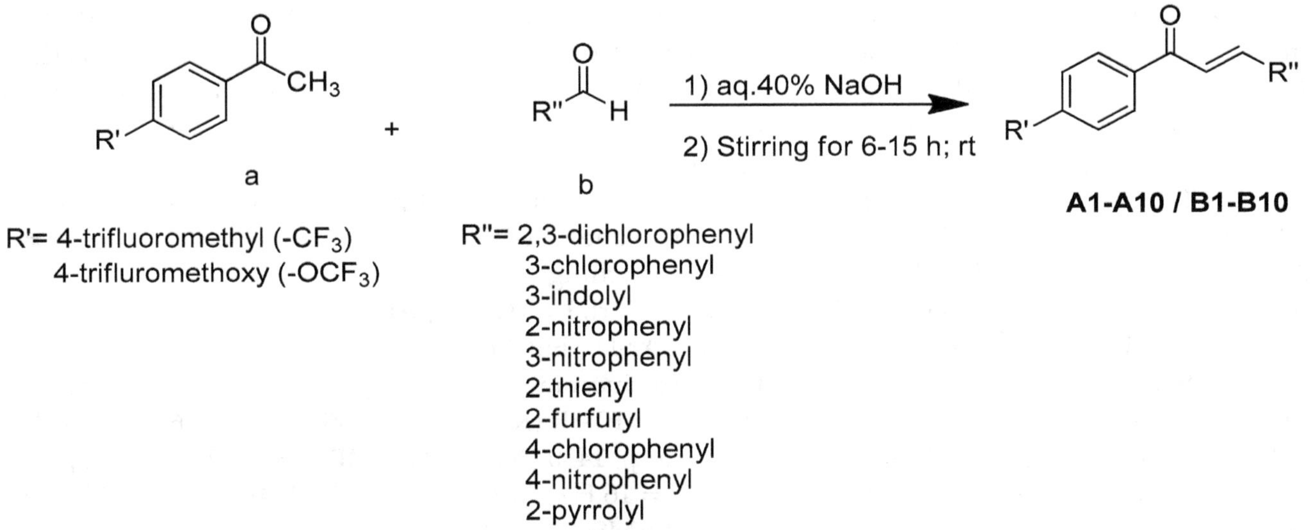

Scheme 1. Synthesis of series-A (**A1–A10**) and series-B (**B1–B10**) fluorinated chalcones.

A1: Synthesis of (*E*)-3-(2″,3″-dichlorophenyl)-1-[4′-(trifluoromethyl)phenyl]prop-2-en-1-one: Yield: 95%; m.p. 76 °C; R_f = 0.81 (30% Ethyl acetate in Hexane); FT-IR (KBr, cm^{-1}): 1660 (C=O), 1602 (C=C Ar), 1502 (CH=CH), 1255 (-CF$_3$), 3011 (Ar C-H stretching), 832 (C-Cl); ^{1}H NMR (400 MHz, CDCl$_3$, ppm), δ: 7.76 (1H, d, *J* = 16.3 CO-CH=), 8.11 (1H, d, *J* = 16.3, Ar-CH=), 8.12–8.22 (4H, m, C-2′, 3′, 5′, 6′, Ar-H), 6.97–7.74 (3H, m, C- 4″, 5″, 6″, Ar-H); ESI-MS: 346.13 [M + H]$^+$.

A2: Synthesis of (*E*)-3-(3″-chlorophenyl)-1-[4′-(trifluoromethyl)phenyl]prop-2-en-1-one: Yield: 90%; m.p. 68 °C; R_f = 0.8 (30% Ethyl acetate in Hexane); FT-IR (KBr, cm^{-1}): 1651 (C=O), 1611 (C=C Ar), 1507 (CH=CH), 1252 (-CF$_3$), 3010 (Ar C-H stretching), 846 (C-Cl); ^{1}H NMR (400 MHz, CDCl$_3$, ppm), δ: 7.77 (1H, d, *J* = 16.3 Hz CO-CH=), 8.11 (1H, d, *J* = 16.2 Hz, Ar-CH=), 8.12–8.22 (4H, m, C-2′, 3′, 5′, 6′, Ar-H), 7.09–7.74 (4H, m, C-3″, 4″, 5″, 6″, Ar-H); ESI-MS: 311.13 [M + H]$^+$.

A3: Synthesis of (*E*)-3-(1″H-indol-3″-yl)-1-[4′-(trifluoromethyl)phenyl]prop-2-en-1-one: Yield: 50%; m.p. 62 °C; R_f = 0.9 (30% Ethyl acetate in Hexane); FT-IR (KBr, cm^{-1}): 1695 (C=O), 1611 (C=C Ar), 1573 (CH=CH), 1263 (-CF$_3$), 3010 (Ar C-H stretching), 3230 (-NH); ^{1}H NMR (400 MHz, CDCl$_3$, ppm): δ: 7.77 (1H, d, *J* = 16.3 Hz, -CO-CH=), 8.13 (1H, d, *J* = 15.9 Hz, Ar-CH=), 8.78 (1H, s, -NH), 7.94-8.14 (4H, m, C-2′, 3′, 5′, 6′, Ar-H), 7.05-7.61 (5H, m, C-2″, 4″, 5″, 6″, 7″, Ar-H); ^{13}C NMR (125 MHz, CDCl3, ppm): 189.93 (C-1), 128.60 (C-2), 142.02 (C-3), 140.11 (C-1′), 128.60 (C-2′ and 6′), 125.59 (C-3′ and 5′), 137.30 (C-4′), 123.77 (C-4,′), 129.52 (C-6′), 112.06 (C-1″), 125.30 (C-2″), 130.30 (C-4″), 114.06 (C-5″), 120.71 (C-6″), 122.02 (C-7″), 117.44 (C-8″), 125.56 (C-9″); ESI-MS: 316.30 [M + H]$^+$; ^{19}F NMR (376 MHz, CDCl$_3$): δ: 63.27 (3F, s).

A4: Synthesis of (*E*)-3-(2″-nitrophenyl)-1-[4′-(trifluoromethyl)phenyl]prop-2-en-1-one: Yield: 60%; m.p. 70 °C; R_f = 0.7 (30% Ethyl acetate in Hexane); FT-IR (KBr, cm^{-1}): 1646 (C=O), 1602 (C=C Ar), 1514 (CH=CH), 1249 (-CF$_3$), 3010 (Ar C-H stretching), 1461 (NO$_2$); ^{1}H NMR (400 MHz, CDCl$_3$, ppm): δ: 7.77 (1H, d, *J* = 17.1 Hz, -CO-CH=), 8.11 (1H, d, *J* = 16 Hz, Ar-CH=), 8.12–8.51 (4H, m, C-2′, 3′, 5′, 6′, Ar-H), 7.70–8.01 (4H, m, C-3″, 4″, 5″, 6″, Ar-H); ESI-MS: 322.11 [M + H]$^+$.

A5: Synthesis of (*E*)-3-(3″-nitrophenyl)-1-[4′-(trifluoromethyl)phenyl]prop-2-en-1-one: Yield: 60%; m.p. 85 °C; R_f = 0.5 (30% Ethyl acetate in Hexane); FT-IR (KBr, cm^{-1}): 1659 (C=O), 1623 (C=C Ar), 1536 (CH=CH), 1250 (-CF$_3$), 3010 (Ar C-H stretching), 1446 (NO$_2$); ^{1}H NMR (400 MHz, CDCl$_3$, ppm): 7.92 (1H, d, *J* = 15.7 Hz, -CO-CH=), 8.15 (1H, d, *J* = 16 Hz, Ar-CH=), 7.82–8.65 (4H, m, C-2′, 3′, 5′, 6′, Ar-H), 7.68–7.89 (4H, m, C-2″, 3″, 5″, 6″, Ar-H); ESI-MS: 322.25 [M + H]$^+$.

A6: Synthesis of (*E*)-3-(thiophen-2″-yl)-1-[4′-(trifluoromethyl)phenyl]prop-2-en-1-one: Yield: 80%; m.p. 86 °C; R_f = 0.76 (30% Ethyl acetate in Hexane); FT-IR (KBr, cm^{-1}): 1658 (C=O), 1504 (CH=CH), 1614 (C=C Ar), 3121 (Ar C-H stretching), 1250 (-CF$_3$), 621 (C-S); ^{1}H NMR (400 MHz, CDCl$_3$, ppm): δ: 7.79 (1H, d, *J* = 16 Hz, -CO-CH=), 8.14 (1H, d, *J* = 16.2, 4.9 Ar-CH=), 7.80–8.12 (4H, m, C-2′, 3′, 5′, 6′, Ar-H), 7.17–7.77 (4H, m, C-3″, 4″, 5″, Ar-H); ESI-MS: 283.36 [M + H]$^+$.

A7: Synthesis of (E)-3-(furan-2″-yl)-1-[4′-(trifluoromethyl)phenyl]prop-2-en-1-one: Yield: 80%; m.p. 72 °C; R_f = 0.71 (30% Ethyl acetate in Hexane); FT-IR (KBr, cm^{-1}): 1658 (C=O), 1514 (CH=CH), 1631 (C=C Ar), 3111 (Ar C-H stretching), 1254 (-CF$_3$), 1700 (C-O); ^{1}H NMR (400 MHz, CDCl$_3$, ppm), δ: 7.75 (1H, d, J = 16.1 Hz, -CO-CH=), 8.14 (1H, d, J = 16.1 Hz, Ar-CH=), 7.59–8.12 (4H, m, C-2′, 3′, 5′, 6′, Ar-H), 6.52–7.53 (3H, m, C-3″, 4″, 5″, Ar-H); ESI-MS: 227.68 [M + H]$^+$.

A8: Synthesis of (E)-3-(4″-chlorophenyl)-1-[4′-(trifluoromethyl)phenyl]prop-2-en-1-one: Yield: 90%; m.p. 68 °C; R_f = 0.72 (30% Ethyl acetate in Hexane); FT-IR (KBr, cm^{-1}): 1656 (C=O), 1609 (C=C Ar), 1505 (CH=CH), 1247 (-CF$_3$), 3001 (Ar C-H stretching), 841 (C-Cl); ^{1}H NMR (400 MHz, CDCl$_3$, ppm): δ: 7.78 (1H, d, J = 16.3 Hz, -CO-CH=), 8.14 (1H, d, J = 16.2 Hz, Ar-CH=), 7.77–8.13 (4H, m, C-2′, 3′, 5′, 6′, Ar-H), 7.43–7.61 (4H, m, C-2″, 4″, 5″, 6″, Ar-H); ESI-MS: 311.62 [M + H]$^+$.

A9: Synthesis of (E)-3-(4″-nitrophenyl)-1-[4′-(trifluoromethyl)phenyl]prop-2-en-1-one: Yield: 61%; m.p. 82 °C; R_f = 0.7 (30% Ethyl acetate in Hexane); FT-IR (KBr, cm^{-1}): 1654 (C=O), 1621 (C=C Ar), 1512 (CH=CH), 1252 (-CF$_3$), 3010 (Ar C-H stretching), 1430 (NO$_2$); ^{1}H NMR (400 MHz, CDCl$_3$, ppm): δ: 7.85 (1H, d, J = 17 Hz, -CO-CH=), 8.11 (1H, d, J = 16 Hz, Ar-CH=), 7.68–7.82 (4H, m, C-2′, 3′, 5′, 6′, Ar-H), 8.12–8.32 (4H, m, C-2″, 3″, 5″, 6″, Ar-H); ESI-MS: 322.11 [M + H]$^+$.

A10: Synthesis of (E)-3-(1″H-pyrrol-2-yl)-1-[4′-(trifluoromethyl)phenyl]prop-2-en-1-one: Yield: 80%; m.p. 75 °C; R_f = 0.68 (30% Ethyl acetate in Hexane); FT-IR (KBr, cm^{-1}): 1650 (C=O), 1501 (CH=CH), 1618 (C=C Ar), 1242 (-CF$_3$), 1370 (C-N), 3115 (Ar C-H stretching); ^{1}H NMR (400 MHz, CDCl$_3$, ppm), δ: 7.77 (1H, d, J = 16 Hz, -CO-CH=), 8.11 (1H, d, J = 16 Hz, Ar-CH=), 7.74–8.23 (4H, m, C-2′, 3′, 5′, 6′, Ar-H), 6.08–6.96 (3H, m, C-3″, 4″, 5″, Ar-H), 9.93 (1H, s, -NH); ESI-MS: 266.23 [M + H]$^+$.

B1: Synthesis of (E)-3-(2″,3″-dichlorophenyl)-1-[4′-(trifluoromethoxy)phenyl]prop-2-en-1-one: Yield: 86%; m.p. 70 °C; R_f = 0.8 (30% Ethyl acetate in Hexane); FT-IR (KBr, cm^{-1}): 1664 (C=O), 1624 (Ar C=C), 1520 (CH=CH), 1242 (-CF$_3$), 3023 (Ar C-H stretching), 1166 (-C-O-) 838 (C-Cl); ^{1}H NMR (400 MHz, CDCl$_3$, ppm), δ: 7.58 (1H, d, J = 16.3 Hz, CO-CH=), 8.03 (1H, d, J = 16.3 Hz, Ar-CH=), 7.64–8.22 (4H, m, C-2′, 3′, 5′, 6′, Ar-H), 6.97–7.62 (3H, m, C- 4″, 5″, 6″, Ar-H); ESI-MS: 362.12 [M + H]$^+$.

B2: Synthesis of (E)-3-(3″-chlorophenyl)-1-[4′-(trifluoromethoxy)phenyl]prop-2-en-1-one: Yield: 84%; m.p. 65 °C; R_f = 0.81 (30% Ethyl acetate in Hexane); FT-IR (KBr, cm^{-1}): 1648 (C=O), 1607 (Ar C=C), 1512 (CH=CH), 1232 (-CF3), 3015 (Ar C-H stretching), 1156 (-C-O-), 840 (C-Cl); ^{1}H NMR (400 MHz, CDCl$_3$, ppm), δ: 7.37 (1H, d, J = 16.3 Hz, -CO-CH=), 8.02 (1H, d, J = 16.2 Hz, Ar-CH=), 7.70–8.22 (4H, m, C-2′, 3′, 5′, 6′, Ar-H), 7.05–7.68 (4H, m, C-3″, 4″, 5″, 6″, Ar-H); ESI-MS: 343.58 [M + H]$^+$.

B3: Synthesis of (E)-3-(1″H-indol-3″-yl)-1-[4′-(trifluoromethoxy)phenyl]prop-2-en-1-one: Yield: 45%; m.p. 67 °C; R_f = 0.74 (30% Ethyl acetate in Hexane); FT-IR (KBr, cm^{-1}): 1651 (C=O), 1602 (Ar C=C), 1595 (CH=CH), 1521 (C-N), 3681 (-NH), 1206 (-OCF$_3$), 3362 (Ar C-H stretching), 1248 (-C-O-); ^{1}H NMR (400 MHz, CDCl$_3$, ppm): δ 7.53 (1H, d, J = 16.3 Hz, -CO-CH=), 8.05 (1H d, J = 15.9, Ar-CH=), 8.78 (1H, s, -NH), 7.38–8.02 (4H, m, C-2′, 3′, 5′, 6′, Ar-H), 7.05–7.66 (5H, m, C-2″, 4″, 5″, 6″, 7″, Ar-H); ^{13}C NMR (125 MHz, CDCl3, ppm): 189.97 (C-1), 125.33 (C-2), 137.37 (C-3), 130.23 (C-1′), 130.71 (C-2′ and 6′), 121.88 (C-3′ and 5′), 139.61 (C-4′), 121.88 (C-4,′), 112.08 (C-1″), 123.63 (C-2″), 137.35 (C-4″),114.41 (C-5″), 120.47 (C-6″), 122.69 (C-7″), 117.81 (C-8″), 123.63 (C-9″); ESI-MS: 332.20 [M + H]$^+$; ^{19}F NMR (376 MHz, CDCl$_3$): δ, 58.64 (3F, s).

B4: Synthesis of (E)-3-(2″-nitrophenyl)-1-[4′-(trifluoromethoxy)phenyl]prop-2-en-1-one: Yield: 56%; m.p. 69 °C; R_f = 0.87 (30% Ethyl acetate in Hexane); FT-IR (KBr, cm^{-1}): 1640 (C=O), 1632 (Ar C=C), 1504 (CH=CH),1232 (-CF$_3$), 3012 (Ar C-H stretching), 1126 (-C-O-), 1462 (NO$_2$); ^{1}H NMR (400 MHz, CDCl$_3$, ppm): δ: 7.85 (1H, d, J = 17 Hz, -CO-CH=), 8.28 (1H, d, J = 16 Hz, Ar-CH=), 8.27–8.51 (4H, m, C-2′, 3′, 5′, 6′, Ar-H), 7.05–8.25 (4H, m, C-3″, 4″, 5″, 6″, Ar-H); ESI-MS: 338.08 [M + H]$^+$.

B5: Synthesis of (E)-3-(3″-nitrophenyl)-1-[4′-(trifluoromethoxy)phenyl]prop-2-en-1-one: Yield: 55%; m.p. 71 °C; R_f = 0.72 (30% Ethyl acetate in Hexane); FT-IR (KBr, cm^{-1}): 1659 (C=O), 1626 (Ar C=C), 1532 (CH=CH), 1248 (-CF$_3$), 3019 (Ar C-H stretching), 1127 (-C-O-), 1448 (NO$_2$); ^{1}H NMR (400 MHz, CDCl$_3$, ppm): δ: 7.06 (1H, d, J = 16.3 Hz, CO-CH=), 8.05 (1H, d, J = 16.2 Hz, Ar-CH=), 7.76–8.03 (4H, m, C-2′, 3′, 5′, 6′, Ar-H), 7.08–7.79 (4H, m, C-2″, 4″, 5″, 6″, Ar-H); ESI-MS: 338.35 [M + H]$^+$.

B6: Synthesis of (E)-3-(thiophen-2"-yl)-1-[4'-(trifluoromethoxy)phenyl]prop-2-en-1-one: Yield: 76%; m.p. 82 °C; R_f = 0.68 (30% Ethyl acetate in Hexane); FT-IR (KBr, cm^{-1}): 1656 (C=O), 1512 (CH=CH), 1610 (Ar C=C), 3126 (Ar C-H stretching), 1262 (-CF$_3$), 1156 (-C-O-), 620 (C-S); ^{1}H NMR (400 MHz, CDCl$_3$, ppm): δ:), 7.05 (1H, d, J = 16, -CO-CH=), 8.05 (1H, d, J = 6.2, 4.9 Ar-CH=), 7.20–8.02 (4H, m, C-2', 3', 5', 6', Ar-H), 7.17–7.79 (3H, m, C-3", 4", 5", Ar-H); ESI-MS: 299.16 [M + H]$^+$.

B7: Synthesis of (E)-3-(furan-2"-yl)-1-[4'-(trifluoromethoxy)phenyl]prop-2-en-1-one: Yield: 78%; m.p. 68 °C; R_f = 0.66 (30% Ethyl acetate in Hexane); FT-IR (KBr, cm^{-1}): 1651 (C=O), 1524 (CH=CH), 1635 (Ar C=C), 3111 (Ar C-H stretching), 1250 (-CF$_3$), 1159 (-C-O-); ^{1}H NMR (400 MHz, CDCl$_3$, ppm), δ: 7.07 (1H, d, J = 16.1 Hz, -CO-CH=), 8.05 (1H, d, J = 16.1 Hz, Ar-CH=), 7.47–8.05 (4H, m, C-2', 3', 5', 6', Ar-H), 6.52–7.59 (3H, m, C-3", 4", 5", Ar-H); ESI-MS: 283.47 [M + H]$^+$.

B8: Synthesis of (E)-3-(4"-chlorophenyl)-1-[4'-(trifluoromethoxy)phenyl]prop-2-en-1-one: Yield: 84%; m.p. 75 °C; R_f = 0.64 (30% Ethyl acetate in Hexane); FT-IR (KBr, cm^{-1}): 1645 (C=O), 1629 (Ar C=C), 1512 (CH=CH), 1237 (-CF$_3$), 3011 (Ar C-H stretching), 1155 (-C-O-), 837 (C-Cl); ^{1}H NMR (400 MHz, CDCl$_3$, ppm): δ: 8.33 (1H, d, J = 16 Hz, Ar-CH=), 7.05 (1H d, J = 15.7 Hz, -CO-CH=), 7.92–8.65 (4H, m, C-2', 3', 5', 6', Ar-H), 7.06–7.89 (4H, m, C-2", 3", 5", 6", Ar-H); ESI-MS: 343.19 [M + H]$^+$.

B9: Synthesis of (E)-3-(4"-nitrophenyl)-1-[4'-(trifluoromethoxy)phenyl]prop-2-en-1-one: Yield: 57%; m.p. 68 °C; R_f = 0.68 (30% Ethyl acetate in Hexane); FT-IR (KBr, cm^{-1}): 1652 (C=O), 1614 (Ar C=C), 1510 (CH=CH), 1242 (-CF$_3$), 3016 (Ar C-H stretching), 1122 (-C-O-), 1436 (NO$_2$); ^{1}H NMR (400 MHz, CDCl$_3$, ppm): δ: 7.06 (1H, d, J = 16 Hz, -CO-CH=), 8.03 (1H, d, J = 16 Hz, Ar-CH=), 7.05–8.04 (4H, m, C-2', 3', 5', 6', Ar-H), 7.82–8.32 (4H, m, C-2", 3", 5", 6", Ar-H); ESI-MS [M + H]$^+$: 338.72 and 339.72.

B10: Synthesis of (E)-3-(1"H-pyrrol-2-yl)-1-[4'-(trifluoromethoxy)phenyl]prop-2-en-1-one: Yield: 67%; m.p. 59 °C; R_f = 0.70 (30% Ethyl acetate in Hexane); FT-IR (KBr, cm^{-1}): 1646 (C=O), 1516 (CH=CH), 1621 (Ar-C=C-), 1232 (-CF$_3$), 1336 (C-N), 3121 (Ar C-H stretching), 1166 (-C-O-); ^{1}H NMR (400 MHz, CDCl$_3$, ppm), δ: 7.07 (1H, d, J = 16.6 Hz, -CO-CH=), 8.03 (1H, d, J= 16.6 Hz, Ar-CH=), 7.08–8.23 (4H, m, C-2', 3', 5', 6', Ar-H), 6.09–7.06 (3H, m, C-3", 4", 5", Ar-H), 9.93 (1H, s, -NH); ESI-MS: 282.02 [M + H]$^+$.

3.3. Biological Activity Studies

3.3.1. Antimicrobial Screening

The antimicrobial activity was performed against six different antimicrobial strains. The organisms selected are listed below:

Gram-positive bacteria	Bacillus subtilis (NCIM-2079), Staphylococcus aureus (NCIM-2079)
Gram-negative bacteria	Escherichia coli (NCIM-2065), Proteus vulgaris (NCIM-2027)
Fungi	Candida albicans (MDCC-227), Aspergillus niger (MTCC 5889)

Glassware was cleaned and kept in a hot air oven at 160 °C for 2 h. The media were sterilized and the solutions of standard drugs (Benzyl penicillin and fluconazole) and A and B series of compounds were kept ready. In the meantime, nutrient agar medium was prepared (composition: peptone 0.5%, meat extract 0.3%, sodium chloride 0.5%, agar 2%, distilled water to make up to 100 mL, and pH adjusted to 7.2). The weighed quantities of peptone, meat extract, and sodium chloride were dissolved in 1000 mL of distilled water and the pH of the medium was adjusted to 7.2. After the dissolution of agar, the medium was distributed into conical flask each containing 25 mL. The media and sterile water were sterilized by autoclaving at 121 °C temperature and 15 lbs/sq. inch pressure for 20 min. Petri plates, test tubes, pipettes, and borer required for experiment were sterilized by dry heat sterilization using hot air oven. Cultures of respective organisms (18 h old) were taken and suspension of these microorganisms was made using sterile water. Later, 0.5 mL of this suspension was used as inoculum and pour plate technique was used for estimation of bacterial load in each sample. The inoculated agar medium was poured into sterile 10 cm-diameter petri dishes and the medium in the plates was allowed to solidify. The solutions of the test compounds in concentrations of 0.1 µg/mL were prepared in DMSO. The cups of 5 mm diameter were prepared using a borer in the corresponding medium. In each plate, 5 wells were prepared. Three wells were for test compounds, one for standard compound and another one was used as control. In each well, samples were poured and then plates were left for 45 min in a refrigerator for diffusion. After incubation for 18 h at 37 °C, the plates were examined for inhibition zones. The experiments were done in triplicate on the same day with the same conditions in order to minimize the experimental errors. The zone of inhibition values was calculated using vernier caliper and represented as a mean of three values and standard deviation was applied [10].

3.3.2. Determination of Minimum Inhibitory Concentration (MIC)

MIC has become the current standard test for antibiotic sensitivity testing because it produces more pertinent information on minimal dosages. Hence, we determined the MIC of selected compounds, i.e., **A3** and **B3** employing the protocol prescribed in our previously published papers [37].

3.3.3. Cytotoxicity Studies

The most potent compounds **A3** and **B3** out of the 20 compounds were tested in vitro for their cytotoxic activity on L02 (human normal liver cell line) by employing MTT assay according to Mosmann's method as described in our previous paper [38]. The MTT assay is based on the reduction of the soluble MTT (0.5 mg mL^{-1}, 100 µL) into a blue–purple formazan product, mainly by mitochondrial reductase activity inside living cells (Mosmann T et al., 1983). The cells used in cytotoxicity assay were cultured in RPMI 1640 medium supplemented with 10% fetal calf serum, penicillin, and streptomycin at 37 °C and humidified at 5% CO_2. Briefly, cells were placed on 96-well plates at 100 µL total volume with a density of $1–2.5 \times 10^4$ cells per mL and were allowed to adhere for 24 h before treatment with tested drugs in DMSO solution (10^{-5}, 10^{-6}, 10^{-7} mol L^{-1} final concentration). Triplicate wells were treated with media and agents. Cell viability was assayed after 96 h of continuous drug exposure with a tetrazolium compound. The supernatant medium was removed, and 150 µL of DMSO solution was added to each well. The plates were gently agitated using mechanical plate mixer until the color reaction was uniform and OD570 was determined using micro plate reader. The 50% inhibitory concentration (IC_{50}) was defined as the concentration that reduced the absorbance of the untreated wells by 50% of the vehicle in the MTT assay. Assays were performed in triplicate on three independent experiments. The results showed good reproducibility between replicate wells with standard errors below 10%.

4. Conclusions

In this paper, we described the design, synthesis, characterization, and antimicrobial screening of 20 new fluorinated chalcones. Most of the compounds displayed promising antibacterial and antifungal activities and two compounds bearing indolyl scaffold, i.e., **A3** and **B3**, showed potential activities and were also non-toxic on the normal human liver cell lines (L02). Additionally, compounds bearing electron-withdrawing nitro or the chloro substituents at the ortho or the meta position showed valuable antimicrobial activity. Hence, these compounds are novel lead compounds identified through our study for the development of novel agents against bacterial and fungal infections. Although the present study gave us some lead molecules, future investigation needs to be done by synthesizing analogues of **A3** and **B3** by replacing the indole scaffold of **A3** and **B3** with benzofuran and benzothiophene moieties as well as by substituting more lipophilic -SCF$_3$ for -OCF$_3$ in **B3**. Further, a plausible mode of action for the proposed activities needs to be investigated.

Author Contributions: Conceptualization, R.P.Y. and A.B.S.; methodology, S.B.L., R.P.Y., R.R.B. and A.B.S.; software, S.B.L. and A.B.S.; validation, S.B.L., R.P.Y. and A.B.S.; formal analysis, R.P.Y., R.R.B. and A.B.S.; investigation, S.B.L., R.P.Y. and A.B.S.; resources, S.B.L., R.P.Y. and A.B.S.; data curation, S.B.L., R.P.Y. and A.B.S.; writing—original draft preparation, S.B.L., R.P.Y., R.R.B. and A.B.S.; writing—review and editing, S.B.L., R.P.Y., R.R.B. and A.B.S.; visualization, S.B.L., R.P.Y. and A.B.S.; supervision, R.P.Y. and A.B.S.; project administration, S.B.L., R.P.Y. and A.B.S.; funding acquisition, S.B.L., R.P.Y., R.R.B. and A.B.S. All authors have read and agreed to the published version of the manuscript.

Acknowledgments: L.S.B. and Y.R.P. would like to acknowledge Department of Pharmaceutical Sciences, Pharmaceutical Chemistry Division, A.U. College of Pharmaceutical Sciences Andhra Pradesh, India for providing the lab facilities and chemicals for this work. R.R.B. and A.B.S. would like to thank the Dean's office of College of Pharmacy and Health Sciences, Ajman University, UAE and Vignan Pharmacy College, Vadlamudi, Andhra Pradesh, India for their support.

References

1. Richard, J.F.; Yitzhak, T. Antibiotics and bacterial resistance in the 21st century. *Perspect. Med. Chem.* **2014**, *6*, S14459. [CrossRef]

2. Halling-Sørensen, B. Inhibition of aerobic growth and nitrification of bacteria in sewage sludge by antibacterial agents. *Arch. Environ. Contam. Toxicol.* **2001**, *40*, 451–460. [CrossRef]

3. Harish, C.; Parul, B.; Archana, Y.; Babita, P.; Abhay, P.M.; Anant, R.N. Antimicrobial resistance and the alternative resources with special emphasis on plant-based antimicrobials-a review. *Plants* **2017**, *6*, 16. [CrossRef]

4. Francesca, P.; Patrizio, P.; Annalisa, P. Antimicrobial resistance: A global multifaceted phenomenon. *Pathog. Glob. Health* **2015**, *109*, 309–318. [CrossRef]

5. Bingyun, L.; Thomas, J.W. Bacteria antibiotic resistance: New challenges and opportunities for implant-associated orthopedic infections. *J Orthop. Res.* **2018**, *36*, 22–32. [CrossRef]

6. Novel Drug Approvals for 2017. Available online: https://www.fda.gov/drugs/new-drugs-fda-cders-new-molecular-entities-and-new-therapeutic-biological-products/novel-drug-approvals-2017 (accessed on 2 November 2020).

7. Novel Drug Approvals for 2018. Available online: https://www.fda.gov/drugs/new-drugs-fda-cders-new-molecular-entities-and-new-therapeutic-biological-products/novel-drug-approvals-2018 (accessed on 2 November 2020).

8. Wang, W.; Sun, Q. Novel targeted drugs approved by the NMPA and FDA in 2019. *Sig. Transduct. Target Ther.* **2020**, *65*, 1–4. [CrossRef]

9. Nurken, B.; Mohamad, A. An overview of drug discovery and development. *Future Med. Chem.* **2020**, *12*, 939–947.

10. Lagu, S.B.; Rajendra, P.Y.; Srinath, N.; Afzal, B.S. Synthesis. antibacterial, antifungal antitubercular activities and molecular docking studies of nitrophenyl derivatives. *Int. J. Life Sci. Pharma Res.* **2019**, *9*, 54–64. [CrossRef]

11. Zhuang, C.; Zhang, W.; Sheng, C.; Zhang, W.; Xing, C.; Miao, Z. Chalcone: A Privileged Structure in Medicinal Chemistry. *Chem. Rev.* **2017**, *117*, 7762–7810. [CrossRef] [PubMed]

12. Maya, Z.G.; Minh, A.N.; Sarah, K.Z. Design, synthesis and evaluation of (2-(Pyridinyl)methylene)-1-tetralone chalcones for Anticancer and Antimicrobial Activity. *Med. Chem.* **2018**, *14*, 333–343. [CrossRef]

13. Mei, L.; Prapon, W.; Mei-Lin, G. Antimalarial alkoxylated and hydroxylated chalones: Structure-activity relationship analysis. *J. Med. Chem.* **2001**, *44*, 4443–4452.

14. Serdar, B.; Oztekin, A.; Derya, A.A.; Arzu, G.; Gulay, G.D.; Ronak, H.E.; Nizami, D. Synthesis and anti-proliferative activity of fluoro-substituted chalcones. *Bioorg. Med. Chem. Lett.* **2016**, *26*, 3172–3176. [CrossRef]

15. Ramesh, C.K.; Rita, A.; Geeta, S.; Dinesh, K.; Chetan, S.; Radhika, J.; Aneja, K.R. Ecofriendly synthesis and antimicrobial activity of chalcones. *Der. Pharma. Chem.* **2010**, *2*, 157–170.

16. Zhang, X.; Zhao, D.-H.; Quan, Y.-C.; Sun, L.; Yin, X.-M.; Guan, L.-P. Synthesis and evaluation of antiinflammatory activity of substituted chalcone derivatives. *Med. Chem. Res.* **2010**, *19*, 403–412. [CrossRef]

17. Khaled, R.A.A.; Heba, A.H.E.; Samir, A.S.; Hany, A.O. Synthesis, characterization and biological evaluation of novel 4-fluoro-2-hydroxychalcone derivatives as antioxidant, anti-inflammatory, analgesic agents. *J Enzyme*

Inhib Med Chem. **2015**, *30*, 484–491. [CrossRef]

18. Shen-Jew, W.; Cheng-Tsung, L.; Lo-Ti, T.; Jing-Ru, W.; Horng-Huey, K.; Jih-Pyang, W.; Chun-Nan, L. Synthetic chalcones as potential anti-inflammatory and cancer chemo preventive agents. *Eur. J. Med. Chem.* **2005**, *40*, 103–112. [CrossRef]

19. Nazifi, S.I.; Farediah, A. Antimicrobial activities of some synthetic flavonoids. *J. App. Chem.* **2014**, *7*, 1–6.

20. Pinki, Y.; Kashmiri; Lokesh, K.; Ashwani, K.; Anil, K.; Avijit, K.P.; Rajnish, K. Synthesis, crystal structure and antimicrobial potential of some fluorinated chalcones-1,2,3-triazole conjugates. *Eur. J. Med. Chem.* **2018**, *155*, 263–274. [CrossRef]

21. Francesca, B.; Giovanna, A.G.; Francesca, B.; Silvia, G.; Angela, R.; Alessandra, B.; Federica, B. Functionalization of the Chalcone Scaffold for the Discovery of Novel Lead Compounds Targeting Fungal Infections. *Molecules* **2019**, *24*, 372. [CrossRef]

22. Man, X.; Piye, W.; Fan, S.; Jiayou, J.; Rakesh, K.P. Chalcone derivatives and their antibacterial activities: Current development. *Bioorg. Chem.* **2019**, *91*, 103133. [CrossRef]

23. Afzal, B.S.; Yejella, R.P.; Shaik, S. Synthesis, Antimicrobial, and Computational Evaluation of Novel Isobutylchalcones as Antimicrobial Agents. *Int. J. Med. Chem.* **2017**, *2017*, 1–14. [CrossRef]

24. Afzal, B.S.; Lohitha, S.V.K.; Puttagunta, S.B.; Shaik, A.; Supraja, K.; Sai, H.K. Synthesis and screening of novel lipophilic diarylpropeones as prospective antitubercular, antibacterial and antifungal agents. *Biointerface Res. Appl. Chem.* **2019**, *9*, 3912–3918.

25. Serdar, B.; Oztekin, A.; Arzu, G.; Derya, A.A.; Mahmut, U.; Busra, G.E.; Engin, K.; Aylin, D.; Gönül, A. Design of potent fluoro-substituted chalcones as antimicrobial agents. *J. Enzyme Inhib. Med. Chem.* **2017**, *32*, 490–495. [CrossRef]

26. Kayode, L.A.; Issac, A.B.; Adebayo, O.O. Synthesis, Characterization and Antibacterial Activities of New Fluorinated Chalcones. *Chem. Afr.* **2019**, *2*, 47–55.

27. Prasad, Y.R.; Rao, A.L.; Rambabu, R. Synthesis and antimicrobial activity of some chalcone derivatives. *J. Chem.* **2008**, *5*, 461–466. [CrossRef]

28. Afzal, S.; Richie, R.B.; Palleapati, K.; Srinath, N.; Venkata, K.; Shaik, S. Antimicrobial, antioxidant, and anticancer activities of some novel isoxazole ring containing chalcone and dihydropyrazole derivatives. *Molecules* **2020**, *25*, 1047. [CrossRef]

29. Marcelo, N.G.; Eugene, N.M.; Maristela, P.; Josana, C.P.; Lucimar, P.R.; Pedro, V.L.C.; Carolina, H.A.; Bruno, J.N. Chalcone derivatives: Promising starting points for drug design. *Molecules* **2017**, *22*, 1210. [CrossRef]

30. Selvakumar, N.; Sunil, K.G.; Malar, A.A.; Govinda, R.G.; Shikha, S.; Sitaram, K.M.; Jagattaran, D.; Javed, I.; Sanjay, T. Synthesis, SAR and antibacterial studies on novel chalcone oxazolidinone hybrids. *Eur. J. Med. Chem.* **2007**, *42*, 538–543. [CrossRef] [PubMed]

31. Hans, J.B.; David, B.; Stefanie, B.; Manfred, K.; Bernd, K.; Klaus, M.; Ulrike, O.; Martin, S. Fluorine in Medicinal Chemistry. *Chem. Bio. Chem.* **2004**, *5*, 637–643. [CrossRef]

32. Poonam, S.; Andrew, D.W. The role of fluorine in medicinal chemistry. *J. Enzyme Inhib. Med. Chem.* **2007**, *22*, 527–540. [CrossRef]

33. Sophie, P.; Peter, R.M.; Steve, S.; Veronique, G. Fluorine in Medicinal Chemistry. *Chem. Soc. Rev.* **2008**, *37*, 320–330. [CrossRef]

34. William, K.H. The Many Roles for Fluorine in Medicinal Chemistry. *J. Med. Chem.* **2008**, *51*, 4359–4369. [CrossRef]

35. Eric, P.G.; Kyle, J.E.; Matthew, D.H.; David, J.D.; Nicholas, A.M.E.; Matthew, D.H.; David, J.D.; Nicholas, A.M. Applications of Fluorine in Medicinal Chemistry. *J. Med. Chem.* **2015**, *58*, 8315–8359. [CrossRef]

36. Claisen, L.; Claparede, B.A. Condensationen von Ketonen mit Aldehyden. *Berichte Deutschen Chemischen Gesellschaft.* **1881**, *14*, 2463. [CrossRef]

37. Shaik, A.B.; Bhandare, R.R.; Nissankararao, S.; Edis, Z.; Tangirala, N.R.; Shahanaaz, S.; Rahman, M.M. Design, facile synthesis and characterization of dichloro substituted chalcones and dihydropyrazole derivatives for their antifungal, antitubercular and antiproliferative activities. *Molecules* **2020**, *25*, 3188. [CrossRef] [PubMed]

38. Lokesh, B.V.S.; Prasad, Y.R.; Shaik, A.B. Novel pyrimidine derivatives from 2,5-dichloro-3-acetylthienyl chalcones as antifungal, antitubercular and cytotoxic agents: Design, synthesis, biological activity and docking study. *Asian J. Chem.* **2019**, *19*, 310–321.

3

Cytotoxicity Effects of Water-Soluble Multi-Walled Carbon Nanotubes Decorated with Quaternized Hyperbranched Poly(ethyleneimine) Derivatives on Autotrophic and Heterotrophic Gram-Negative Bacteria

Nikolaos S. Heliopoulos [1,2], Georgia Kythreoti [1,3], Kyriaki Marina Lyra [1], Katerina N. Panagiotaki [1], Aggeliki Papavasiliou [1], Elias Sakellis [1], Sergios Papageorgiou [1], Antonios Kouloumpis [4], Dimitrios Gournis [4], Fotios K. Katsaros [1], Kostas Stamatakis [3] and Zili Sideratou [1,*]

[1] Institute of Nanoscience and Nanotechnology, National Centre of Scientific Research "Demokritos", 15310 Aghia Paraskevi, Greece; nikosheliopoulos@gmail.com (N.S.H.); geokyth@bio.demokritos.gr (G.K.); kymarin@gmail.com (K.M.L.); knpanagiotaki@gmail.com (K.N.P.); a.papavasiliou@inn.demokritos.gr (A.P.); e.sakellis@inn.demokritos.gr (E.S.); s.papageorgiou@inn.demokritos.gr (S.P.); f.katsaros@inn.demokritos.gr (F.K.K.)
[2] Department of Industrial Design & Production Engineering, University of West Attica, 12241 Egaleo, Attiki, Greece
[3] Institute of Biosciences and Applications, National Centre of Scientific Research "Demokritos", 15310 Aghia Paraskevi, Greece; kstam@bio.demokritos.gr
[4] Department of Material Science & Engineering, University of Ioannina, 45110 Ioannina, Greece; antoniokoul@gmail.com (A.K.); dgourni@uoi.gr (D.G.)
* Correspondence: z.sideratou@inn.demokritos.gr

Abstract: Oxidized multi-walled carbon nanotubes (oxCNTs) were functionalized by a simple non-covalent modification procedure using quaternized hyperbranched poly(ethyleneimine) derivatives (QPEIs), with various quaternization degrees. Structural characterization of these hybrids using a variety of techniques, revealed the successful and homogenous anchoring of QPEIs on the oxCNTs' surface. Moreover, these hybrids efficiently dispersed in aqueous media, forming dispersions with excellent aqueous stability for over 12 months. Their cytotoxicity effect was investigated on two types of gram(−) bacteria, an autotrophic (cyanobacterium *Synechococcus* sp. PCC 7942) and a heterotrophic (bacterium *Escherichia coli*). An enhanced, dose-dependent antibacterial and anti-cyanobacterial activity against both tested organisms was observed, increasing with the quaternization degree. Remarkably, in the photosynthetic bacteria it was shown that the hybrid materials affect their photosynthetic apparatus by selective inhibition of the Photosystem-I electron transport activity. Cytotoxicity studies on a human prostate carcinoma DU145 cell line and 3T3 mouse fibroblasts revealed that all hybrids exhibit high cytocompatibility in the concentration range, in which they also exhibit both high antibacterial and anti-cyanobacterial activity. Thus, QPEI-functionalized oxCNTs can be very attractive candidates as antibacterial and anti-cyanobacterial agents that can be used for potential applications in the disinfection industry, as well as for the control of harmful cyanobacterial blooms.

Keywords: carbon nanotubes; quaternary ammonium groups; hyperbranched dendritic polymers; antibacterial properties; anti-cyanobacterial properties

1. Introduction

Carbon nanotubes (CNTs) have attracted significant scientific and technological interest due to their unique structural characteristics and their excellent electronic, mechanical, and thermal properties [1,2]. Based on these properties, they have been used in a wide range of applications, including fillers in composite materials, sensors, drug delivery systems, antibacterial agents, and others [3,4]. However, their poor dispersibility in solvents, especially in water, has prevented their widespread industrial use, and reduced their great potential. Attempts to overcome this problem have focused on the functionalization of their surface, using a variety of covalent and non-covalent modification strategies [5]. On one hand, various organic molecules, such as dendritic and linear polymers, have been covalently conjugated onto the CNT's convex surfaces and tips by chemical reactions [6–8] in order to reduce aggregates and size polydispersity. However, covalent functionalization causes damage to the conjugated π-electrons, leading to degradation of their properties. On the other hand, non-covalent functionalization, based on π–π stacking and ionic interactions between various molecules and the CNTs graphitic surface [9–11] does not affect their electronic structure, and has been achieved using a multitude of surfactants [6,7] and polymers [8,10], resulting in modified CNTs, compatible with specific solvents or targeted applications. In this context, their functionalization with dendritic polymers such as dendrons, dendrimers, and hyperbranched polymers, is expected to be a very promising strategy, when aiming to achieve increased water solubility. This strategy has already been applied to single-walled carbon nanotubes (SWCNTs) that were functionalized using dendritic polymers through non-covalent interactions, achieving enhanced water solubility [8,12,13]. However, only a few studies have addressed the non-covalent functionalization of multi-walled carbon nanotubes (MWCNTs) with dendritic polymers for increased water solubility [14].

Dendritic polymers are highly branched macromolecules of nanosized dimensions, consisting of repeating units and surface end groups [15]. Their properties depend on both the structural characteristics of the branches in their interior, and the large number of surface end groups. These polymers can incorporate a variety of organic compounds as well as inorganic ions in their interior, while the surface end groups are primarily susceptible to functionalization or even multi-functionalization, to yield a variety of novel materials with diversified, tailor-made properties such as drug delivery systems, antibacterial agents, etc. [16–18]. Additionally, these terminal groups exhibit the so-called polyvalency effect [19], which enhances their binding with various substrates, due to their close proximity to the dendritic polymers' scaffold.

Recently, several studies have focused on the potential applications of carbon nanomaterials (CNMs), taking advantage of their antibacterial properties [20–22]. Specifically, functionalized single-walled carbon nanotubes (SWCNTs) and multi-walled carbon nanotubes (MWCNTs) were found to exhibit significant antibacterial activity towards both gram-positive and gram-negative bacteria [23,24]. CNTs' properties, such as carbon nanotube diameter [25], length [26], aggregation [27], concentration [28], surface functionalization [29–31], etc. have been reported to influence their antibacterial activity. To that respect, aqueous dispersibility can critically influence antibacterial efficiency, as highly dispersed CNTs enhance their interaction with cells, leading to increased antibacterial properties. Indeed, it was found [32] that individually dispersed CNTs were more toxic to bacteria than CNTs aggregates, due to increased contact with bacterial cells.

Nowadays, there is a growing concern about the possible effects of nanomaterials, as end of life products, on organisms and ecosystems [33,34]. Apart from studies investigating the mechanisms of interaction between CNTs and various biomacromolecules (DNA, RNA, etc.), to identify possible causes of undesired effects, [35] research efforts have also focused on the possible impact of MWCNTs on photosynthetic pathways. Remarkably, in photosynthetic organisms, unlike bacteria, a favorable effect of MWCNTs was observed, e.g., in the development of cereals, and the production of vegetative biomass [36]. Studies on algae revealed that MWCNTs did not influence photosynthesis, and any negative effects were due to turbidity and the resulting reduction of the available light [37]. However, oxidized MWCNTs were found to be toxic to the marine green alga *Dunaliella tertiolecta*, as at concentrations between 1–10 mg/L they reduced algal growth, and affected the Photosystem (PS) II photochemical process and the cellular glutathione redox status [38]. Moreover, although cyanobacterial blooms have become a serious environmental problem, only recently, a novel nanomaterial based on MWCNTs, called Taunit, loaded with antibiotic chloramphenicol or herbicide diuron, was investigated as an effective anti-cyanobacterial agent [39]. It was found that the Taunit-diuron complex exhibited high biocide action against cyanobacterium *Synechocystis* sp. PCC 6803, higher than that of a Taunit-chloramphenicol complex.

In this study, aiming to develop water soluble MWCNTs with enhanced antibacterial/anti-cyanobacteria properties, oxidized multi-walled carbon nanotubes (oxCNTs) were non-covalently functionalized using a series of partially quaternized hyperbranched poly(ethyleneimine) derivatives, yielding novel water-soluble hybrid materials. Specifically, three positively charged derivatives of hyperbranched poly(ethyleneimine) (PEI) with a different degree of quaternization at the primary amino groups of PEI were prepared and interacted with the negatively charged oxidized CNTs through electrostatic interactions and van der Waals attraction forces. The obtained hybrid materials were physicochemically characterized by various techniques (FTIR, Raman, SEM, TEM, AFM, etc.). Their excellent aqueous stability was demonstrated using ζ-potential measurements, dynamic light scattering, and UV-vis spectroscopy. Additionally, their antibacterial and anti-cyanobacterial activity was investigated against two types of gram negative bacteria, an autotrophic (cyanobacterium *Synechococcus* sp. PCC 7942) and a heterotrophic (bacterium *Escherichia coli*), while their cytocompatibility was investigated on eukaryotic cell lines.

2. Results and Discussion

2.1. Synthesis and Characterization of QPEI-Functionalized oxCNTs

Positively charged stable aqueous suspensions of carbon nanotubes were prepared, applying quaternized hyperbranched poly(ethyleneimine) derivatives (QPEIs). A series of partially quaternized hyperbranched poly(ethyleneimine) derivatives with 30%, 50%, and 80% substitution degree of primary amino groups was prepared, following a method analogous to one previously described [40,41]. Initially, PEI was characterized by inverse-gate decoupling ^{13}C NMR. According to the literature [42] and comparing the integration of carbons of α-CH$_2$ relative to primary, secondary, and tertiary amine groups, the ratio of primary to secondary and to tertiary amines of PEI was found to be 1.00:1.18:1.01. The branching degree was found to be 0.68, and the average number of primary amine groups was determined to be 183. Based on the above, the introduction of α-hydroxyamine moieties, together with the trimethylammonium groups, to PEI was achieved by the reaction of the PEI primary amines with appropriate amounts of glycidyltrimethylammonium chloride, yielding three PEI derivatives, i.e., 30-QPEI, 50-QPEI, and 80-QPEI (Scheme 1). Their structures were confirmed by ^{1}H and ^{13}C NMR spectroscopy. Specifically, the new quintet appearing at 4.25 ppm was attributed to the proton of α-CH group relative to hydroxyl group, which was formed after an oxiran ring opening. Additionally, the α-CH$_2$ protons relative to the quaternary group appeared as a triplet at 3.45 ppm, and the protons of the quaternary methyl groups at 3.25 ppm, while a multiplet in the region 2.50–2.70 ppm was attributed to the PEI scaffold protons. Comparing the integration of peaks at 3.45 ppm and 2.70–2.50 ppm, the degree of quaternization at the primary amino group of PEI was calculated, and was found to be 30%, 50%, and 80% for 30-QPEI, 50-QPEI, and 80-QPEI, respectively.

Furthermore, ^{13}C NMR spectroscopy provided insights into the structure of QPEIs. The attachment of the α-hydroxyamine moiety at the PEI scaffold was confirmed by the peaks at 51.0 and 48.0 ppm, attributed to the α carbon of PEI, and relative to the newly formed amino group (α-CH$_2$NH-Q), close to secondary (known as C$_{1,2}$) and tertiary (known as C$_{1,3}$) amines, respectively. Additionally, the α-methylene and methyl groups, attached at the quaternary center, were observed at 71.5 and 57.0 ppm, respectively, while a peak at 67.5 ppm was attributed to the α carbon relative to the newly formed hydroxyl group (CH–OH).

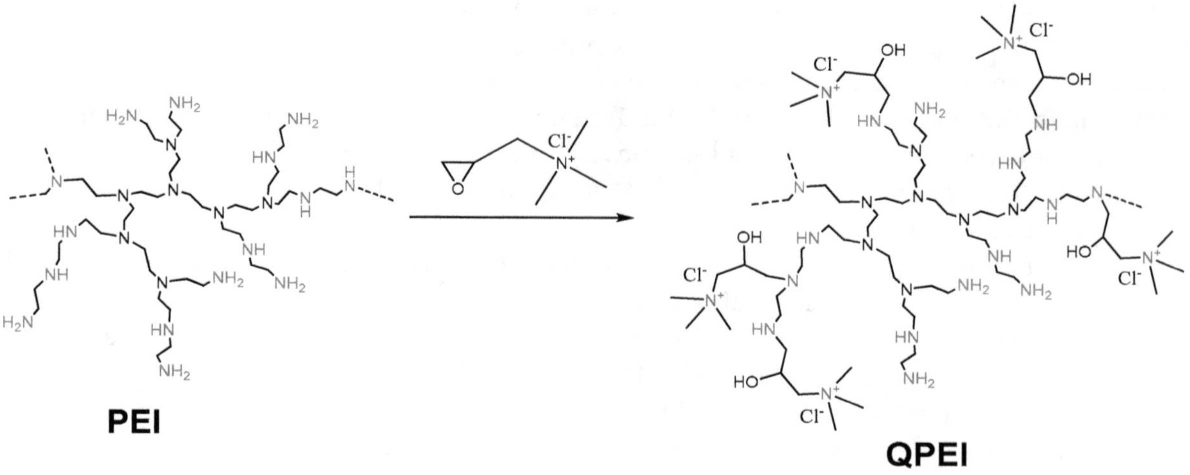

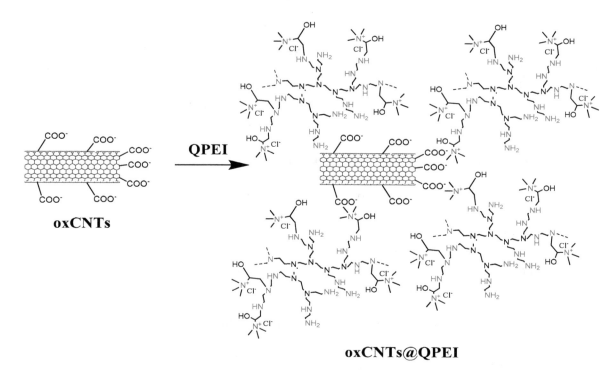

Scheme 1. Schematic representation of poly(ethyleneimine) (PEI) and the reaction scheme of quaternization.

Subsequently, these dendritic derivatives were interacted with oxidized CNTs in aqueous media (Scheme 2). The final hybrid nanomaterials, oxCNTs@30-QPEI, oxCNTs@50-QPEI, and oxCNTs@80-QPEI, were obtained after ultracentrifugation to remove the excess QPEIs, and physicochemically characterized using a variety of techniques, such as FTIR, RAMAN, TGA, SEM, TEM, AFM, etc.

Scheme 2. Schematic representation of oxidized multi-walled carbon nanotubes (oxCNTs) decorated with quaternized hyperbranched poly(ethyleneimine) derivative (QPEI).

To investigate the successful attachment of QPEIs on the oxCNTs, initially, FTIR spectroscopy was employed. In Figures 1A and S1, the FTIR spectra of QPEIs, oxCNTs, and QPEI-functionalized oxCNTs are shown. The spectrum of oxCNTs shows a C=C stretching band at 1650 cm^{-1}, attributed to the CNTs graphite structure. Additionally, the presence of oxygen containing groups (carboxylates, carbonyl, hydroxyl, and epoxy groups) on the oxCNTs was confirmed by the appearance of a C=O stretching band at 1740 cm^{-1}, a broad OH stretching band centered at 3370 cm^{-1}, and a strong C–OH stretching band at 1100 cm^{-1}, as well as two peaks at 1565 and 1380 cm^{-1}, which are associated with the carboxylate anion stretch mode (asymmetrical and symmetrical vibrations of COO$^-$, respectively). Furthermore, the peaks at 2750 and 1255 cm^{-1}, attributed to the stretching vibrations of OC–H and C–O–C, respectively, revealed the presence of aldehydes and epoxy groups on oxCNTs [43]. On the other hand, as expected, the FTIR spectra of all QPEIs exhibited the sample characteristic bands. Those included the characteristic vibrations of PEI, i.e., at 3360 and 3270 cm^{-1}, attributed to the stretching vibration of primary and secondary amino groups, at 2940 and 2835 cm^{-1}, assigned to the asymmetrical and symmetrical vibrations of CH$_2$, at 1600 and 1560 cm^{-1}, attributed to the NH deformation mode of the primary and secondary amino groups, respectively, at 1455 and 760 cm^{-1}, corresponding to the bending and rocking mode of CH$_2$, respectively, and at 1115 and 1050 cm^{-1}, assigned to the asymmetrical and symmetrical vibrations of C–N [44]. Additionally, the most important stretching and deformation vibrations of CH$_3$ in the quaternary ammonium group (CH$_3$)$_3$N$^+$ at 3030 cm^{-1} and 1485 cm^{-1}, the asymmetrical stretching vibration of the whole (CH$_3$)$_3$N$^+$ group at 970 cm^{-1}, and the stretching vibrations of C–OH groups at 1100 cm^{-1} were observed [45]. The FTIR spectra of the QPEI-functionalized oxCNTs (Figures 1A and S1) revealed the existence of both oxCNTs and QPEIs, confirming their successful interaction.

The successful functionalization of oxCNTs was also confirmed by Raman measurements. The spectra of oxCNTs and QPEI-functionalized oxCNTs presented in Figure 1B, display the two main typical graphite bands at 1585 cm^{-1} (G band) and 1345 cm^{-1} (D band), attributed to the in-plane vibration of the sp^2-bonded carbon atoms in graphite layers, and to the defects presented in carbon nanotubes due to the conversion of carbon atoms from an sp^2 to an sp^3 hybridization state, respectively. Additionally, a band at ~2700 cm^{-1} (G' band) is shown in Figure 1B, attributed to the D band overtone. As observed in Figure 1B, the Raman shifts of QPEI-functionalized oxCNTs compared to those of oxCNTs did not change, revealing that the graphitic structure of oxCNTs does not significantly alter after functionalization. Only the value of the intensity ratio of D- to G- bands (I$_D$/I$_G$), a measure of the defects present in a graphene structure during functionalization, slightly increased from 1.03 to 1.16, revealing successful polymer wrapping all over the graphite layer of CNTs [46]. In analogous studies involving covalent functionalization of multi-walled carbon nanotubes via third-generation dendritic poly(amidoamine) or amphiphilic poly(propyleneimine) dendrimers, a larger increase of the intensity ratio (I$_D$/I$_G$), was reported indicating that functionalization caused a larger defect of the graphitic network [47,48]. In contrast, in the present study oxCNTs were non-covalently functionalized with QPEI derivatives, retaining their surface almost intact.

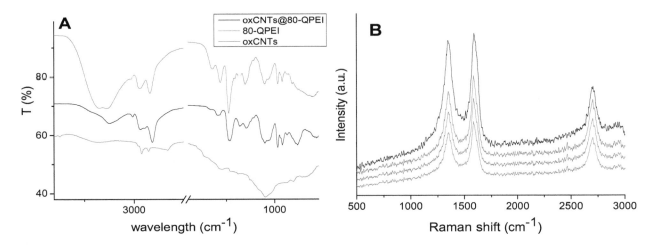

Figure 1. (**A**) FTIR spectra of oxCNTs, oxCNTs@80-QPEI, and 80-QPEI. (**B**) Raman spectra of oxCNTs (black), oxCNTs@30-QPEI (red), oxCNTs@50-QPEI (blue), and oxCNTs@80-QPEI (magenta).

    The results of thermogravimetric analysis (TGA) provided further information on the QPEI content on the surfaces of oxCNTs (Figure 2). In the TGA curve of oxCNTs, two distinct decomposition regions were observed. Specifically, a weight loss corresponding to ~4% of the initial weight was recorded in the temperature range of 180–400 °C, due to the removal of oxygen-containing functional groups present on the graphitic framework. A second significant loss was observed at higher temperatures (>500 °C), and was attributed to the thermal degradation of the graphitic framework. In contrast, the QPEI-functionalized oxCNTs exhibited a significant weight loss (10–20%) up to 250 °C, due to both the removal of oxCNTs' oxygen-containing groups, and the partial PEI degradation. The weight loss for QPEI-functionalized oxCNTs in the temperature range 250–400 °C was significantly higher in comparison to oxCNTs (up to 60%), since together with the decomposition of graphitic lattice, QPEI molecules were removed from the graphitic framework. Therefore, TGA measurements provided further qualitative experimental evidence that functionalization had occurred, however, due to the oxCNT contribution to the thermal phenomena, the polymer content could not be quantified. Again, above ~500 °C, the sharp weight loss indicated the total thermal destruction of the graphitic network.

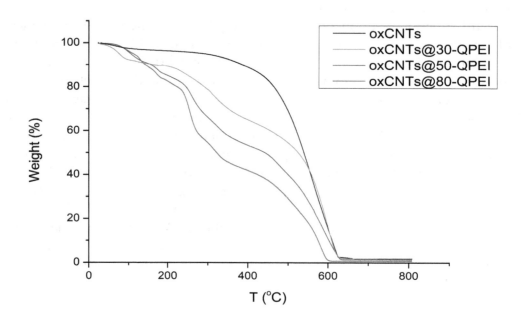

Figure 2. Thermogravimetric curves of oxCNTs and QPEI-functionalized oxCNTs.

    Elemental analysis measurements were additionally performed to confirm and quantify the polymer content in the QPEI-functionalized oxCNTs. Given that the nitrogen signal in the final hybrid originated mainly from QPEI, the difference compared to the starting oxCNTs represented the amount of polymer attached to the CNTs. Therefore, the QPEI content in hybrids was calculated from the following formula:

$$\text{QPEI } (\% \ w/w) = (N_s - N_{\text{CNTs}})/(N_{\text{QPEI}} - N_{\text{CNTs}}) \times 100$$

where N_s, N_{QPEI}, and N_{CNTs}, were the nitrogen elemental mass fraction in QPEI-functionalized oxCNTs, QPEI, and oxCNTs, respectively [49]. The results are summarized in Table S1. According to the elemental analysis results, the actual value of QPEI weight fraction in oxCNTs@30-QPEI, oxCNTs@50-QPEI, and oxCNTs@80-QPEI was found to be 16.05%, 19.92%, and 23.23%, respectively.

    The morphology of the QPEI-functionalized oxCNTs was studied by scanning electron (SEM), transmission electron (TEM), and atomic force (AFM) microscopies. Representative SEM micrographs are shown in Figure 3. It is clear that after functionalization with QPEIs, the morphology of the oxCNTs did not change significantly. Additionally, oxCNTs@QPEIs are shown to be well-dispersed and no aggregation of nanotubes was observed, as in the case of oxCNTs (Figure S2). Especially, functionalization of oxCNTs with 80-QPEI rendered them fully isolated, as shown in Figure 3 (images C and D).

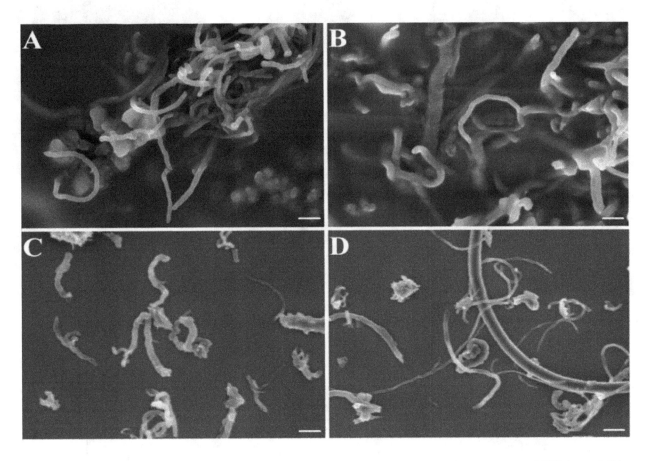

Figure 3. SEM images of oxCNTs@30-QPEI (**A**), oxCNTs@50-QPEI (**B**), and oxCNTs@80-QPEI (part **C,D**). The scale bar is 100 nm.

The morphology of QPEI-functionalized oxCNTs, as well as the presence of QPEIs on their surface, was studied by combining TEM bright-field imaging, EFTEM elemental mapping, and EELS spectroscopy. In Figure 4A functionalized carbon nanotubes are observed isolated, without any aggregation, as in the SEM images. These observations suggest that the QPEIs covered the surface of the nanotubes, improving their aqueous dispersibility and debundling. In the HRTEM images the structured graphite walls of oxCNTs can be observed, covered with an amorphous layer of QPEI polymer (Figure 4D,E). For this reason, electron energy loss spectroscopy (EELS) was employed to investigate the spatial distribution of nitrogen, observed in the bright field images of oxCNTs. An energy-filtered TEM (EFTEM) image (utilizing the three-window method), using the nitrogen K-edge at 401 eV electron energy loss, can be seen in Figure 4C, while Figure 4B is the bright field image of the same area. It is obvious that since the intensity of the maps corresponds to the concentration of N (red) that exclusively originated from QPEI, it can be concluded that oxCNTs were uniformly covered by QPEI. Additionally, in a typical background subtracted EELS spectrum the nitrogen K-edges recorded for oxCNTs@80-QPEI (Figure 4) are evidence for the presence of nitrogen atoms and the successful attachment of QPEI on the surface of oxCNTs.

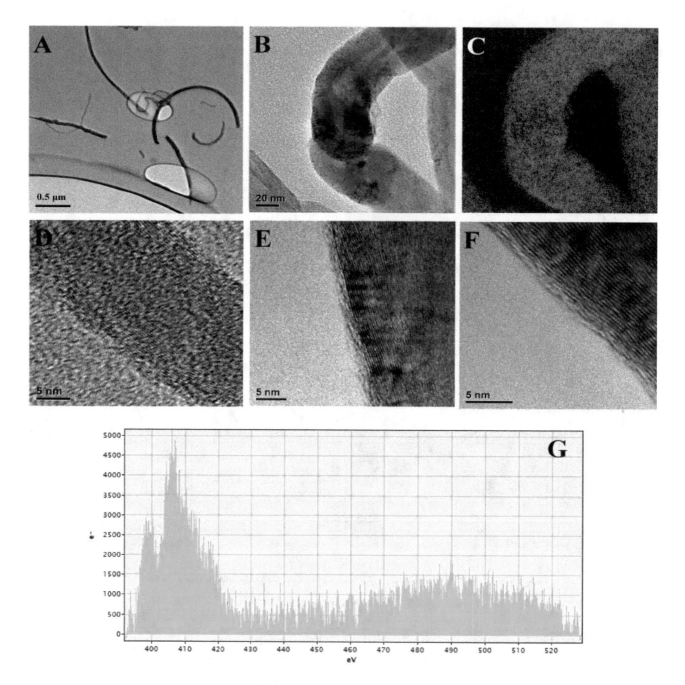

Figure 4. TEM bright field image of oxCNTs@50-QPEI (**A**). Bright field image (**B**) and the corresponding EFTEM compositional nitrogen N map (red, **C**) of oxCNTs@50-QPEI, HRTEM images: images of oxCNTs@80-QPEI (**D–F**) and a typical background subtracted EELS spectrum of nitrogen K- edges, recorded for oxCNTs@80-QPEI (**G**).

AFM images of oxCNTs@50-QPEI and oxCNTs@80-QPEI, deposited on Si-wafer (Figure 5) show the morphological features of oxCNTs at the nanoscale after the interaction with the polymers. The AFM images (height and 3D) of nanocomposites reveal the successful attachment (wrapping) of polymer on the oxCNTs sidewalls. As derived from topographical section analysis, an overlay of 10–25 nm is observed from each side of nanotube in the case of oxCNTs@50-QPEI, while the size of the polymeric coating is much higher, and easily distinguishable in the case of oxCNTs@80-QPEI, corresponding to an average of 25–40 nm (Figure 5). Moreover, the average diameter of oxCNTs@80-QPEI, as derived from height analysis, is about 40–50 nm, a value much higher than that of oxCNTs in the absence of 80-QPEI, which ranges between 15 and 25 nm (Figure S2).

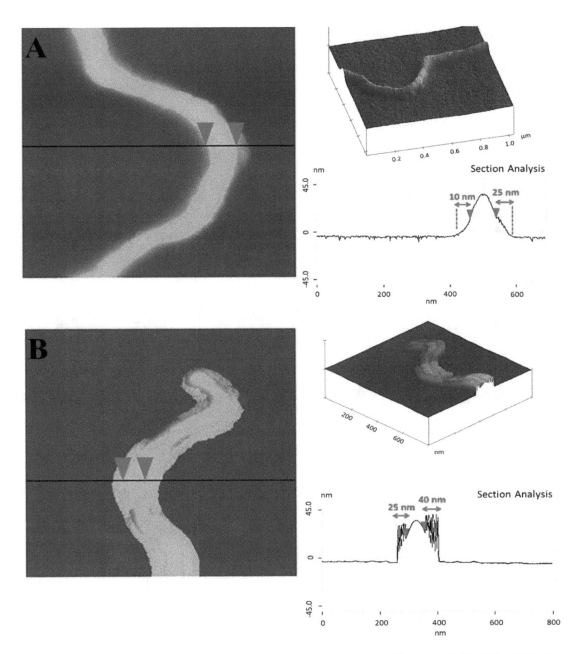

Figure 5. AFM images (height, profile section analysis, and 3D) of oxCNTs@50-QPEI (**A**) and oxCNTs@80-QPEI (**B**), showing the coverage of QPEI derivatives in the sidewalls of oxCNTs.

2.2. Colloidal Stability of the CNTs Dispersions

CNTs have an extremely strong tendency to aggregate in water due to their high surface energy, making them difficult to disperse in aqueous media resulting in the formation of large bundles [50]. Although the dispersibility of CNTs in aqueous media has been shown to increase following (i) various oxidation processes [51], and (ii) using high concentrations of various surfactants [6,7] or polymers [8,9], the resulting dispersions are only stable for short time. In this study, the negatively charged oxidized CNTs, modified with positively charged QPEIs through electrostatic interactions and van der Waals attraction forces, resulted in functionalized oxCNTs with high positive charge contents, and able to form stable aqueous dispersions. All QPEIs derivatives enhance the aqueous dispersibility of oxCNTs, as revealed by visual observation over time (Figure 6, upper part). It is obvious that stable dispersions of oxCNTs were obtained after functionalization with QPEIs for at least twelve months (Figure 6, upper part), while oxCNTs had precipitated within one month after the sonication process. This was achieved thanks to the presence of quaternary ammonium groups on the surface of the oxCNTs that provide a high compatibility with aqueous media due to their strong hydrophilicity, while preventing the CNTs' aggregation due to electrostatic repulsion. In an analogous study, involving SWCNTs, Grunlan, J.C. et al. observed that after non-covalent functionalization with PEI, SWCNTs exhibited poor aqueous stability, attributed to PEIs hyperbranched structure that sterically reduced electrostatic interactions [52]. The same behavior was observed in this study for PEI functionalized oxCNTs. In contrast, quaternized PEI derivatives behave differently, probably due to their higher positively charged moieties content.

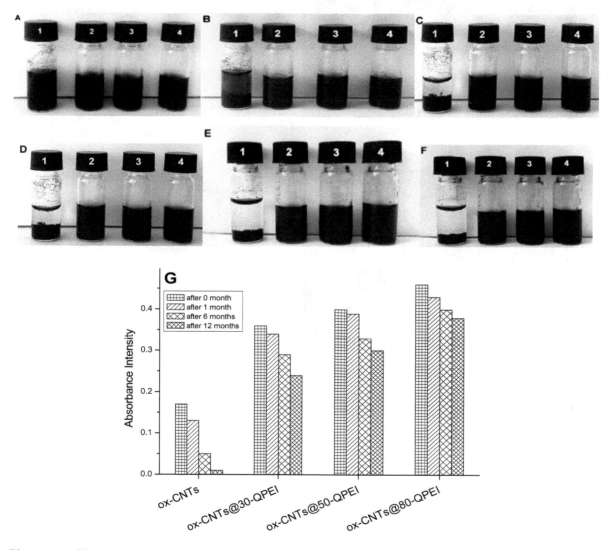

Figure 6. Dispersion state of (1) oxCNTs, (2) oxCNTs@30-QPEI, (3) oxCNTs@50-QPEI, and (4) oxCNTs@80-QPEI in water (5 mg/mL), (**A**) immediately after sonication, and after quiescent settling for (**B**) 2 weeks, (**C**) 1 month, (**D**) 3 months, (**E**) 6 months, and (**F**) 12 months (upper part). (**G**) Sedimentation behavior of oxCNTs and QPEI-functionalized oxCNTs at different aging times (lower part).

It is known that bundled CNTs, unlike individual ones, are not active in the UV–vis region [53] allowing the investigation of their dispersibility using UV–vis absorption spectroscopy. Figure S3 shows the UV–vis spectra of the oxCNTs@30-QPEI, oxCNTs@50-QPEI, and oxCNTs@80-QPEI aqueous dispersions. The dispersions have a characteristic absorption peak at 263 nm, affected by the p-plasmon absorption of carbon nanomaterials. The higher absorption, caused by the p-plasmon from the oxCNTs@80-QPEI, demonstrates more efficient debundling of oxCNTs by 80-QPEI, compared to other carbon nanomaterials [54]. Furthermore, the evaluation of colloidal stability of the CNTs was attained by UV–vis spectroscopy, again after investigation of the characteristic absorption of CNTs at 263 nm. Figure 6G presents the optical density (O.D.) of the oxCNTs and QPEI-functionalized oxCNTs dispersed in water within the storage periods. It was obvious that the dispersions of all QPEI-functionalized oxCNTs were stable for at least twelve months, since their optical densities were reduced only by 10–20% compared to the initial O.D. On the other hand, the O.D. of the oxCNTs dispersion was reduced by 90% after 12 months storage. The O.D. reduction of oxCNTs dispersion was attributed to the gradual formation of CNTs agglomerates, some of which subsequently aggregated and finally precipitated. These findings are in line with the visual inspection of the CNT dispersions presented in Figure 6A–F. Moreover, the dispersion of oxCNTs@80-QPEI is the most stable since only a 10% reduction of O.D. was observed after 12 months storage. To the best of our knowledge the stability achieved is one of the highest reported in the literature, and its importance lies in the fact that the aqueous stability of such hybrid nanomaterials is of paramount importance in several industrial applications.

2.3. Characterization of the QPEI-Functionalized oxCNTs Dispersions

Dynamic light scattering (DLS) and ζ-potential measurements can provide information on nanomaterials regarding their size distribution, and also their surface charge. Although, DLS measurement is appropriate for determination of the spherical particle diameter, it can also be used to determine the hydrodynamic diameter of nanotubes, based on the assumption that an equivalent hydrodynamic diameter (D_h) of a sphere has the same diffusion properties as the CNT. [55] Even though one cannot determine absolute values, a relative size comparison can be obtained for similarly shaped materials [56]. Thus, comparing the aggregate size of oxCNTs to those of QPEI-functionalized oxCNTs, it is obvious that debundling of the oxCNTs took place after their interaction with the QPEIs, since the value of hydrodynamic diameter of the oxCNTs decreased from 1300 nm to 150 nm when 80-QPEI was used (Figure 7).

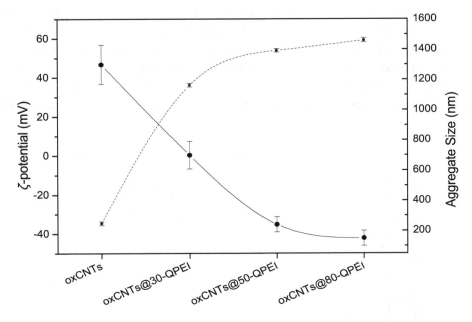

Figure 7. Mean hydrodynamic diameter (solid line) and ζ-potential values (dot line) of oxCNTs and QPEI-functionalized oxCNTs dispersions (0.05 mg/mL, pH = 7.0).

Zeta potential values of the oxCNTs dispersions at pH = 7.0 are given in Figure 7. As expected, the aqueous dispersion of oxCNTs has a ζ-potential value around −34 mV, due to their negative surface charges. After modification with QPEI, the ζ-potential values of the QPEI-functionalized oxCNTs dispersions increased to positive, reaching the value of +60 mV for oxCNTs@80-QPEI, offering further evidence that the positively charged QPEIs were successfully attached onto the oxCNTs surface. It should be noted that all ζ-potential values were higher than +30 mV, indicating stable aqueous colloidal suspensions, in which the CNTs' aggregation was prevented due to electrostatic repulsion, in line with the results of UV–vis and DLS measurements (see above) [57].

2.4. Evaluation of Antibacterial and Anti-Cyanobacterial Activity

The cytotoxicity of QPEI-functionalized oxCNTs was assessed against two types of Gram-negative bacteria, i.e., the heterotrophic bacterial strain *Escherichia coli* XL1-blue and the autotrophic cyanobacterium *Synechococcus* sp. PCC 7942.

2.4.1. Cytotoxicity Effects of oxCNTs@QPEIs on *Escherichia coli* XL1-Blue Bacteria

Escherichia coli growth was investigated by monitoring the fluorescence intensity of bacterial cells suspensions at 37 °C that express red fluorescent protein (RFP). The excellent dispersibility of oxCNTs@QPEIs renders the commonly used turbidity measurement inapplicable, as functionalized CNTs, especially at high concentrations, contribute to the final measurement. Thus, by employing the inherent fluorescence of RFP, the antibacterial activity can be precisely assessed, even in the presence of nanoparticle dispersions, as in the case of oxCNTs@QPEIs. Comparing the fluorescence intensity of each bacterial suspension containing oxCNTs@QPEIs at a certain time, with the initial fluorescence intensity corresponding to the initial *Escherichia coli* population (at OD_{600} = 0.4), bacterial growth could be directly determined. Figure 8 depicts the *Escherichia coli* growth after 6 h incubation in the presence of oxCNTs and oxCNTs@QPEIs at different concentrations, ranging from 5 to 400 μg/mL, as a function of the fluorescence intensity of RFP at 590 nm (excitation: 545 nm), and normalized with the initial fluorescence intensity of control (100% fluorescence intensity). Contrary to the increase of the fluorescence intensity upon untreated bacteria growth (Figure S4), a decrease in the intensity was observed, for all samples, revealing bacterial growth inhibition. However, as shown in Figure 8, the oxCNTs exhibited low antibacterial activity, which is in accordance with the literature [58]. On the other hand, all QPEI-functionalized oxCNTs inhibited bacterial growth in a dose-dependent manner, displaying significantly higher antibacterial activity than the oxCNTs, and which increased upon substitution of PEI from 30% to 80%. In a further attempt to quantify the antibacterial activity of oxCNTs@QPEIs, the 50% inhibitory concentrations (IC-50) were calculated (Table 1). It was found that the lowest IC-50 was observed in the case of oxCNTs@80-QPEI (28.4 μg/mL), which showed that oxCNTs@80-QPEI exhibited the highest antibacterial activity amongst the other hybrid materials, due to both the increased aqueous dispersibility and the higher positive quaternary ammonium group content.

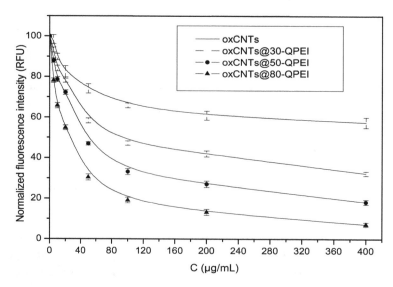

Figure 8. Cytotoxicity of oxCNTs and QPEI-functionalized oxCNTs against gram-negative *Escherichia coli* XL1-blue bacteria. Fluorescence intensity of RFP at 590 nm (excitation: 545 nm) after bacteria incubation for 6 h with oxCNTs@QPEIs at concentrations ranging from 5 to 400 μg/mL, normalized with the initial fluorescence intensity, corresponding to initial *E.coli* population (at OD_{600} = 0.4). Error bars represent mean ± SD for at least three independent experiments.

Table 1. IC-50 values of QPEI-functionalized oxCNTs on *Escherichia coli* XL1-blue bacteria.

Samples	IC-50 (µg/mL)
oxCNTs@30-QPEI	93.2
oxCNTs@50-QPEI	50.1
oxCNTs@80-QPEI	28.4

The morphology of *Escherichia coli* after 6-h incubation at 37 °C with oxCNTs@QPEIs was investigated by scanning electron microscopy (SEM). In Figure 9, SEM images of control (untreated cells) and cells treated with oxCNTs@QPEIs at 50% inhibitory concentrations are presented, showing significant changes in cell morphology. Specifically, the treated cells lost their cellular integrity, and are shown more clustered, while their cell walls seem rougher and damaged in all cases (Figure 9B–D) compared to the untreated cells (Figure 9A), which appear to be intact, with a smooth surface. Moreover, Figure 9D shows the most severe effect of oxCNTs@80-QPEI on the bacterial cell wall and membrane, in which the cell walls seem to be ruptured and bacterial cell lysis is clearly observed probably due to membrane damage.

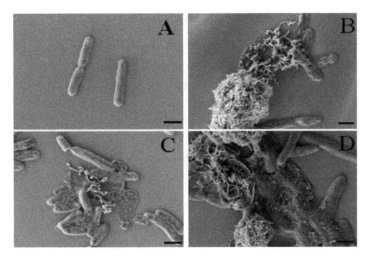

Figure 9. SEM images of *Escherichia coli* bacteria: untreated cells (**A**) and cells after 6-h incubation time at 37 °C with oxCNTs@30-QPEI (**B**), oxCNTs@50-QPEI (**C**), and oxCNTs@80-QPEI (**D**) at 50% inhibitory concentrations. The scale bar is 1 µm.

It is known that highly dispersed carbon nanotubes, mainly single wall carbon nanotubes, are able to interact strongly with bacteria through van der Waals forces, forming bacteria-CNTs aggregations [20,25]. This fact results in bacterial death due to either inhibition of transmembrane electron transfer, or to penetration leading to rupture or deformation of cell walls and membranes, which alter the bacterial metabolic processes [59]. Moreover, SWCNTs and MWCNTs containing various types of surface groups were investigated [29] regarding their antibacterial activity towards gram-negative and gram-positive bacteria. It was found that SWCNTs functionalized with hydroxyl and carboxyl surface groups exhibited improved antimicrobial activity against both gram-positive and gram-negative bacteria. However, MWCNTs containing the same functional surface groups did not exhibit any significant antibacterial effect [29]. On the contrary, covalently functionalized MWCNTs with positive moieties such as amines, arginines, and lysines, [60,61] or MWCNTs combined with surfactant molecules, such as dioctyl sodium sulfosuccinate [32], hexadecyltrimethylammonium bromide, triton X-100, and sodium dodecyl sulfate [7], exhibited enhanced antibacterial properties, due to enhanced interactions with bacterial membranes and the improved aqueous dispersibility and stability. In this study, similar antibacterial behavior of QPEI-functionalized oxCNTs was observed due to the high positive quaternary ammonium group content. These positive groups, as in the case of surfactant molecules or other positive functional groups, not only improved the debundling of

MWCNTs, which favors the strong interaction between the bacteria and MWCNTs, but also enhanced the penetration of MWCNTs though cell membranes, resulting in cell lysis and death.

Moreover, it is known that the quaternary ammonium moieties efficiently interact with the negatively charged groups of bacterial walls or cytoplasmic membranes, mainly through electrostatic as well as with secondary hydrophobic interactions, leading to dysfunction in cellular processes and probably to cell death [62]. Highly functionalized polymers with quaternary ammonium groups have been found to be more effective antibacterial agents than their low molecular weight analogues, as their higher charge densities lead to stronger interactions with the negatively charged bacteria walls [63]. For example, poly(propylene imine) dendrimers bearing 16 quaternary ammonium groups per molecule were found to exhibit two orders of magnitude greater antimicrobial activity than their mono-functional counterparts [64]. In agreement with this, the 80-QPEI derivative containing the highest content of quaternary ammonium groups provided the highest polycationic character to oxCNTs, in regards to the other QPEI derivatives. This effect probably induces the strongest interaction with bacteria, and the highest permeability of the cell membrane, and thus oxCNTs@80-QPEI exhibited the best antibacterial activity against the *Escherichia coli* bacteria compared to the other hybrid materials.

2.4.2. Cytotoxicity Effects of oxCNTs@QPEIs on *Synechococcus* sp. PCC 7942 Cyanobacteria

The antibacterial activity of oxCNTs@QPEIs was further assessed against the cyanobacterium *Synechococcus* sp. PCC 7942, a very widespread bacterial strain in the aquatic environment. In general, cyanobacteria (gram negative bacteria) are prokaryotic organisms that perform oxygenic photosynthesis similar to higher plants. They are the oldest and one of the largest and most important groups of bacteria on earth. Cyanobacteria (except prochlorophytes) contain only Chl α, the molecule which makes photosynthesis possible, by passing its energized electrons on to molecules during sugar synthesis [65]. However, several cyanobacterial strains are known to produce a wide range of toxic secondary metabolites (hepatotoxins, neurotoxins, cytotoxins, dermatotoxins, and irritant toxins), which could be harmful to animals and potentially dangerous to humans [66].

In this study, cyanobacteria *Synechococcus* sp. PCC 7942 cell proliferation was monitored by measurement of the Chl α concentration every 24 h, for seven days. Figure 10 shows the cell proliferation of the unicellular cyanobacterium *Synechococcus* sp. PCC 7942 cells in the presence of increasing concentrations of oxCNTs@30-QPEI, oxCNTs@50-QPEI, and oxCNTs@80-QPEI. For comparison reasons, analogous experiments were performed using oxCNTs, and their effect on the cyanobacteria cell proliferation is shown in Figure S5. It is clear that oxCNTs did not inhibit the cyanobacterial cell proliferation in contrast to all oxCNTs@QPEIs. This can be attributed again to the strong positive character of oxCNTs@QPEIs that intensified the interaction with the cyanobacteria membrane, and resulted in higher cell penetration compare to oxCNTs. In order to quantify these results, the effective concentration for 50% inhibition (IC-50), which shows the ability of cells to proliferate under the toxic effect of the oxCNTs@QPEIs, was calculated from the cyanobacterial cell proliferation curves in the presence of each hybrid material (Figure S6 and Table 2). Based on the interpretation of the experimental data using a non-linear regression of the four-parameter logistic function (Figure S6), it is obvious that cell proliferation is concentration dependent, while oxCNTs@80-QPEI exhibited the most promising anti-cyanobacterial activity, compared to the other two hybrid materials. This implies that upon increasing the degree of quaternization, the proliferation rate of cyanobacteria cells decreases. Therefore the anti-cyanobacterial properties, as in case of *Escherichia coli*, depend, not only on the concentration, but also on the degree of quaternization.

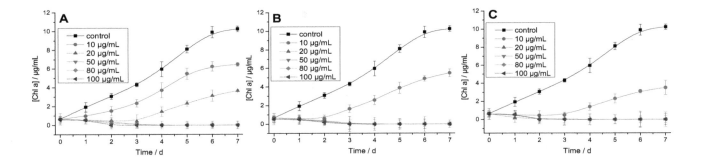

Figure 10. Effect of oxCNTs@QPEIs on cell proliferation of cyanobacteria *Synechococcus* sp. PCC 7942. Growth curves of cyanobacteria in the presence of different concentrations of: oxCNTs@30-QPEI (**A**), oxCNTs@50-QPEI (**B**), and oxCNTs@80-QPEI (**C**). Error bars represent mean ± SD for at least three independent experiments.

Table 2. IC-50 values of oxCNTs@QPEIs on cyanobacterium *Synechococcus* sp. PCC 7942.

Samples	IC-50 (μg/mL)
oxCNTs@30-QPEI	12.4
oxCNTs@50-QPEI	≤10
oxCNTs@80-QPEI	<10

Triggered by these results, it was interesting to evaluate the effect of oxCNTs@QPEIs on the photosynthetic apparatus of cyanobacteria. Therefore, the activity of Photosystem (PS) I and II was assessed in the presence of oxCNTs@80-QPEI, the material exhibiting the best antibacterial performance, to investigate the consequences of oxCNTs@QPEIs on the integrity of the photosynthetic apparatus in terms of photoinduced electron transport.

Specifically, selective detection of the PSII [67] and PSI electron transporting activities [68] was performed on *Synechococcus* sp. PCC 7942 bacteria treated with lysozyme (permeaplasts) at room temperature [69]. Using *Synechococcus* permeaplasts, oxymetrically photoinduced electron transport activities, across both PSII (electron donor: water; post-PSII electron acceptor: p-benzoquinone) and PSI (post- PSII inhibitor: DCMU; post-PSII electron donor: diaminodurene and ascorbate; post-PSI electron acceptor: methyl viologen) were measured. It was found that upon increase in concentration of oxCNTs@80-QPEI, the rate of oxygen evolution decreases (Table S2), indicating that PSII and PSI electron transport activities depend on the QPEI-functionalized oxCNT concentration. The inhibition of PSI and PSII by oxCNTs and oxCNT@80-QPEI is shown in Figure 11. Similarly to results previously reported in the literature, [70], at high concentrations (250 μg/mL) the oxCNTs used in this study inhibited the PSII and PSI by 37.6% and 95.7%, respectively, while at lower concentrations (20 μg/mL) the PSII is practically unaffected and the PSI activity is reduced by almost 44.8%. However, the impact of oxCNT@80-QPEI was much higher. The novel hybrid with an 80% quaternization degree inhibited the PSII by 16.7% at concentration 20 μg/mL, and by around 53.9% at 250 μg/mL. In the case of the PSI, the effect was even more significant, exhibiting almost complete inhibition (more than 97%), even at low concentrations (20 μg/mL).

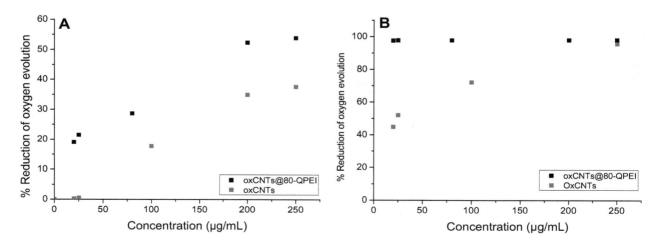

Figure 11. Effect of oxCNTs and oxCNTs@80-QPEI on the photosynthetic electron transport activities of PSII (**A**) and PSI (**B**) in *Synechococcus* sp. PCC 7942 permeaplasts.

The remarkable decrease in the IC-50 values of oxCNTs@QPEIs on cyanobacterial cell proliferation (Table 2) indicates that photosynthetic electron transport of both PSII and PSI is functionally impaired in cyanobacterial cells. Although, oxCNTs inhibit the photosynthetic redox reactions, and in the case of PSI almost fully prevent its activity, the effect of QPEI is significant. This may be attributed to the polycationic character of QPEI, as such compounds are known to completely inhibit PSI reactions, while leaving PSII relatively unaffected [71]. However, under the test conditions oxCNTs did not inhibit cyanobacterial cell proliferation (Figure S5), implying that the oxCNTs could not penetrate the cyanobacteria membranes. On the contrary, as mentioned above, the oxCNTs@QPEIs, exhibited high toxicity against cyanobacteria as a result of their efficient cell penetration (Figure 10).

Furthermore, to elucidate the potential alternative patterns for electron flow to and from PSI, the $P700^+$ transients in the presence of oxCNTs@80-QPEI were investigated. Table S3 shows the amounts of functional PSI complexes, estimated as the photooxidizable form of the PSI ($P700^+$) reaction center, measured as $\Delta A820/A820$ [72], where an 80% inhibition by oxCNTs@80-QPEI at high concentrations (250 µg/mL) can be observed. In a previous study, MWCNTs were successfully applied for direct transfer of electrons in isolated spinach thylakoids and cyanobacteria Nostoc sp. [73], pointing out that the results obtained in this study may also be associated with an interruption of the electron transport, due to the presence of oxCNTs. Concomitantly, the lower steady state photooxidation of P700 by far red light, might also be considered as an indication that oxCNTs@QPEIs quench the $P700^+$. Based on the above, the observed enhanced anti-cyanobacterial effect of QPEI-functionalized oxCNTs on cyanobacterium *Synechococcus* sp. PCC 7942 is ascribed to the selective inhibition of PSI.

2.5. Cell Viability Assay

To investigate the cytotoxicity of QPEI-functionalized oxCNTs, the human prostate carcinoma DU145 cell line and the 3T3 mouse fibroblasts were employed. For this purpose, these cells were incubated for 24 h with oxCNTs and oxCNTs@QPEIs at concentrations below and above their IC-50 values and cell viability was assessed, employing the standard MTT assay. The percent cell viability caused by all derivatives is presented in Figure 12. It is obvious that all oxCNTs@QPEIs were not toxic at their IC-50 values, and significantly less lethal than the parent oxCNTs, while at higher concentrations (100–200 µg/mL) only oxCNTs@30-QPEI exhibited slight toxicity (~70% cell survival). It should be noted that at 200 µg/mL, a concentration much higher than their IC-50 values, oxCNTs@50-QPEI and oxCNTs@80-QPEI did not display any cytotoxicity. These results suggest that all oxCNTs@QPEIs simultaneously exhibited both low cytotoxicity and enhanced antibacterial/anti-cyanobacterial properties.

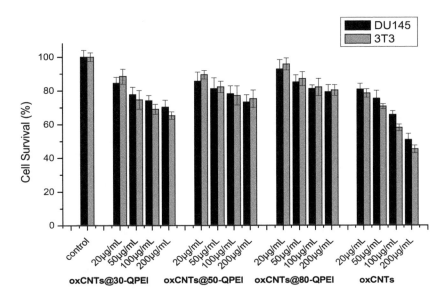

Figure 12. Cytotoxicity of oxCNTs and QPEI-functionalized oxCNTs on DU145 and 3T3 cells following incubation at various concentrations for 24 h, as determined by MTT assays. Data are expressed as mean ± SD of eight independent values obtained from at least three independent experiments.

3. Materials and Methods

3.1. Chemicals and Reagents

Hyperbranched poly(ethyleneimine) (PEI) with molecular weight 25 KDa (Lupasol® WF, water-free, 99%) and oxidized multi-walled carbon nanotubes were kindly donated by BASF (Ludwigshafen, Germany) and Glonatech S.A. (Athens Greece), respectively. Glycidyltrimethylammonium chloride, dialysis tubes (molecular weight cut-off: 1200) and triethylamine were obtained from Sigma-Aldrich (St. Louis, MA, USA). D-MEM low glucose with phenol red, L-glutamine, phosphate buffer saline (PBS), fetal bovine serum (FBS), penicillin/streptomycin, and trypsin/EDTA were purchased from BIOCHROM (Berlin, Germany). Thiazolyl blue tetrazolium bromide (MTT) and isopropanol were purchased from Merck KGaA (Calbiochem®, Darmstadt, Germany).

3.2. Synthesis of Quaternized Hyperbranched Poly(ethyleneimine) Derivatives

Quaternized derivatives of hyperbranched poly(ethyleneimine), with different substitution degrees of primary amino groups were prepared by a method previously described [40,41]. In brief, to an aqueous solution (20 mL) of PEI (5 mM), an aqueous mixture (10 mL) containing, 8, 12, or 18 mmol glycidyltrimethylammonium chloride and 16, 24, or 36 mmol triethylamine, respectively, was added. The reaction was completed after two days at room temperature and the final quaternized derivatives with 30% (30-QPEI), 50% (50-QPEI), and 80% (80-QPEI) degree substitution of primary amino groups were received after dialysis against deionized water and lyophilization. The introduction of the quaternary moieties at the external surface of the parent PEI was confirmed by ^{1}H and ^{13}C NMR spectroscopy. Additionally, the degree of quaternization at the primary amino groups of PEI was calculated by the integration of peaks at 3.45 ppm and 2.70–2.50 ppm in the ^{1}H NMR spectra.

^{1}H NMR: (500 MHz, D$_2$O) δ (ppm) = 4.25 (broad s, CH–OH), 3.45 (m, CH$_2$N$^+$(CH$_3$)$_3$), 3.25 (s, CH$_3$), 2.70–2.50 (m, CH$_2$ of PEI scaffold).

^{13}C NMR (125.1 MHz, D$_2$O): δ (ppm) = 71.5 (CH$_2$N$^+$CH$_3$)$_3$), 67.5 (CH–OH), 57.0 (CH$_3$), 55–51.0 (CH$_2$ of PEI scaffold), 51.0 and 48.0 (CH$_2$NH-Q primary and secondary, respectively), 42.0 and 40.0 (CH$_2$NH$_2$ close to secondary (C$_{1,2}$) and tertiary (C$_{1,3}$) amine, respectively).

3.3. Preparation of QPEI-Functionalized oxCNTs

The functionalization of oxCNTs was achieved by a method previously described [41]. Specifically, 50 mg of oxCNT powder was dispersed in 50 mL of an aqueous solution, containing an excess quantity (150 mg) of each quaternized derivative, and the resulting dispersions were ultrasonicated for 15 min (Hielscher UP200S high intensity ultrasonic processor equipped with a standard sonotrode (3 mm tip-diameter) at 50% amplitude and 0.5 cycles) and stirred for a further 12 h, at room temperature. The final hybrid materials, oxCNTs@30-QPEI, oxCNTs@50-QPEI, and oxCNTs@80-QPEI, were received after ultracentrifugation at 45,000 rpm, followed by thorough washing with water to remove the unreacted QPEI derivatives and lyophilization.

3.4. Characterization of QPEI-Functionalized oxCNTs

FTIR spectra were recorded using a Nicolet 6700 spectrometer (Thermo Scientific, Waltham, MA, USA) equipped with an attenuated total reflectance accessory with a diamond crystal (Smart Orbit, Thermo Electron Corporation, Madison, WI, USA). Raman spectra were obtained using a micro-Raman system RM 1000 Renishaw (laser excitation line at 532 nm, Nd-YAG) in the range of 400–2000 cm^{-1}. AFM images were obtained in tapping mode, with a 3D Multimode Nanoscope, using Tap-300G silicon cantilevels with a <10 nm tip radius and a ≈20–75 N/m force constant. Samples were deposited onto silicon wafers (P/Bor, single side polished) by drop casting from ethanol solutions. Scanning electron microscopy (SEM) images were recorded using a Jeol JSM 7401F field emission scanning electron microscope equipped with a gentle beam mode. Transmission electron micrographs were taken using a Philips C20 TEM instrument equipped with a Gatan GIF 200 energy filter for electron energy loss elemental mapping. For the sample preparation, a drop of oxCNTs@QPEIs aqueous solution (0.1 mg/mL) was casted on a PELCO® Formvar grid and was left to evaporate. Thermogravimetric analyses (TGA) were carried out on a Setaram SETSYS Evolution 17 system at a 5 °C/min heating rate under oxygen atmosphere. Elemental analysis (EA) was measured by a Perkin Elmer 240 CHN elemental analyzer.

3.5. Preparation and Characterization of QPEI-Functionalized oxCNTs Aqueous Dispersions

The suspensions of polymer-functionalized oxCNTs were prepared by adding 10 mg of oxCNTs@30-QPEI, oxCNTs@50-QPEI, or oxCNTs@80-QPEI into 2 mL pure water. The suspensions were then ultra-sonicated for 5 min using a Hielscher UP200S high intensity ultrasonic processor at 40% amplitude and 0.5 cycles. Each sample was centrifuged at 1500 rpm for 15 min, and then the supernatant was diluted with pure water before measurement.

ζ-potential measurements were performed using a ZetaPlus -Brookhaven Instruments Corp. In a typical experiment, an aqueous 0.05 mg/mL dispersion of QPEI-functionalized oxCNTs was used, ten ζ-potential measurements were collected, and the results were averaged. Dynamic light scattering studies were carried out on an AXIOS-150/EX (Triton Hellas) system equipped with a 30 mW laser source, and an avalanche photodiode detector at 90° angle. In a typical experiment, an aqueous 0.05 mg/mL dispersion of QPEI-functionalized oxCNTs was used, at least ten measurements were collected, and the data were analyzed using the CONTIN algorithm to obtain the hydrodynamic radii distribution.

UV-vis spectra of the aqueous dispersions (1 mg/mL) were obtained by a Cary 100 Conc UV-visible spectrophotometer (Varian Inc., Mulgrave, Australia) in the range of 200–600 nm. Additionally, the colloid stability of the functionalized carbon nanotubes was evaluated at static conditions for 1, 6, and 12 months. Specifically, the dispersions obtained as described previously, were placed in vertically standing tubes and stored at room temperature. At each time point, 100 μL of the stock solutions from the very upper part was taken diluted in 1 mL water and the optical density (O.D.) of these dispersions was measured using UV-vis spectroscopy.

3.6. Escherichia coli Growth Inhibition Assay

The antibacterial activity of QPEI-functionalized oxCNTs was obtained by a bacteria growth inhibition assay. *Escherichia coli* XL1-blue bacteria expressing red fluorescent protein (RFP), from a plasmid-encoded gene, were grown in Luria–Bertani (LB) broth at 37 °C overnight, in a Stuart SI500 orbital shaker at approximately 200 rpm shaking speed in aerobic conditions. The culture was subsequently diluted to an optical density (O.D.) of 0.4 at 600 nm. The QPEI-functionalized oxCNTs were homogeneously dispersed in distilled water by sonication and added to the bacterial culture at concentrations ranging from 5 to 400 µg/mL. The assay was performed in a 96-well plate format in a 200 µL final volume. Fluorescence intensity over growth of untreated bacteria revealed that the optimum incubation time was 6 h, as the intensity reached a plateau (Figure S4). Thus, plates were incubated at 37 °C, shaking at 100 rpm in aerobic conditions for 6 h, and bacterial growth was monitored using the fluorescence intensity of red fluorescent protein, which was recorded at an emission wavelength of 590 nm by an Infinite M200 plate reader (Tecan group Ltd., Männedorf, Switzerland) at an excitation wavelength of 545 nm. In order to eliminate the effect of CNTs in the measured intensities, the initial values (at 0 h), although minor compared to those obtained after 6 h, were subtracted from the final measurements. For each treatment eight replicates were used and three independent experiments were performed. Untreated bacteria were used as control, representing 100% fluorescence intensity in Figure 8.

3.7. SEM Analysis of the Cellular Morphology

The morphology of the *Escherichia coli* bacteria after treatment with QPEI-functionalized oxCNTs was characterized by scanning electron microscopy (Jeol JSM 7401F Field Emission SEM). Specifically, cells were incubated with QPEI-functionalized oxCNTs at their 50% inhibitory concentration (IC-50), fixed with 3% glutaraldehyde in sodium cacodylate buffer (100 mM, pH = 7.1) for 6 h, transferred to a poly(L-lysine) coated glass cover slip, dehydrated using ethanol gradient (twice of 50%, 70%, 95%, and 100% ethanol for 10 min each), drying, and coated with gold in a sputter coater [74].

3.8. Synechococcus sp. PCC7942 Cyanobacteria Growth Inhibition Assay

In vitro anti-cyanobacterial activity of QPEI-functionalized oxCNTs was screened against *Synechococcus* sp. PCC 7942 bacteria. The unicellular cyanobacterium *Synechococcus* sp. PCC7942 was purchased from the Collection Nationale de Cultures de Microorganismes (CNCM), Institut Pasteur, Paris, France. The cyanobacterial cells were cultured in BG11 that additionally contained 20 mM HEPES-NaOH (pH = 7.5). The cultures were illuminated with white light from fluorescent lamps, providing a photosynthetic active radiation (PAR) of 100 µmol photons m^{-2} s^{-1}, and were aerated with air containing 5% (*v/v*) CO_2 in an orbital incubator (Galenkamp INR-400) at 31 °C [75]. QPEI-functionalized oxCNTs dispersed in distilled water using ultrasonication were added to the bacterial culture at concentrations ranged from 10 to 100 µg/mL. Cyanobacterial cell proliferation was monitored in terms of concentration of Chl α, determined in *N,N*-dimethylformamide (DMF) extracts [76]. To extract Chl α, the cell suspensions were centrifuged, DMF was added to the residue, and the resulting clear supernatant DMF extract was obtained after a second centrifugation.

Toxicity tests were performed in three replicate experiments using at least five geometrically scaled dilutions for each compound concentration. The cyanobacteria culture was inoculated in each test solution in the exponential growth phase at concentrations of approximately 1 µg Chl α/mL. The toxicity of the oxCNTs@QPEIs was evaluated as the effective concentrations (µg/mL) of the test substance inhibiting cell proliferation by 50% (IC-50) relative to the control cultures; in this test, the IC-50 values were calculated by the area under the growth curves (biomass) for each concentration of the hybrid materials, using non-linear regression of a 4-parameters logistic function. The related data are presented in Figure S6.

3.9. Measurements of Photosystem I and II Electron Transport Activities

Photo-induced electron transport rates were determined in *Synechococcus* permeaplasts [68] at room temperature oxymetrically (for each Photosystem) with a Clark-type oxygen electrode (DW1; Oxygraph, Hansatech, King's Lynn, UK). *Synechococcus* sp. PCC 7942 bacteria were treated with lysozyme to obtain permeaplasts before the measurement of the photosynthetic electron transport activities [69]. The instrument was fitted with a slide projector to provide actinic illumination of samples. PSI activity was determined by measuring the rate of oxygen uptake, in the presence of the post-PSII electron transfer inhibitor 3-(3,4-dichlorophenyl)-1,10-dimethylurea (DCMU), using Na ascorbate/diaminodurene as an electron donor to PSI and methyl viologen as a post-PSI electron acceptor and mediator of oxygen uptake [77]. The reaction mixture (1 mL, in buffered BG11) contained permeaplasts (5 μg Chl α), diaminodurene (1 mM), Na-ascorbate (2 mM), methyl viologen (0.15 mM), and DCMU (0.01 mM). PSII activity was determined by measuring the rate of oxygen evolution, with water as electron donor and p-benzoquinone as post-PSII electron acceptor. The reaction mixture (1 mL in buffered BG11) contained permeaplasts (5 μg Chl α/mL) and p-benzoquinone (1 mM).

The redox state of P700 was determined *in vivo* using a PAM-101-modulated fluorometer (Heinz Walz GmbH, Effeltrich, Germany), equipped with an ED-800T emitter-detector, and PAM-102 units, following the procedure of Schreiber at al. [64]. The redox state of P700 was evaluated as the absorbance change around 820 nm (ΔA820/A820).

3.10. Cell Cytotoxicity

In this study, human prostate carcinoma cell line DU145 and 3T3 mouse fibroblasts, obtained from the American Type Culture Collection (ATCC, Manassas, VA, USA), were used. Cells were grown in low glucose supplemented D-MEM, containing 10% FBS, penicillin/streptomycin solution (100 U/mL + 100 μg/mL), and 2 mM L-Glutamine. Cells were incubated at 37 °C in a humidified atmosphere, containing 5% CO_2 and sub-cultured, twice a week after detaching with a solution containing 0.05% (*w/v*) trypsin and 0.02% (*w/v*) EDTA. The cytotoxicity of oxCNTs and the QPEI functionalized oxCNTs was assessed employing MTT assay. DU145 cancer cells and 3T3 mouse fibroblasts were inoculated (10^4 cells/well) into 96-well plates and incubated in complete media for 24 h. Cells were then treated with various concentrations of oxCNTs@QPEIs for 24 h. The mitochondrial redox function (translated as cell viability) of all cell groups was measured by the MTT assay. In brief, cell media was replaced with complete media containing MTT (10 μg/mL) and incubated at 37 °C in a 5% CO_2 humidified atmosphere for 3 h. Then, the supernatant containing MTT was discarded and the produced formazan crystals were dissolved in isopropyl alcohol (100 μL per well) under shaking for 10 min at 100 rpm in a Stuart SI500 orbital shaker. Finally, the endpoint absorbance measurements at 540 nm were carried out, employing an Infinite M200 plate reader (Tecan group Ltd., Männedorf, Switzerland). Eight replicates were performed for each concentration, and the experiment was repeated in triplicate. The relative cell viability was calculated as cell survival percentage compared to cells that were treated only with complete media (control). Blank values measured in wells with isopropyl alcohol and no cells, were in all cases subtracted.

4. Conclusions

In this study, negatively charged oxidized multi-walled carbon nanotubes (oxCNTs) were modified with positively charged quaternized hyperbranched poly(ethyleneimine) derivatives (QPEIs), through non-covalent functionalization. Specifically, three derivatives of hyperbranched poly(ethyleneimine), with a 30, 50, and 80% substitution degree of primary amino groups, were prepared and, subsequently, physically interacted with oxCNTs, yielding three novel QPEI functionalized oxCNTs, with QPEI loading ranged between 16–23%, approximately. Structural characterization of these hybrid materials using a variety of techniques, such as FTIR, RAMAN, SEM, TEM, AFM, etc., revealed the successful and homogenous anchoring of QPEIs on the oxCNTs surface. Furthermore, the microscopic techniques revealed the effective wrapping of the QPEI over the ox-CNTs. Contrary to previous studies on non-covalent functionalization of CNTs with PEI, the obtained hybrids efficiently dispersed in aqueous media, forming dispersions with excellent aqueous stability for over 12 months. To evaluate the antibacterial and anti-cyanobacterial properties of these hybrids, two types of gram(−) bacteria, an autotrophic (cyanobacterium *Synechococcus* sp. PCC 7942) and a heterotrophic (bacterium *Escherichia coli*), were used. It was found that all materials exhibited an enhanced, dose-dependent antibacterial and anti-cyanobacterial activity against both test organisms. The obtained IC-50 values were much lower compared to oxidized MWCNTs, revealing that the non-covalent attachment of QPEIs strongly induces the antibacterial/anti-cyanobacterial properties of the hybrid materials. These improved properties were attributed to the polycationic character of the oxCNTs@QPEIs, which enables the effective interaction of the hybrids with the bacteria membranes, facilitating their internalization into the cells. Moreover, the excellent aqueous dispersibility and stability of the hybrids, upon increasing the quaternization degree, further enhanced their activity. Indeed, the QPEI derivative containing the highest content of quaternary ammonium groups (80-QPEI) exhibited the highest performance, compared to the other QPEI derivatives. In the case of the photosynthetic bacteria, it was shown that the hybrid materials affect their photosynthetic apparatus by selective inhibition of the Photosystem (PS) I electron transport activity, while also reducing the photosynthetic electron transport in PSII. To the best of our knowledge, the QPEI functionalized hybrids are the first materials exhibiting strong anti-cyanobacterial properties, without the use of any antibiotic/herbicide. Furthermore, cytotoxicity studies on human prostate carcinoma DU145 cell line and the 3T3 mouse fibroblasts were performed, revealing that all hybrids exhibit high cytocompatibility in the concentration range in which they also exhibit high antibacterial and anti-cyanobacterial properties. These results suggest that QPEI-functionalized oxCNTs can be very attractive candidates as antibacterial and anti-cyanobacterial agents that can be used for potential applications in the disinfection industry, as well as for control of harmful cyanobacterial blooms.

Supplementary Materials:
Figure S1: FTIR spectra of oxCNTs, 30-QPEI, oxCNTs@30-QPEI, 50-QPEI and oxCNTs@50-QPEI, Figure S2: SEM images (upper part), AFM image and profile section (lower part) of oxCNTs, Figure S3: UV–vis absorption spectra of oxCNTs (a), oxCNTs@30-QPEI (b), oxCNTs@50-QPEI (c) and oxCNTs@80-QPEI (d) in aqueous solution (1 mg/mL), Figure S4: Fluorescence intensity change of RFP at 590 nm (excitation: 545 nm) upon *Escherichia coli* XL1-blue bacteria growth. Figure S5: Effect of oxCNTs on cell proliferation of cyanobacteria *Synechococcus* sp. PCC 7942 in the presence of different concentrations. Error bars represent mean ± SD for at least three independent experiments. Figure S6: Plot of the area under the growth curves of *Synechococcus* sp. PCC 7942 cells for each concentration of oxCNTs@PEIs versus the corresponding concentration as well as the relevant IC-50 calculations. Table S1: Elemental analysis results of ox-CNTs, QPEI and QPEI-functionalized ox-CNTs. Table S2: Photosystem II and I electron transport activities measured on *Synechococcus* sp. PCC 7942 permeaplasts in the presence of oxCNTs@80-QPEI. Table S3: Effects of oxCNTs@80-QPEI on the steady state oxidation of P700 (ΔA820/A820) by FR light in *Synechococcus* sp. PCC 7942 cells.

Author Contributions: Conceptualization, Z.S.; Data curation, N.S.H., G.K., K.M.L., K.N.P., A.P., E.S. and A.K.; Formal analysis, N.S.H., G.K., K.M.L., K.N.P., A.P., E.S., S.P. and A.K.; Investigation, D.G. and F.K.K.; Methodology, N.S.H., G.K., K.M.L., K.N.P., A.P., E.S., S.P., A.K., F.K.K. and K.S.; Project administration, D.G. and Z.S.; Resources, K.S.; Supervision, F.K.K. and Z.S.; Validation, K.N.P.; Visualization, S.P.; Writing—original draft, F.K.K., K.S. and Z.S.; Writing—review & editing, S.P., D.G., F.K.K. and Z.S. All authors have read and agreed to the published version of the manuscript.

Acknowledgments: This research was supported by the Greek General Secretariat for Research and Technology, under the frame of EuroNanoMed III, ANNAFIB project (MIS 5053890) and by the internal project entitled: "Synthesis and characterization of nanostructured materials for environmental applications" (EE11968). K.M.L. acknowledges financial support from the Greek State Scholarships Foundation, program "Enhancement of human scientific resources through implementation of PhD research" with resources of the European program "Development of human resources, Education and lifelong learning", 2014–2020, co-funded by the European Social Fund and Greek State (MIS 5000432, contract number: 2018-050-0502-13820).

References

1.   Dresselhaus, M.S.; Dresselhaus, G.; Avouris, P. *Carbon Nanotubes: Synthesis, Structure, Properties and Applications*; Springer: Berlin, Germany, 2001.

2. Novoselov, K.S.; Fal, V.; Colombo, L.; Gellert, P.; Schwab, M.; Kim, K. A roadmap for graphene. *Nature* **2012**, *490*, 192–200. [CrossRef] [PubMed]
3. Ji, H.; Sun, H.; Qu, X. Antibacterial applications of graphene-based nanomaterials: Recent achievements and challenges. *Adv. Drug Deliv. Rev.* **2016**, *105*, 176–189. [CrossRef] [PubMed]
4. Goenka, S.; Sant, V.; Sant, S. Graphene-based nanomaterials for drug delivery and tissue engineering. *J. Control. Release* **2014**, *173*, 75–88. [CrossRef] [PubMed]
5. Breuer, O.; Uttandaraman, S. Big returns from small fibers: A review of polymer/carbon nanotube composites. *Polym. Compos.* **2004**, *25*, 630–645. [CrossRef]
6. Soleyman, R.; Hirbod, S.; Adeli, M. Advances in the biomedical application of polymer-functionalized carbon nanotubes. *Biomater. Sci.* **2015**, *3*, 695–711. [CrossRef]
7. Baia, Y.; Park, I.S.; Lee, S.J.; Bae, T.S.; Watari, F.; Uo, M.; Lee, M.H. Aqueous dispersion of surfactant-modified multiwalled carbon nanotubes and their application as an antibacterial agent. *Carbon* **2011**, *49*, 3663–3671. [CrossRef]
8. Sun, J.-T.; Hong, C.-Y.; Pan, C.-Y. Surface modification of carbon nanotubes with dendrimers or hyperbranched polymers. *Polym. Chem.* **2011**, *2*, 998–1007. [CrossRef]
9. Tuncel, D. Non-covalent interactions between carbon nanotubes and conjugated polymers. *Nanoscale* **2011**, *3*, 3545–3554. [CrossRef]
10. Bilalis, P.; Katsigiannopoulos, D.; Avgeropoulos, A.; Sakellariou, G. Non-covalent functionalization of carbon nanotubes with polymers. *RSC Adv.* **2014**, *4*, 2911–2934. [CrossRef]
11. Ata, M.S.; Poon, R.; Syed, A.M.; Milne, J.; Zhitomirsky, I. New developments in non-covalent surface modification, dispersion and electrophoretic deposition of carbon nanotubes. *Carbon* **2018**, *130*, 584–598. [CrossRef]
12. Star, A.; Stoddart, J.F. Dispersion and Solubilization of Single-Walled Carbon Nanotubes with a Hyperbranched Polymer. *Macromolecules* **2002**, *35*, 7516–7520. [CrossRef]
13. Caminade, A.-M.; Majoral, J.-P. Dendrimers and nanotubes: A fruitful association. *Chem. Soc. Rev.* **2010**, *39*, 2034–2047. [CrossRef] [PubMed]
14. Chen, M.-L.; Chen, M.-L.; Chen, X.-W.; Wang, J.-H. Functionalization of MWNTs with Hyperbranched PEI for Highly Selective Isolation of BSA. *Macromol. Biosci.* **2010**, *10*, 906–915. [CrossRef]
15. Fréchet, J.M.J.; Tomalia, D.A. *Dendrimers and Other Dendritic Polymers*; J Wiley & Sons: Chichester, UK, 2001.
16. Pedziwiatr-Werbicka, E.; Milowska, K.; Dzmitruk, V.; Ionov, M.; Shcharbin, D.; Bryszewska, M. Dendrimers and hyperbranched structures for biomedical applications. *Eur. Polym. J.* **2019**, *119*, 61–73. [CrossRef]
17. Paleos, C.M.; Tsiourvas, D.; Sideratou, Z. Triphenylphosphonium decorated liposomes and dendritic polymers: Prospective second generation drug delivery systems for targeting mitochondria. *Mol. Pharm.* **2016**, *13*, 2233–2241. [CrossRef] [PubMed]
18. Yudovin-Farber, I.; Golenser, J.; Beyth, N.; Weiss, E.I.; Domb, A.J. Quaternary ammonium polyethyleneimine: Antibacterial activity. *J. Nanomater.* **2010**, *2010*. [CrossRef]
19. Mammen, M.; Choi, S.-K.; Whitesides, G.M. Polyvalent interactions in biological systems: Implications for design and use of multivalent ligands and inhibitors. *Angew. Chem. Int. Ed.* **1998**, *37*, 2755–2794. [CrossRef]
20. Maleki Dizaj, S.; Mennati, A.; Jafari, S.; Khezri, K.; Adibkia, K. Antimicrobial activity of carbon-based nanoparticles. *Adv. Pharm. Bull.* **2015**, *5*, 19–23.
21. Al-Jumaili, A.; Alancherry, S.; Bazaka, K.; Jacob, M.V. Review on the antimicrobial properties of carbon nanostructures. *Materials* **2017**, *10*, 1066. [CrossRef]
22. Maas, M. Carbon Nanomaterials as Antibacterial Colloids. *Materials* **2016**, *9*, 617. [CrossRef]
23. Kang, S.; Pinault, M.; Pfefferle, L.D.; Elimelech, M. Single-walled carbon nanotubes exhibit strong antimicrobial activity. *Langmuir* **2007**, *23*, 8670–8673. [CrossRef] [PubMed]
24. Mocan, T.; Matea, C.T.; Pop, T.; Mosteanu, O.; Buzoianu, A.D.; Suciu, S.; Puia, C.; Zdrehus, C.; Iancu, C.; Mocan, L. Carbon nanotubes as anti-bacterial agents. *Cell. Mol. Life Sci.* **2017**, *74*, 3467–3479. [CrossRef] [PubMed]
25. Kang, S.; Herzberg, M.; Rodrigues, D.F.; Elimelech, M. Antibacterial effects of carbon nanotubes: Size does matter! *Langmuir* **2008**, *24*, 6409–6413. [CrossRef] [PubMed]
26. Yang, C.; Mamouni, J.; Tang, Y.; Yang, L. Antimicrobial activity of single-walled carbon nanotubes: Length effect. *Langmuir* **2010**, *26*, 16013–16019. [CrossRef]
27. Kang, S.; Mauter, M.S.; Elimelech, M. Physicochemical determinants of multiwalled carbon nanotube

bacterial cytotoxicity. *Environ. Sci. Technol.* **2008**, *42*, 7528–7534. [CrossRef]

28. Arias, L.R.; Yang, L.J. Inactivation of bacterial pathogens by carbon nanotubes in suspensions. *Langmuir* **2009**, *25*, 3003–3012. [CrossRef]

29. Baek, S.; Joo, S.H.; Su, C.; Toborek, M. Antibacterial effects of graphene- and carbon-nanotube-based nanohybrids on *Escherichia coli*: Implications for treating multidrug-resistant bacteria. *J. Environ. Manag.* **2019**, *247*, 214–223. [CrossRef]

30. Xia, L.; Xu, M.; Cheng, G.; Yang, L.; Guo, Y.; Li, D.; Fang, D.; Zhang, Q.; Liu, H. Facile construction of Ag nanoparticles encapsulated into carbon nanotubes with robust antibacterial activity. *Carbon* **2018**, *130*, 775–781. [CrossRef]

31. Atiyah, A.A.; Haider, A.J.; Dhahi, R.M. Cytotoxicity properties of functionalised carbon nanotubes on pathogenic bacteria. *IET Nanobiotechnol.* **2019**, *13*, 597–601. [CrossRef]

32. Baia, Y.; Park, I.S.; Lee, S.J.; Wen, P.S.; Bae, T.S.; Lee, M.H. Effect of AOT-assisted multi-walled carbon nanotubes on antibacterial activity. *Colloids Surf. B* **2012**, *89*, 101–107. [CrossRef]

33. Deng, R.; Zhu, Y.; Hou, J.; White, J.C.; Gardea-Torresdey, J.L.; Lin, D. Antagonistic toxicity of carbon nanotubes and pentachlorophenol to *Escherichia coli*: Physiological and transcriptional responses. *Carbon* **2019**, *145*, 658–667. [CrossRef]

34. Trompeta, A.-F.A.; Preiss, I.; Ben-Ami, F.; Benayahu, Y.; Charitidis, C.A. Toxicity testing of MWCNTs to aquatic organisms. *RSC Adv.* **2019**, *9*, 36707–36716. [CrossRef]

35. Ganguly, P.; Breen, A.; Pillai, S.C. Toxicity of nanomaterials: Exposure, pathways, assessment, and recent advances. *ACS Biomater. Sci. Eng.* **2018**, *4*, 2237–2275. [CrossRef]

36. Wang, X.P.; Han, H.Y.; Liu, X.Q.; Gu, X.X.; Chen, K.; Lu, D.L. Multi-walled carbon nanotubes can enhance root elongation of wheat (*Triticum aestivum*) plants. *J. Nanopart. Res.* **2012**, *14*, 841–850. [CrossRef]

37. Schwab, F.; Bucheli, T.D.; Lukhele, L.P.; Magrez, A.; Nowack, B.; Sigg, L.; Knauer, K. Are carbon nanotube effects on green algae caused by shading and agglomeration? *Environ. Sci. Technol.* **2011**, *45*, 6136–6144. [CrossRef]

38. Wei, L.; Thakkar, M.; Chen, Y.; Ntim, S.A.; Mitra, S.; Zhang, X. Cytotoxicity effects of water dispersible oxidized multiwalled carbon nanotubes on marine alga *Dunaliella Tertiolecta*. *Aquat. Toxicol.* **2010**, *100*, 194–201. [CrossRef]

39. Timofeeva, A.V.; Tashlitsky, V.N.; Tkachev, A.G.; Baratova, L.A.; Koksharova, O.A. Nanocomplexes on the basis of taunit associated with biocides as effective anti-cyanobacterial agents. *Russ. J. Plant Physiol.* **2017**, *64*, 833–838. [CrossRef]

40. Sideratou, Z.; Tsiourvas, D.; Paleos, C.M. Quaternized poly(propylene imine) dendrimers as novel pH-sensitive controlled-release systems. *Langmuir* **2000**, *16*, 1766–1769. [CrossRef]

41. Sapalidis, A.; Sideratou, Z.; Panagiotaki, K.N.; Sakellis, E.; Kouvelos, E.P.; Papageorgiou, S.; Katsaros, F. Fabrication of antibacterial PVA nanocomposite films containing dendritic polymer functionalized multi-walled carbon nanotubes. *Front. Mater.* **2018**, *5*. [CrossRef]

42. Cao, X.; Li, Z.; Song, X.; Cui, X.; Cao, P.; Liu, H.; Cheng, F.; Chen, Y. Core-shell type multiarm star poly(ε-caprolactone) with high molecular weight hyperbranched polyethylenimine as core: Synthesis, characterization and encapsulation properties. *Eur. Polym. J.* **2008**, *44*, 1060–1070. [CrossRef]

43. Bellamy, L. *The Infra-Red Spectra of Complex Molecules*; Springer: Amsterdam, The Netherlands, 1975. [CrossRef]

44. Arkas, M.; Tsiourvas, D. Organic/inorganic hybrid nanospheres based on hyperbranched poly(ethyleneimine) encapsulated into silica for the sorption of toxic metal ions and polycyclic aromatic hydrocarbons from water. *J. Hazard. Mater.* **2009**, *170*, 35–42. [CrossRef] [PubMed]

45. Pigorsch, E. Spectroscopic characterisation of cationic quaternary ammonium starches. *Starke* **2009**, *61*, 129–138. [CrossRef]

46. Wepasnick, K.A.; Smith, B.A.; Bitter, J.L.; Fairbrother, D.H. Chemical and structural characterization of carbon nanotube surfaces. *Anal. Bioanal. Chem.* **2010**. [CrossRef] [PubMed]

47. Yuan, W.; Jiang, G.; Che, J.; Qi, X.; Xu, R.; Chan-Park, M.B. Deposition of Silver Nanoparticles on Multiwalled Carbon Nanotubes Grafted with Hyperbranched Poly(amidoamine) and Their Antimicrobial Effects. *J. Phys. Chem. C* **2008**, *112*, 18754–18759. [CrossRef]

48. Murugan, E.; Vimala, G. Effective functionalization of multiwalled carbon nanotube with amphiphilic poly(propyleneimine) dendrimer carrying silver nanoparticles for better dispersability and antimicrobial

activity. *J. Colloid Interface Sci.* **2011**, *357*, 354–365. [CrossRef] [PubMed]

49. Zhou, X.; Chen, Z.; Yan, D.; Lu, H. Deposition of Fe–Ni nanoparticles on polyethyleneimine-decorated graphene oxide and application in catalytic dehydrogenation of ammonia borane. *J. Mater. Chem.* **2012**, *22*, 13506–13516. [CrossRef]

50. Zhang, N.; Xie, J.; Guers, M.; Varadan, V.K. Chemical bonding of multiwalled carbon nanotubes to SU-8 via ultrasonic irradiation. *Smart Mater. Struct.* **2003**, *12*, 260–263. [CrossRef]

51. Schierz, A.; Zänker, H. Aqueous suspensions of carbon nanotubes: Surface oxidation, colloidal stability and uranium sorption. *Environ. Pollut.* **2009**, *157*, 1088–1094. [CrossRef] [PubMed]

52. Etika, K.C.; Cox, M.A.; Grunlan, J.C. Tailored dispersion of carbon nanotubes in water with pH-responsive polymers. *Polymer* **2010**, *51*, 1761–1770. [CrossRef]

53. Yu, J.; Grossiord, N.; Koning, C.E.; Loos, J. Controlling the dispersion of multi-wall carbon nanotubes in aqueous surfactant solution. *Carbon* **2007**, *45*, 618–623. [CrossRef]

54. Zhang, W.; Chen, M.; Gong, X.; Diao, G. Universal water-soluble cyclodextrin polymer–carbon nanomaterials with supramolecular recognition. *Carbon* **2013**, *61*, 154–163. [CrossRef]

55. Moon, Y.K.; Lee, J.; Lee, J.K.; Kim, T.K.; Kim, S.H. Synthesis of length-controlled aerosol carbon nanotubes and their dispersion stability in aqueous solution. *Langmuir* **2009**, *25*, 1739–1743. [CrossRef] [PubMed]

56. Schwyzer, I.; Kaegi, R.; Sigg, L.; Nowack, B. Colloidal stability of suspended and agglomerate structures of settled carbon nanotubes in different aqueous matrices. *Water Res.* **2013**, *47*, 3910–3920. [CrossRef] [PubMed]

57. Bhattacharjee, S. DLS and zeta potential—What they are and what they are not? *J. Control. Release* **2016**, *235*, 337–351. [CrossRef] [PubMed]

58. Chen, H.; Wang, B.; Gao, D.; Guan, M.; Zheng, L.; Ouyang, H.; Chai, Z.; Zhao, Y.; Feng, W. Broad-Spectrum Antibacterial Activity of Carbon Nanotubes to Human Gut Bacteria. *Small* **2013**, *9*, 2735–2746. [CrossRef] [PubMed]

59. Liu, D.; Mao, Y.; Ding, L. Carbon nanotubes as antimicrobial agents for water disinfection and pathogen control. *J. Water Health* **2018**, *16*, 171–180. [CrossRef]

60. Zardini, H.Z.; Amiri, A.; Shanbedi, M.; Maghrebi, M.; Baniadam, M. Enhanced antibacterial activity of amino acids-functionalized multi walled carbon nanotubes by a simple method. *Colloids Surf. B* **2012**, *92*, 196–202. [CrossRef]

61. Zardini, H.Z.; Davarpanah, M.; Shanbedi, M.; Amiri, A.; Maghrebi, M.; Ebrahimi, L. Microbial toxicity of ethanolamines—Multiwalled carbon nanotubes. *J. Biomed. Mater. Res. Part A* **2014**, *102*, 1774–1781. [CrossRef]

62. Gottenbos, B.; van der Mei, H.C.; Klatter, F.; Nieuwenhuis, P.; Busscher, H.J. In Vitro and In Vivo antimicrobial activity of covalently coupled quaternary ammonium silane coatings on silicone rubber. *Biomaterials* **2002**, *23*, 1417–1423. [CrossRef]

63. Tamayo-Belda, M.; González-Pleiter, M.; Pulido-Reyes, G.; Martin-Betancor, K.; Leganés, F.; Rosal, R.; Fernández-Piñas, F. Mechanism of the toxic action of cationic G5 and G7 PAMAM dendrimers in the cyanobacterium Anabaena sp. PCC7120. *Environ. Sci. Nano* **2019**, *6*, 863–878. [CrossRef]

64. Chen, C.Z.S.; Beck-Tan, N.C.; Dhurjati, P.; van Dyk, T.K.; LaRossa, R.A.; Cooper, S.L. Quaternary ammonium functionalized poly(propylene imine) dendrimers as effective antimicrobials: Structure-activity studies. *Biomacromolecules* **2000**, *1*, 473–480. [CrossRef] [PubMed]

65. Herrero, A.; Flores, E. *The Cyanobacteria: Molecular Biology, Genomics and Evolution*; Caister Academic Press: Norfolk, UK, 2008.

66. Wieg, C.; Pflugmacher, S. Ecotoxicological effects of selected cyanobacterial secondary metabolites a short review. *Toxicol. Appl. Pharmacol.* **2005**, *203*, 201–218.

67. Vernon, L.P.; Shaw, E.R. Photoreduction of 2,6-dichlorophenolindophenol by diphenylcarbazide: A Photosystem 2 reaction catalyzed by tris-washed chloroplasts and subchloroplast fragments. *Plant Physiol.* **1969**, *44*, 1645–1649. [CrossRef] [PubMed]

68. Papageorgiou, G.C. Rapid permeabilization of anacystis nidulans to electrolytes. *Meth. Enzymol.* **1988**, *167*, 259–262.

69. Kumazawa, S.; Mitsui, A. Photosynthetic activities of a synchronously grown aerobic N_2-fixing unicellular cyanobacterium, *Synechococcus* sp. Miami BG 043511. *J. Gen. Microbiol.* **1992**, *138*, 467–472. [CrossRef]

70. Zheng, M.; Diner, B.A. Solution Redox Chemistry of Carbon Nanotubes. *J. Am. Chem. Soc.* **2004**, *126*, 15490–15494. [CrossRef]

71. Brand, J.; Baszynski, T.; Crane, F.L.; Krogmann, D.W. Selective inhibition of photosynthetic reactions by polycations. *J. Biol. Chem.* **1972**, *247*, 2814–2819.

72. Schreiber, U.; Klughammer, C.; Neubauer, C. Measuring P700 absorbance changes around 830 nm with a new type of pulse modulation system. *Z. Naturforsch. C* **1988**, *43*, 686–698. [CrossRef]

73. Sekar, N.; Umasankar, Y.; Ramasamy, R.P. Photocurrent generation by immobilized cyanobacteria via direct electron transport in photo-bioelectrochemical cells. *Phys. Chem. Chem. Phys.* **2014**, *16*, 7862–7871. [CrossRef]

74. Goldbeck, J.C.; Victoria, F.N.; Motta, A.; Savegnago, L.; Jacob, R.G.; Perin, G.; Lenardão, E.J.; da Silva, W.P. Bioactivity and morphological changes of bacterial cells after exposure to 3-(p-chlorophenyl)thio citronellal. *LWT* **2014**, *59*, 813–819. [CrossRef]

75. Stamatakis, K.; Papageorgiou, G.C. The osmolality of the cell suspension regulates phycobilisome-to-photosystem I excitation transfers in Cyanobacteria. *Biochim. Biophys. Acta* **2001**, *1506*, 172–181. [CrossRef]

76. Moran, P. Formulae for determination of chlorophyllous pigments extracted with N,N- Dimethylformamide. *Plant Physiol.* **1982**, *69*, 1376–1381. [CrossRef] [PubMed]

77. Trebst, A.; Pistorius, E. Photosynthetische reaktionen in UV-bestrahlten chloroplasten. *Z. Naturforsch.* **1965**, *20b*, 885–889. [CrossRef]

4

3-Pentylcatechol, a Non-Allergenic Urushiol Derivative, Displays Anti-*Helicobacter pylori* Activity In Vivo

Hang Yeon Jeong [1], Tae Ho Lee [1], Ju Gyeong Kim [1], Sueun Lee [2], Changjong Moon [2], Xuan Trong Truong [3], Tae-Il Jeon [3] and Jae-Hak Moon [1,*]

[1] Department of Food Science and Technology, Chonnam National University, 77 Yongbongro, Gwangju 61186, Korea; wjdgkddus@naver.com (H.Y.J.); xogh9954@naver.com (T.H.L.); wnrud0610@naver.com (J.G.K.)
[2] Department of Veterinary Anatomy, College of Veterinary Medicine and BK21 FOUR Program, Chonnam National University, Gwangju 61186, Korea; leese@kiom.re.kr (S.L.); moonc@chonnam.ac.kr (C.M.)
[3] Department of Animal Science, Chonnam National University, Gwangju 61186, Korea; trongxuan.vp@gmail.com (X.T.T.); tjeon@jnu.ac.kr (T.-I.J.)
* Correspondence: nutrmoon@jnu.ac.kr

Abstract: We previously reported that 3-pentylcatechol (PC), a synthetic non-allergenic urushiol derivative, inhibited the growth of *Helicobacter pylori* in an in vitro assay using nutrient agar and broth. In this study, we aimed to investigate the in vivo antimicrobial activity of PC against *H. pylori* growing in the stomach mucous membrane. Four-week-old male C57BL/6 mice (n = 4) were orally inoculated with *H. pylori* Sydney Strain-1 (SS-1) for 8 weeks. Thereafter, the mice received PC (1, 5, and 15 mg/kg) and triple therapy (omeprazole, 0.7 mg/kg; metronidazole, 16.7 mg/kg; clarithromycin, 16.7 mg/kg, reference groups) once daily for 10 days. Infiltration of inflammatory cells in gastric tissue was greater in the *H. pylori*-infected group compared with the control group and lower in both the triple therapy- and PC-treated groups. In addition, upregulation of cytokine mRNA was reversed after infection, upon administration of triple therapy and PC. Interestingly, PC was more effective than triple therapy at all doses, even at 1/15th the dose of triple therapy. In addition, PC demonstrated synergism with triple therapy, even at low concentrations. The results suggest that PC may be more effective against *H. pylori* than established antibiotics.

Keywords: urushiol; 3-pentylcatechol; 3-pentadecylcatechol; *Helicobacter pylori*; antimicrobial; triple therapy

---

1. Introduction

Helicobacter pylori infection is a major public health concern worldwide. This infection occurs in the gastric mucosa of more than 50% of the world's population [1] and it is directly associated with gastrointestinal disorders, including chronic gastritis, peptic ulcer disease, mucosa-associated lymphoid tissue (MALT) lymphoma, and gastric cancer [2–5]. Gastric cancer is the second leading cause of cancer-related mortality worldwide, following only lung cancer [6]. Furthermore, *H. pylori* infection is also associated with numerous extra-gastric disorders, such as cardiovascular, neurologic, hematologic, dermatologic, head and neck, and urogynecologic diseases, as well as diabetes mellitus and metabolic syndrome [7,8].

The international gold-standard treatment for *H. pylori* infection is triple therapy, comprising two antibiotics (usually selected from clarithromycin, metronidazole, amoxicillin, and tetracycline) and a proton-pump inhibitor, for 7–14 days [9–11]. However, the success rates of these *H. pylori* eradication therapies are less than 80%, and the failure rate of *H. pylori* eradication therapy has increased, primarily due to increased antibiotic resistance [12–14]. Another reason for treatment failure is patient non-adherence, owing to the complexity of the treatment: it involves the repeat administration of at least three drugs over a long period [15]. In addition, these drugs are associated with several side effects, including abdominal pain, nausea, and diarrhea [16]. The high cost of *H. pylori* treatment may also be a disadvantage [15]. Therefore, there is an urgent need for the development of safe and effective therapeutic agents for *H. pylori* infections.

Lacquer tree (*Toxicodendron vernicifluum* (Stokes) F.A. Barkley, Anacardiaceae) has been used for thousands of years as a protective surface-coating material and in traditional medicine in China, Japan, and Korea [17]. It is particularly effective for treating gastrointestinal disorders, such as gastritis and gastric cancer [17]. Urushiols are a group of compounds with alkyl side chains comprising 15 or 17 carbon atoms at the C-3 position of catechol. They are the major constituents of lacquer tree sap, accounting for 60–70% of the total content [18]. In addition to their various biological activities [19–23], urushiols display antimicrobial activity against *H. pylori* [24]. However, urushiols can also cause serious contact dermatitis [25–27], which is a limitation associated with their use.

Previously, we chemically synthesized catechol-type urushiol derivatives with different alkyl side chain lengths of $-C_5H_{11}$, $-C_{10}H_{21}$, $-C_{15}H_{31}$, and $-C_{20}H_{41}$ at the C-3 position (Figure 1) [28]. Among these compounds, 3-decylcatechol ($-C_{10}H_{21}$) and 3-pentadecylcatechol (PDC, natural type, $-C_{15}H_{31}$) induced contact dermatitis; however, 3-pentylcatechol (PC, $-C_5H_{11}$) and 3-eicosylcatechol (EC, $-C_{20}H_{41}$) did not [28]. In addition, PC and EC exhibited strong antioxidative activity and high affinity for phospholipid membranes [28]. Notably, PC demonstrated enhanced antimicrobial effects in agar and broth cultures against various microorganisms involved in food spoilage and pathogenicity [29]. In addition, PC inhibited *H. pylori* to a greater extent than nalidixic acid, erythromycin, tetracycline, and ampicillin, which have been used in *H. pylori* eradication therapy [29]. Moreover, unlike PDC (Part I), PC was absorbed in the blood after oral administration [30,31]. Therefore, PC is expected to effectively eradicate *H. pylori* in gastric tissue. In this study, the in vivo antimicrobial activity of PC against *H. pylori* was evaluated and compared to that of triple therapy.

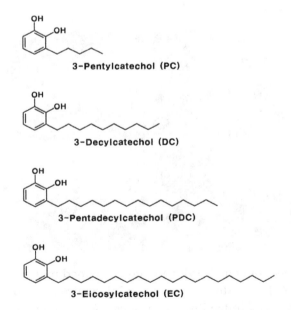

3-Pentylcatechol (PC)

3-Decylcatechol (DC)

3-Pentadecylcatechol (PDC)

3-Eicosylcatechol (EC)

Figure 1. Structures of synthesized urushiol derivatives.

2. Results

2.1. *Confirmation of Infection and Associated Gastric Disorders after H. pylori Inoculation*

After 30 days of *H. pylori* Sydney Strain-1 (SS-1) inoculation, the colonization of *H. pylori* and associated gastric disorders in mouse gastric tissue were confirmed via quantitative polymerase chain reaction (qPCR) and histological analysis. The relative mRNA expression of the inflammatory cytokines, tumor necrosis factor alpha (Tnfα) and interleukin-1 beta (Il-1β) was upregulated to a greater extent in mice in the infected group than in mice in the control group (Figure 2). In addition, the expression of *H. pylori*-related genes, urease subunit alpha (ureA) and cytotoxin-associated gene A (cagA), was detected in mice in the infected group, but not in mice in the control group (Figure 2). Histological analysis revealed characteristics of gastritis, including inflammatory cell infiltration, erosion, and catarrhal inflammation in the gastric tissue of the infected group (Figure 3). These results indicate that *H. pylori* successfully colonized the stomachs of mice after inoculation and induced gastric disorders. Therefore, this animal model was used to investigate the in vivo antimicrobial activity of PC against *H. pylori*.

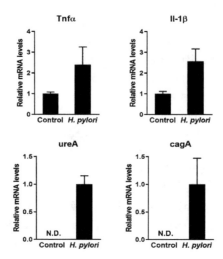

Figure 2. Expression levels of tumor necrosis factor alpha (Tnfα), interleukin-1 beta (Il-1β), urease subunit alpha (ureA), and cytotoxin-associated gene A (cagA) mRNA in mouse gastric tissue following *Helicobacter pylori* Sydney Strain-1 (SS-1) inoculation. *H. pylori* SS-1 was administered to C57BL/6 mice for 30 days. N.D., not detected.

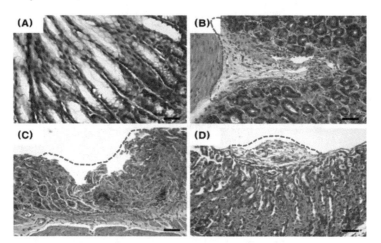

Figure 3. Histological analysis of hematoxylin and eosin-stained mouse gastric tissue after *H. pylori* SS-1 inoculation. *H. pylori* SS-1 was administered to C57BL/6 mice for 30 days. (**A**) uninfected control; (**B**) inflammatory cell infiltration (dotted line) in an *H. pylori*-infected mouse; (**C**) erosion (dotted line) in an *H. pylori*-infected mouse; (**D**) catarrhal inflammation (dotted line) in an *H. pylori*-infected mouse. Scale bar = 20 μm.

2.2. Effect of PC on the Gastric Tissue Histology of H. pylori-Infected Mice

We evaluated and graded the level of inflammatory cell infiltration in the gastric mucosa of *H. pylori*-infected mice via hematoxylin and eosin (H&E) staining (Figure 4). Grades of 0 to 3 were assigned, as follows: 0, normal; 1, mild; 2, moderate; 3, marked. All mice in the uninfected control group displayed a score of 0 (no infiltration of inflammatory cells), whereas those in the infected group displayed a score of 2 (moderate infiltration of inflammatory cells) and 3 (marked infiltration of inflammatory cells) in two mice each. The inflammation scores in all treatment groups were lower than those in the infected group. Interestingly, the scores were lower in mice treated with low doses of PC (1 and 5 mg/kg) compared with those treated with triple therapy.

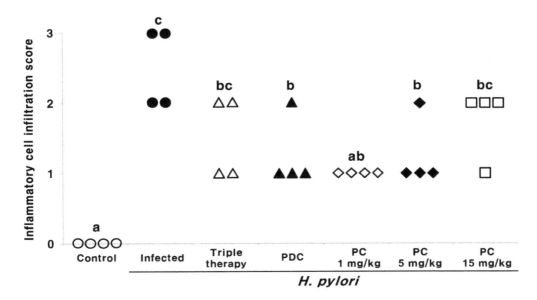

Figure 4. Effect of 3-pentylcatechol (PC) treatment on the histology of gastric tissue from *H. pylori*-infected mice (hematoxylin and eosin staining). Inflammatory cell infiltration was graded from 0 to 3: 0, normal; 1, mild; 2, moderate; 3, marked. ○, inflammatory cell infiltration score of control group; •, inflammatory cell infiltration score of *H. pylori*-infected group; Δ, inflammatory cell infiltration score of *H. pylori* + triple therapy-treated group; ▲, inflammatory cell infiltration score of *H. pylori* + 3-pentadecylcatechol (PDC)-treated group; ◊, inflammatory cell infiltration score of *H. pylori* + 1 mg/kg of PC-treated group; ♦, inflammatory cell infiltration score of *H. pylori* + 5 mg/kg of PC-treated group; □, inflammatory cell infiltration score of *H. pylori* + 15 mg/kg of PC-treated group. Different letters (a, b, and c) indicate a significant difference ($p < 0.05$), ascertained via the Tukey–Kramer test.

2.3. Effect of PC on H. pylori Eradication and Cytokine Expression

To assess the effect of PC therapy on *H. pylori* eradication, the mRNA expression of the *H. pylori* markers cagA, ureA, and neutrophil-activating protein A (napA) was assessed in pyloric antrum tissue via qPCR. As shown in Figure 5, all three *H. pylori*-related transcripts were detected in the infected mice, but not in the uninfected control mice. This suggests that PC can effectively eradicate *H. pylori*, even at a dose at 1/15th of the antibiotics used in triple therapy. This response was also observed when analyzing the mRNA expression of inflammatory cytokines Tnfα and Il-1β in the pyloric antrum tissue (Figure 6). The expression of both Tnfα and Il-1β was markedly upregulated in the infected group compared with the uninfected control group; however, these genes were significantly downregulated upon PC treatment and in the reference groups. Moreover, PC treatment reduced the levels of two inflammatory cytokines more efficiently than triple therapy. Notably, in mice treated with 1 and 5 mg/kg of PC, the mRNA expression of Tnfα and Il-1β was downregulated, similar to the observation in the uninfected control mice. These results suggest that PC effectively eradicates *H. pylori* in the gastric mucosa and also helps alleviate gastrointestinal disorders at much lower concentrations than conventional antibiotics.

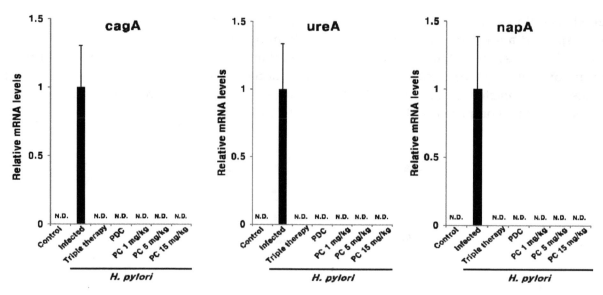

Figure 5. Effect of PC treatment on the expression of *H. pylori* cagA, ureA, and napA in the gastric tissue of the *H. pylori*-infected mice. N.D., not detected.

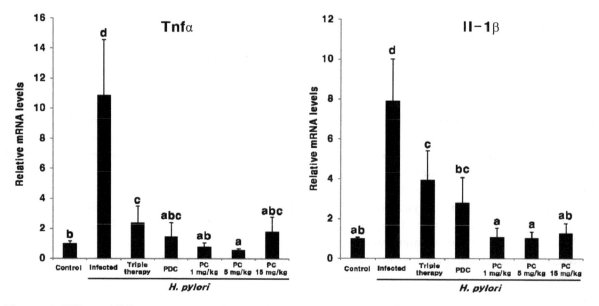

Figure 6. Effect of PC treatment on the expression of Tnfα and Il-1β mRNA in the gastric tissue of the *H. pylori*-infected mice. Different letters (a, b, c, and d) indicate a significant difference ($p < 0.05$), ascertained via the Tukey–Kramer test. PC, 3-pentylcatechol; PDC, 3-pentadecylcatechol.

2.4. Synergistic Effect of PC in Combination with Triple Therapy

Next, we evaluated the in vivo efficacy of PC in combination with triple therapy. The expression of *H. pylori*-related genes (cagA, ureA, and napA) was not completely suppressed in the triple therapy group when the antibiotic concentration was decreased (Figure 7). In contrast, when PC was administered with triple therapy, the expression of the *H. pylori*-related genes was not observed with all concentrations (Figure 7).

Next, we evaluated the synergistic effect of PC and triple therapy on the inflammatory response (Figure 8). When mice were treated with triple therapy alone, inflammation was not completely suppressed. However, when mice were treated with PC and triple therapy, cytokine expression decreased to a level similar to that observed in the uninfected control group. These results indicate that PC demonstrated synergism with conventional antibiotic therapy, suggesting that the use of antibiotics can be reduced in the treatment of *H. pylori*.

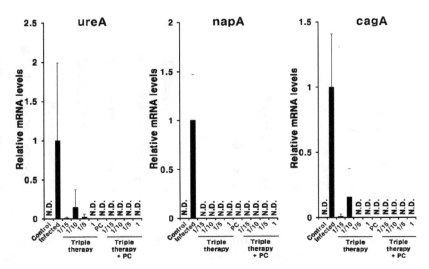

Figure 7. Expression of *H. pylori* ureA, napA, and cagA mRNA in the gastric tissue of the *H. pylori*-infected mice following combination treatment with PC and triple therapy. Different letters indicate a significant difference ($p < 0.05$), ascertained via the Tukey–Kramer test. Triple therapy was administered at four concentrations. 1, Existing concentration of triple therapy (metronidazole and clarithromycin: 16.7 mg/kg; omeprazole: 700 µg/kg); 1/5, one-fifth of the existing concentration of triple therapy; 1/10, one-tenth of the existing concentration of triple therapy; 1/15, one-fifteenth of the existing concentration of triple therapy. PC was administered at 1 mg/kg. N.D., not detected.

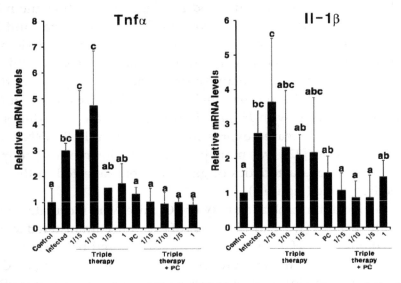

Figure 8. Expression levels of Tnfα and Il-1β mRNA in the gastric tissue of the *H. pylori*-infected mice after combination treatment with PC and triple therapy. Different letters (a, b, and c) indicate a significant difference ($p < 0.05$), ascertained via the Tukey–Kramer test. Triple therapy was administered at four concentrations. 1, Existing concentration of triple therapy (metronidazole and clarithromycin: 16.7 mg/kg; omeprazole: 700 µg/kg); 1/5, one-fifth of the existing concentration of triple therapy; 1/10, one-tenth of the existing concentration of triple therapy; 1/15, one-fifteenth of the existing concentration of triple therapy. PC was administered at 1 mg/kg.

2.5. *Hepatotoxicity of PC*

Plasma glutamate pyruvate transaminase (GPT) and glutamate oxaloacetate transaminase (GOT) levels were determined using commercial ELISA kits to evaluate the in vivo toxicity of PC after oral administration (Figure 9). No significant differences were observed between the PC-treated groups and the uninfected control group. These results indicate that PC does not cause liver toxicity.

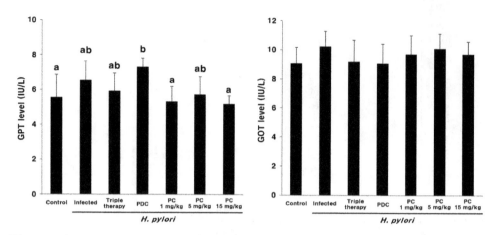

Figure 9. Plasma glutamate pyruvate transaminase (GPT) and glutamate oxaloacetate transaminase (GOT) levels after 3-pentylcatechol treatment. Different letters (a and b) indicate a significant difference ($p < 0.05$), ascertained via the Tukey–Kramer test.

3. Discussion

Urushiols are major constituents present in high concentrations in lacquer tree sap [18], with antimicrobial activity against *H. pylori* [24]. However, urushiols induce contact dermatitis [25–27], thereby limiting their application.

Previously, PC, a non-allergenic urushiol derivative (Figure 1), was chemically synthesized [28], and its antimicrobial activity against various food spoilage and pathogenic microorganisms was determined [29]. PC displayed marked antimicrobial effects in both agar and broth cultures [29]. In addition, PC demonstrated greater anti-*H. pylori* activity than nalidixic acid, erythromycin, tetracycline, and ampicillin, which have been widely used to eradicate *H. pylori* [29]. In the present study, we investigated the in vivo antimicrobial activity of PC against *H. pylori* and compared it with triple therapy, which is considered the international gold-standard treatment for *H. pylori* infections.

C57BL/6 mice were inoculated with *H. pylori* SS-1 to generate a model of *H. pylori* infection. In the pyloric antrum tissue, the increased expression of Tnfα and Il-1β mRNA, which are involved in *H. pylori*-induced inflammation [32], was more prominent in the infected group than in the control group (Figure 2). In addition, characteristics of gastritis were detected in the gastric tissue of the infected mice upon H&E staining (Figure 3).

To determine the in vivo antimicrobial activity of PC, mice were inoculated with *H. pylori* SS-1 for 60 days. Subsequently, three doses (1, 5, and 15 mg/kg) of PC were administered to the *H. pylori*-infected mice once daily for 10 days. Anti-*H. pylori* activity was compared between the PC-treated groups, the positive control group, the triple therapy group, and the group receiving PDC, a natural urushiol derivative. Mortality and inflammation upon *H. pylori* infection were assessed via qPCR and histological analysis of the pyloric antrum tissue, the major habitat of *H. pylori* [33].

Histological analysis of the gastric tissues following H&E staining (Figure 4) revealed that all uninfected mice appeared normal; in contrast, inflammatory cell infiltration increased in the infected group. Inflammation scores were reduced upon PC treatment, which was more effective than triple therapy (Figure 4).

The CagA toxin, encoded by cagA, is one of the most widely studied *H. pylori* virulence factors. The CagA effector protein is injected into host target cells via a type IV secretion system and is highly associated with inflammation and the development of gastric cancer [1]. The napA encodes the NapA protein, which activates neutrophils, prevents oxidative DNA damage [34], and regulates the adhesion of *H. pylori* to stomach mucin and host epithelial cells [35]. The ureA contributes to acid resistance in *H. pylori* via the production of ammonia through the enzymatic degradation of urea in the gastric environment [1]. *H. pylori*-related genes, cagA, ureA, and napA, were analyzed via qPCR to evaluate the extent of *H. pylori* eradication (Figure 5). All three genes were detected in the infected group only and not in the uninfected groups and those receiving treatment (Figure 5).

Therefore, these data indicate that *H. pylori* can be completely eradicated by PC at a much lower concentration than antibiotics. In addition, the expression of *H. pylori*-induced Tnfα and Il-1β mRNA was markedly downregulated following PC treatment (Figure 6). Moreover, the levels of these two inflammatory cytokines were effectively reduced in all the PC-treated groups compared with the triple therapy group (Figure 6).

A recent study showed that epidermal growth factor receptor signaling, implicated in gastric inflammation and carcinogenesis, remains activated following the eradication of *H. pylori* by antibiotics [36]. In addition, clarithromycin does not affect the expression of inflammatory markers in patients with atherosclerosis [37]. Knoop et al. (2016) reported that antibiotic therapy accelerates inflammation via the translocation of native intestinal bacteria [38]. Our results indicate that PC not only eradicates *H. pylori* but also improves *H. pylori*-induced gastritis. Although further studies are required to investigate the underlying mechanism of action, these results reflect the strong antioxidant activity and amphipathic structure of PC [28,39]. In addition, despite using a low concentration of PC, synergistic effects were observed with triple therapy (Figures 7 and 8). Thus, PC can markedly reduce the concentration of antibiotics used and can overcome issues associated with the misuse of antibiotics [16]. In addition, the poor treatment compliance of patients owing to the need to take large amounts of antibiotics, which is a major obstacle in the antibiotic treatment of *H. pylori* infections [15], can be improved.

The plasma levels of liver transaminases, GOT and GPT, are useful biomarkers of liver injury. These enzymes are released in the blood upon hepatocyte necrosis due to acute hepatitis, ischemic injury, or toxic injury [40]. In the present study, plasma GPT and GOT levels were determined following the oral administration of PC. No evidence of liver toxicity was observed following treatment with PC (Figure 9).

4. Materials and Methods

4.1. Chemicals

3-Pentylcatechol (PC) and 3-pentadecylcatechol (PDC) were chemically synthesized in accordance with our previous method [28]. Clarithromycin, metronidazole, and omeprazole were purchased from TCI Chemical Industry (Tokyo, Japan). All other chemicals and solvents were of analytical grade, unless specified otherwise.

4.2. H. pylori Strain and Culture Conditions

Mouse-adapted *H. pylori* Sydney Strain-1 (SS-1) was obtained from the Korean Culture Center of Microorganisms (KCCM, Seoul, Korea) and cultured on Columbia agar or in broth medium (MB cell, Seoul, Korea), containing 5% horse serum (Gibco, Gaithersburg, MD, USA). The culture was incubated at 37 °C in a 10% CO_2 incubator (MCO175, Sanyo, Osaka, Japan), and the bacteria were sub-cultured every 72 h [29]. Culture purity was assessed regularly.

4.3. Animals and Infection

All experimental procedures were approved by the Institutional Animal Care and Use Committee of Chonnam National University (no. CNU IACUC-YB-2012-26). Four-week-old C57BL/6 male mice were purchased from Samtako Bio Korea (Osan, Korea). Mice were reared in an environmentally controlled animal facility, operating on a 12:12 h dark/light cycle at 20 ± 1 °C and 55 ± 5% humidity, with ad libitum access to water and standard laboratory chow (Harlan Rodent diet, 2018S, by Samtako Bio Korea) [24].

Four mice per group were inoculated with *H. pylori* SS-1, which can effectively colonize the mouse gastric mucosa [41]. A total of 100 μL aliquots (10^8 CFU) of Columbia broth were administered to the mice for 60 days, three times every 2 days, using a zonde needle. After 30 days of inoculation, three mice were sacrificed to confirm infection. Blood was withdrawn from the abdominal aorta of the mice under light anesthesia (isoflurane) and collected in heparinized tubes. Plasma was obtained via centrifugation ($2767\times g$, 4 °C, 15 min). The pyloric antrum of the stomach was harvested for quantitative polymerase chain reaction (qPCR) and histological analysis. Uninfected mice were administered the same volume of fresh Columbia broth; this group was considered the negative control. All samples were stored at −80 °C until use.

4.4. PC Treatment after H. pylori Infection

Following 60-day *H. pylori* inoculation, PC was administered to the infected mice with 100 μL of water once daily for 10 days [24]. Triple therapy and PDC, a natural form of urushiol, were used as reference groups. Infected mice were divided into seven experimental groups ($n = 4$): control group (uninfected, negative control); *H. pylori*-infected group; *H. pylori* infection + triple therapy treatment group; *H. pylori* infection + PDC 26.7 mg (83.3 μmol)/kg treatment group; *H. pylori* infection + PC 1 mg (5.6 μmol)/kg treatment group; *H. pylori* infection + PC 5 mg (27.8 μmol)/kg treatment group; and *H. pylori* infection + PC 15 mg (83.3 μmol)/kg treatment group. Triple therapy comprised omeprazole (700 μg/kg), metronidazole (16.7 mg/kg), and clarithromycin (16.7 mg/kg). After 10 days of treatment, the mice were euthanized and samples were harvested as described above.

To confirm the synergistic effect of PC with triple therapy, triple therapy was administered at four concentrations, as follows: existing concentration (metronidazole and clarithromycin: 16.7 mg/kg; omeprazole: 700 μg/kg), one-fifth, one-tenth, and one-fifteenth of the existing concentration. In contrast, PC was administered at the same concentration (1 mg/kg). In accordance with the above conditions, triple therapy and PC were administrated orally to the *H. pylori*-infected mice once daily for 5 days. The control and infection groups received distilled water under the same conditions. After 5 days of treatment, the mice were euthanized and samples were harvested, as described above.

4.5. Histological Examination

Gastric tissue was fixed in 4% (*w/v*) paraformaldehyde (PFA) in phosphate-buffered saline (PBS, pH 7.4) for 24 h, dehydrated in a graded ethanol series (70%, 80%, 90%, 95%, and 100%), cleared in xylene, embedded in paraffin, and sectioned into 5-μm-thick slices. Serial sections were stained with hematoxylin and eosin (H&E) and examined microscopically to determine whether the gastric mucosa contained any pathological lesions [42].

4.6. RNA Analysis

Total RNA was isolated from mouse gastric tissue using the TRI Reagent® (Molecular Research Center, Cincinnati, OH, USA). cDNA was synthesized using the ReverTra Ace® qPCR RT kit (Toyobo, Osaka, Japan), and qPCR amplification was accomplished using a Mx3000P qPCR System (Agilent Technologies, Santa Clara, CA, USA). Primer sequences are listed in Table 1. mRNA expression levels were normalized to those of the mouse ribosomal protein, Large, P0 (Rplp0), as the internal control, determined via the comparative threshold cycle method [43].

Table 1. Primers used in this study.

Gene	Sequence	
	Forward	Reverse
Rplp0	GTGCTGATGGGCAAGAAC	AGGTCCTCCTTGGTGAAC
Tnfα	CGAGTGACAAGCCTGTAGCC	AGCTGCTCCTCCACTTGGT
Il-1β	ATGAGAGCATCCAGCTTCAA	TGAAGGAAAAGAAGGTGCTC
cagA	CCGATCGATCCGAAATTTTA	CGTTCGGATTTGATTCCCTA
ureA	TGTTGGCGACAGACCGGTTCAAATC	GCTGTCCCGCTCGCAATGTCTAAGC
napA	CCATGTGCATAAAGCCACTG	GAGTTTGAGCGCTTCGGATA

Ribosomal protein (Rplp0), Large, P0; tumor necrosis factor alpha (Tnfα); interleukin-1 beta (Il-1β); cytotoxin-associated gene A (cagA); urease subunit alpha (ureA); neutrophil-activating protein A (napA).

4.7. Determination of Plasma Glutamate Oxaloacetate Transaminase (GOT) and Glutamate Pyruvate Transaminase (GPT) Levels

Plasma GPT and GOT levels were determined using GPT and GOT enzyme-linked immunosorbent assay (ELISA) kits (Asan Pharmaceutical, Seoul, Korea) in accordance with the manufacturer's instructions.

4.8. Statistical Analysis

Data are presented as the mean ± standard deviation and were determined using Statistical Package for Social Sciences (SPSS, IBM, Armonk, NY, USA) version 19.0. Statistically significant differences were ascertained using one-way analysis of variance, followed by the Tukey–Kramer and Student's *t*-tests. $p < 0.05$ was considered significant.

5. Conclusions

In summary, we compared the in vivo antimicrobial effects of PC and conventional triple therapy against *H. pylori* using a mouse model of *H. pylori* infection. PC completely eradicated *H. pylori*, even when administered at a dose 1/15th that of conventional antibiotics used for triple therapy. In addition, gastritis was rapidly alleviated upon PC treatment. Thus, PC may be a potential viable alternative to triple therapy for *H. pylori* and gastrointestinal disorders.

Author Contributions: Conceptualization, H.Y.J. and J.-H.M.; methodology, H.Y.J., T.H.L., J.G.K., S.L., C.M., X.T.T., T.-I.J., and J.-H.M.; validation, H.Y.J., T.H.L., J.G.K., S.L., C.M., X.T.T., T.-I.J., and J.-H.M.; formal analysis, H.Y.J., T.H.L., J.G.K., S.L., and X.T.T.; investigation, H.Y.J., T.H.L., and S.L.; resources, T.-I.J., C.M., and J.-H.M.; data curation, H.Y.J., T.-I.J., C.M., and J.-H.M.; writing—original draft preparation, H.Y.J. and T.H.L.; writing—review and editing, T.-I.J., C.M., and J.-H.M.; supervision, J.-H.M.; project administration, J.-H.M.; funding acquisition, J.-H.M. All authors have read and approved the final version of the manuscript.

Acknowledgments: We thank the members of Moon and Jeon's laboratory for their discussions and technical support.

References

1.   Kusters, J.G.; van Vliet, A.H.M.; Kuipers, E.J. Pathogenesis of *Helicobacter Pylori* Infection. *Clin. Microbiol. Rev.* **2006**, *19*, 449–490. [CrossRef] [PubMed]
2.   Marshall, B.J.; Warren, J.R. Unidentified Curved Bacilli in the Stomach of Patients with Gastritis and Peptic Ulceration. *Lancet* **1984**, *1*, 1311–1315. [CrossRef]
3.   Uemura, N.; Okamoto, S.; Yamamoto, S.; Matsumura, N.; Yamaguchi, S.; Yamakido, M.; Taniyama, K.; Sasaki, N.; Schlemper, R.J. *Helicobacter Pylori* Infection and the Development of Gastric Cancer. *N. Engl. J. Med.* **2001**, *345*, 784–789. [CrossRef] [PubMed]
4.   Goodwin, C.S. *Helicobacter Pylori* Gastritis, Peptic Ulcer, and Gastric Cancer: Clinical and Molecular Aspects. *Clin. Infect. Dis.* **1997**, *25*, 1017–1019. [CrossRef] [PubMed]
5.   Parsonnet, J.; Hansen, S.; Rodriguez, L.; Gelb, A.B.; Warnke, R.A.; Jellum, E.; Orentreich, N.; Vogelman, J.H.; Friedman, G.D. *Helicobacter Pylori* Infection and Gastric Lymphoma. *N. Engl. J. Med.* **1994**, *330*, 1267–1271. [CrossRef] [PubMed]
6.   Ferlay, J.; Shin, H.-R.; Bray, F.; Forman, D.; Mathers, C.; Parkin, D.M. Estimates of Worldwide Burden of Cancer in 2008: GLOBOCAN 2008. *Int. J. Cancer* **2010**, *127*, 2893–2917. [CrossRef] [PubMed]
7.   Leontiadis, G.I.; Sharma, V.K.; Howden, C.W. Non-Gastrointestinal Tract Associations of *Helicobacter Pylori* Infection. *Arch. Intern. Med.* **1999**, *159*, 925–940. [CrossRef]
8.   Franceschi, F.; Tortora, A.; Gasbarrini, G.; Gasbarrini, A. *Helicobacter Pylori* and Extragastric Diseases. *Helicobacter* **2014**, *19* (Suppl. 1), 52–58. [CrossRef]
9.   Chey, W.D.; Wong, B.C.Y. American College of Gastroenterology Guideline on the Management of *Helicobacter Pylori* Infection. *Am. J. Gastroenterol.* **2007**, *102*, 1808–1825. [CrossRef]
10.   Delchier, J.C.; Malfertheiner, P.; Thieroff-Ekerdt, R. Use of a Combination Formulation of Bismuth, Metronidazole and Tetracycline with Omeprazole as a Rescue Therapy for Eradication of *Helicobacter Pylori*. *Aliment. Pharmacol. Ther.* **2014**, *40*, 171–177. [CrossRef]

11. Chuah, S.-K.; Tsay, F.-W.; Hsu, P.-I.; Wu, D.-C. A New Look at Anti-*Helicobacter Pylori* Therapy. *World J. Gastroenterol.* **2011**, *17*, 3971–3975. [CrossRef] [PubMed]

12. Vakil, N.; Vaira, D. Treatment for *H. Pylori* Infection: New Challenges with Antimicrobial Resistance. *J. Clin. Gastroenterol.* **2013**, *47*, 383–388. [CrossRef] [PubMed]

13. Gong, E.J.; Yun, S.-C.; Jung, H.-Y.; Lim, H.; Choi, K.-S.; Ahn, J.Y.; Lee, J.H.; Kim, D.H.; Choi, K.D.; Song, H.J.; et al. Meta-Analysis of First-Line Triple Therapy for *Helicobacter Pylori* Eradication in Korea: Is It Time to Change? *J. Korean Med. Sci.* **2014**, *29*, 704–713. [CrossRef] [PubMed]

14. Kawai, T.; Takahashi, S.; Suzuki, H.; Sasaki, H.; Nagahara, A.; Asaoka, D.; Matsuhisa, T.; Masaoaka, T.; Nishizawa, T.; Suzuki, M.; et al. Changes in the First Line Helicobacter Pylori Eradication Rates Using the Triple Therapy-a Multicenter Study in the Tokyo Metropolitan Area (Tokyo Helicobacter Pylori Study Group). *J. Gastroenterol. Hepatol.* **2014**, *29* (Suppl. 4), 29–32. [CrossRef]

15. Ayala, G.; Escobedo-Hinojosa, W.I.; de la Cruz-Herrera, C.F.; Romero, I. Exploring Alternative Treatments for *Helicobacter Pylori* Infection. *World J. Gastroenterol.* **2014**, *20*, 1450–1469. [CrossRef]

16. Myllyluoma, E.; Veijola, L.; Ahlroos, T.; Tynkkynen, S.; Kankuri, E.; Vapaatalo, H.; Rautelin, H.; Korpela, R. Probiotic Supplementation Improves Tolerance to *Helicobacter Pylori* Eradication Therapy—A Placebo-Controlled, Double-Blind Randomized Pilot Study. *Aliment. Pharmacol. Ther.* **2005**, *21*, 1263–1272. [CrossRef]

17. Yang, Y.X.; Lohakare, J.; Chae, B. Effects of Lacquer (*Rhus Verniciflua*) Meal Supplementation on Layer Performance. *Asian-Australas. J. Anim. Sci.* **2007**, *20*. [CrossRef]

18. Hatada, K.; Kitayama, T.; Nishiura, T.; Nishimoto, A.; Simonsick, W.J.; Vogl, O. Structural Analysis of the Components of Chinese Lacquer "Kuro-Urushi". *Macromol. Chem. Phys.* **1994**, *195*, 1865–1870. [CrossRef]

19. Hong, S.H.; Suk, K.T.; Choi, S.H.; Lee, J.W.; Sung, H.T.; Kim, C.H.; Kim, E.J.; Kim, M.J.; Han, S.H.; Kim, M.Y.; et al. Anti-Oxidant and Natural Killer Cell Activity of Korean Red Ginseng (*Panax Ginseng*) and Urushiol (*Rhus Vernicifera* Stokes) on Non-Alcoholic Fatty Liver Disease of Rat. *Food Chem. Toxicol.* **2013**, *55*, 586–591. [CrossRef]

20. Kim, M.; Choi, Y.; Kim, W.; Kwak, S. Antioxidative Activity of Urushiol Derivatives from the Sap of Lacquer Tree (*Rhus Vernicifera* Stokes). *Korean J. Plant Res.* **1997**, *10*, 227–230.

21. Kim, D.; Jeon, S.; Seo, J. The Preparation and Characterization of Urushiol Powders (YPUOH) Based on Urushiol. *Prog. Org. Coat.* **2013**, *76*, 1465–1470. [CrossRef]

22. Kim, H.S.; Yeum, J.H.; Choi, S.W.; Lee, J.Y.; Cheong, I.W. Urushiol/Polyurethane-Urea Dispersions and Their Film Properties. *Prog. Org. Coat.* **2009**, *65*, 341–347. [CrossRef]

23. Choi, J.Y.; Park, C.S.; Choi, J.O.; Rhim, H.S.; Chun, H.J. Cytotoxic Effect of Urushiol on Human Ovarian Cancer Cells. *J. Microbiol. Biotechnol.* **2001**, *11*, 399–405.

24. Suk, K.T.; Baik, S.K.; Kim, H.S.; Park, S.M.; Paeng, K.J.; Uh, Y.; Jang, I.H.; Cho, M.Y.; Choi, E.H.; Kim, M.J.; et al. Antibacterial Effects of the Urushiol Component in the Sap of the Lacquer Tree (*Rhus Verniciflua* Stokes) on *Helicobacter Pylori*. *Helicobacter* **2011**, *16*, 434–443. [CrossRef]

25. Ma, X.M.; Lu, R.; Miyakoshi, T. Recent Advances in Research on Lacquer Allergy. *Allergol. Int.* **2012**, *61*, 45–50. [CrossRef]

26. Zepter, K.; Häffner, A.; Soohoo, L.F.; De Luca, D.; Tang, H.P.; Fisher, P.; Chavinson, J.; Elmets, C.A. Induction of Biologically Active IL-1 Beta-Converting Enzyme and Mature IL-1 Beta in Human Keratinocytes by Inflammatory and Immunologic Stimuli. *J. Immunol.* **1997**, *159*, 6203–6208.

27. Wakabayashi, T.; Hu, D.-L.; Tagawa, Y.-I.; Sekikawa, K.; Iwakura, Y.; Hanada, K.; Nakane, A. IFN-Gamma and TNF-Alpha Are Involved in Urushiol-Induced Contact Hypersensitivity in Mice. *Immunol. Cell Biol.* **2005**, *83*, 18–24. [CrossRef]

28. Kim, J.Y.; Cho, J.Y.; Ma, Y.K.; Lee, Y.G.; Moon, J.H. Nonallergenic Urushiol Derivatives Inhibit the Oxidation of Unilamellar Vesicles and of Rat Plasma Induced by Various Radical Generators. *Free Radic. Biol. Med.* **2014**, *71*, 379–389. [CrossRef]

29. Cho, J.-Y.; Park, K.Y.; Kim, S.-J.; Oh, S.; Moon, J.-H. Antimicrobial Activity of the Synthesized Non-Allergenic Urushiol Derivatives. *Biosci. Biotechnol. Biochem.* **2015**, *79*, 1915–1918. [CrossRef]

30. Lee, Y.G. Absorption and Metabolism of an Urushiol Derivative, 3-Pentylcathechol, in Rat Plasma. Master's Thesis, Chonnam National University, Gwangju, Korea, 2013.

31. Jeong, H.Y. Comparison of Absorption, Metabolism, and Bioactivity among Chemically Synthesized 3-Pentylcatechol and Its Glucosides. Master's Thesis, Chonnam National University, Gwangju, Korea, 2014.

32. Noach, L.A.; Bosma, N.B.; Jansen, J.; Hoek, F.J.; van Deventer, S.J.; Tytgat, G.N. Mucosal Tumor Necrosis Factor-Alpha, Interleukin-1 Beta, and Interleukin-8 Production in Patients with *Helicobacter Pylori* Infection. *Scand. J. Gastroenterol.* **1994**, *29*, 425–429. [CrossRef]

33. Olbe, L.; Hamlet, A.; Dalenbäck, J.; Fändriks, L. A Mechanism by Which *Helicobacter Pylori* Infection of the Antrum Contributes to the Development of Duodenal Ulcer. *Gastroenterology* **1996**, *110*, 1386–1394. [CrossRef] [PubMed]

34. Wang, G.; Hong, Y.; Olczak, A.; Maier, S.E.; Maier, R.J. Dual Roles of *Helicobacter Pylori* NapA in Inducing and Combating Oxidative Stress. *Infect. Immun.* **2006**, *74*, 6839–6846. [CrossRef] [PubMed]

35. Tzouvelekis, L.S.; Mentis, A.F.; Makris, A.M.; Spiliadis, C.; Blackwell, C.; Weir, D.M. *In Vitro* Binding of *Helicobacter Pylori* to Human Gastric Mucin. *Infect. Immun.* **1991**, *59*, 4252–4254. [CrossRef] [PubMed]

36. Sierra, J.C.; Asim, M.; Verriere, T.G.; Piazuelo, M.B.; Suarez, G.; Romero-Gallo, J.; Delgado, A.G.; Wroblewski, L.E.; Barry, D.P.; Peek, R.M.J.; et al. Epidermal Growth Factor Receptor Inhibition Downregulates *Helicobacter Pylori*-Induced Epithelial Inflammatory Responses, DNA Damage and Gastric Carcinogenesis. *Gut* **2018**, *67*, 1247–1260. [CrossRef] [PubMed]

37. Berg, H.F.; Maraha, B.; Scheffer, G.-J.; Peeters, M.F.; Kluytmans, J.A.J.W. Effect of Clarithromycin on Inflammatory Markers in Patients with Atherosclerosis. *Clin. Diagn. Lab. Immunol.* **2003**, *10*, 525–528. [CrossRef]

38. Knoop, K.A.; McDonald, K.G.; Kulkarni, D.H.; Newberry, R.D. Antibiotics Promote Inflammation through the Translocation of Native Commensal Colonic Bacteria. *Gut* **2016**, *65*, 1100–1109. [CrossRef] [PubMed]

39. Farooqui, T.F.; Farooqui, A.A. Molecular Mechanism Underlying the Therapeutic Activities of Propolis: A Critical Review. *Curr. Nutr. Food Sci.* **2010**, *6*, 186–199. [CrossRef]

40. Johnston, D.E. Special Considerations in Interpreting Liver Function Tests. *Am. Fam. Physician* **1999**, *59*, 2223–2230.

41. Lee, A.; O'Rourke, J.; De Ungria, M.C.; Robertson, B.; Daskalopoulos, G.; Dixon, M.F. A Standardized Mouse Model of *Helicobacter Pylori* Infection: Introducing the Sydney Strain. *Gastroenterology* **1997**, *112*, 1386–1397. [CrossRef]

42. Lee, S.; Yang, M.; Kim, J.; Son, Y.; Kim, J.; Kang, S.; Ahn, W.; Kim, S.-H.; Kim, J.-C.; Shin, T.; et al. Involvement of BDNF/ERK Signaling in Spontaneous Recovery from Trimethyltin-Induced Hippocampal Neurotoxicity in Mice. *Brain Res. Bull.* **2016**, *121*, 48–58. [CrossRef]

43. Go, D.-H.; Lee, Y.G.; Lee, D.-H.; Kim, J.-A.; Jo, I.-H.; Han, Y.S.; Jo, Y.H.; Kim, K.-Y.; Seo, Y.-K.; Moon, J.-H.; et al. 3-Decylcatechol Induces Autophagy-Mediated Cell Death through the IRE1α/JNK/P62 in Hepatocellular Carcinoma Cells. *Oncotarget* **2017**, *8*, 58790–58800. [CrossRef] [PubMed]

5

Imidazole and Imidazolium Antibacterial Drugs Derived from Amino Acids

Adriana Valls [1][ID], Jose J. Andreu [1], Eva Falomir [1][ID], Santiago V. Luis [1][ID],
Elena Atrián-Blasco [2,3,*][ID], Scott G. Mitchell [2,3,*][ID] and Belén Altava [1,*]

[1]   Departamento de Química Inorgánica y Orgánica, Universitat Jaume I, Av. Sos Baynat s/n,
      12071 Castellón, Spain; avalls@uji.es (A.V.); al314093@uji.es (J.J.A.); efalomir@uji.es (E.F.); luiss@uji.es (S.V.L.)
[2]   Instituto de Nanociencia y Materiales de Aragón (INMA), Consejo Superior de Investigaciones
      Científicas-Universidad de Zaragoza, 50009 Zaragoza, Spain
[3]   CIBER de Bioingeniería, Biomateriales y Nanomedicina, Instituto de Salud Carlos III, 28029 Madrid, Spain
*   Correspondence: elenaab@unizar.es (E.A.-B.); scott.mitchell@csic.es (S.G.M.); altava@uji.es (B.A.)

Abstract: The antibacterial activity of imidazole and imidazolium salts is highly dependent upon their lipophilicity, which can be tuned through the introduction of different hydrophobic substituents on the nitrogen atoms of the imidazole or imidazolium ring of the molecule. Taking this into consideration, we have synthesized and characterized a series of imidazole and imidazolium salts derived from *L*-valine and *L*-phenylalanine containing different hydrophobic groups and tested their antibacterial activity against two model bacterial strains, Gram-negative *E. coli* and Gram-positive *B. subtilis*. Importantly, the results demonstrate that the minimum bactericidal concentration (MBC) of these derivatives can be tuned to fall close to the cytotoxicity values in eukaryotic cell lines. The MBC value of one of these compounds toward *B. subtilis* was found to be lower than the IC_{50} cytotoxicity value for the control cell line, HEK-293. Furthermore, the aggregation behavior of these compounds has been studied in pure water, in cell culture media, and in mixtures thereof, in order to determine if the compounds formed self-assembled aggregates at their bioactive concentrations with the aim of determining whether the monomeric species were in fact responsible for the observed antibacterial activity. Overall, these results indicate that imidazole and imidazolium compounds derived from *L*-valine and *L*-phenylalanine—with different alkyl lengths in the amide substitution—can serve as potent antibacterial agents with low cytotoxicity to human cell lines.

Keywords: imidazole and imidazolium salts; amino acid; antibacterial agents; aggregation; lipophilicity

1. Introduction

Aromatic heterocycles, particularly the imidazole ring, have been used in the last decades as structural skeletons to obtain different types of bioactive compounds with antibacterial, antifungal, anticancer, antiviral, antidiabetic, and other properties [1–4]. The search for new potent drug molecules derived from imidazole continues to be an intense area of investigation in medicinal chemistry [5–7]. Moreover, pharmaceutical research, manufacture, and regulation are enhancing the development of solid active ingredients, delivered as powders or tablets; however, many solid drugs which perform well in in vitro evaluation remain too insoluble for the body to absorb [8,9]. Most of the bioactive agents sold for pharmaceutical or food industries are salts [10,11], and in this context, ionic liquids (ILs) represent a promising class of drug candidates whose physicochemical and pharmaceutical properties can be easily tuned [12–17]. In this regard, the imidazolium skeleton can be transformed into ionic liquids with promisingly potent pharmacological properties [18–21]. Consequently, monoimidazolium [22–24] and bisimidazolium [25–28] salts have been explored as a new generation of antibacterial agents. In this context, amino acid-based monoimidazolium salts with good bacterial toxicity have been reported in the literature [29].

Our research group has an ongoing interest in the biomimetic and bioactive capacity of imidazole or imidazolium amino acid derivatives [30–33]. Herein, imidazole, monotopic, and ditopic imidazolium salts derived from *L*-valine and *L*-phenylalanine with different alkyl lengths in the amide substitution were synthesized and characterized comprehensively. The antibacterial activity of these amino acid-based imidazolium salts against Gram-negative *Escherichia coli* DH5-α (herein *E. coli*) and Gram-positive *Bacillus subtilis* 1904-E (herein *B. subtilis*) were evaluated and their cytotoxicity was also studied using a human embryonic kidney cell line (HEK-293). Finally, due to the amphiphilic character of these compounds and the strong tendency towards self-aggregation of ionic liquid-related surfactants based on imidazolium salts [34–37], we investigated the spontaneous aggregation behavior of these compounds in water and in bacterial cell culture medium. Through optical and scanning electron microscopy, as well as UV-vis and fluorescence spectroscopy, we have extracted structure-property relationships between the degree of aggregation/self-assembly of the *L*-valine and *L*-phenylalanine derivatives and their corresponding antibacterial activity and cytotoxicity [38].

2. Results

2.1. Synthesis

The imidazole-amino acid derivatives **1a**, **2a**, and **3a** were obtained from the corresponding α-amino amide as previously described [31]. Monotopic and ditopic -imidazolium salts **1b–3b** and **1c–3c** were obtained in high yield by treatment of the corresponding imidazole with benzyl bromide or 1,3-bromomethylbenzene, respectively, as described in our previous publications (Scheme 1) [30,32].

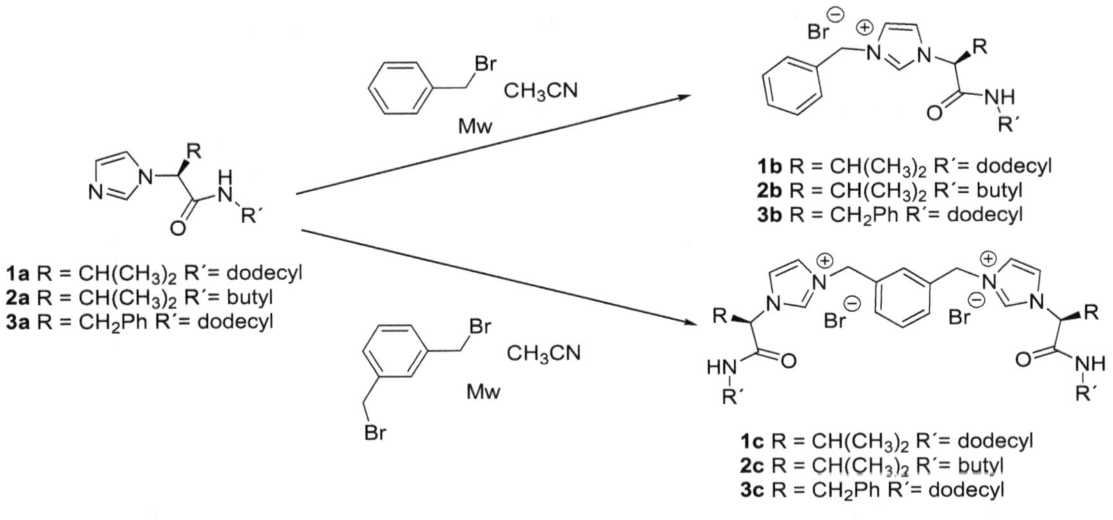

Scheme 1. Synthesis of the amino acid-based imidazolium salts in this report.

2.2. Antibacterial and Cytotoxicity Studies

The in vitro antibacterial activities of the synthesized compounds were examined against *E. coli* and *B. subtilis*. Bacteria were incubated in culture media with varying concentrations of the examined compound and the antibacterial properties were determined by observation of the optical density at 560 nm (bacteriostatic activity) and by the Resazurin cell viability assay (bactericidal activity). The corresponding minimal bactericidal concentration (MBC) and minimum inhibitory concentration (MIC) values that were obtained are summarized in Table 1 (please refer to Table S1 for MIC and MBC values in μM).

The outer membrane of Gram-negative bacteria such as *E. coli* includes porins, which allow the passage of small hydrophilic molecules across the membrane, and lipopolysaccharide molecules that extend into extracellular space. Thus, the observed trend in the activity results could be explained by the relative lipophilicity of the compounds combined with their capacity to disrupt the cell membrane [39,40]. The relative lipophilicity of the compounds was determined theoretically using VCCLab and Molinspiration softwares (LogP values Table 1) and experimentally (retention time values from HPLC, Table 1, Figures S3–S8). The HPLC method used was first validated using different lipophilic commercial compounds with LogP values from 1 to 4.5 (Figure S3a). The structure-activity relationships of the compounds will be further discussed in Section 3.

Table 1. Minimum inhibitory concentration (MIC, µg/mL), minimal bactericidal concentration (MBC, µg/mL), the half maximal inhibitory concentration IC_{50} (µg/mL) values and the partition coefficient log P values and HPLC retention times for the different compounds.

Entry	Compound	LogP [a]	Retention Time (min) [b]	E. coli MIC µg/mL [e]	E. coli MBC µg/mL [e]	B. subtilis MIC µg/mL [e]	B. subtilis MBC µg/mL [e]	HEK-293 IC_{50} µg/mL
1	**1a**	3.01 [c]	6.1	>2000	>2000	16	16	3.2 ± 0.5
2	**1b**	3.63 [d]	6.2	128	256	4	8	0.8 ± 0.2
3	**1c**	4.83 [d]	7.7	256	256	16	32	18 ± 4
4	**2a**	−0.67 [c]	3.4	>2000	>2000	>2000	>2000	>45
5	**2b**	−0.20 [d]	3.7	>2000	>2000	>1000	>1000	>79
6	**2c**	−1.34 [d]	3.1	1000	>2000	128	256	>142
7	**3a**	3.50 [c]	6.7	1000	>2000	16	16	7.3 ± 1.2
8	**3b**	4.26 [d]	8.8	32	128	4	4	61 ± 6
9	**3c**	5.96 [d]	10.0	2000	2000	64	64	37 ± 5
10	Alamethicin [41]	–	–			16	–	62.5 [f] [42]

[a] Average of values calculated using VCCLab and Molinspiration software. [b] Retention time in HPLC C18 reverse phase, CH_3CN/H_2O 70/30 (0.1% HCO_2H). [c] Value for the protonated forms. [d] Calculated for the imidazolium cations. [e] MIC/MBC values were obtained from a minimum of three separate experiments. Please refer to Supporting Information for MIC/MBC/IC_{50} values in µM. [f] Cytotoxicity against MRC-5 cells.

The MBC values obtained were plotted against the logP values of the corresponding compounds to study the possible correlation between activity and lipophilicity (Figure 1).

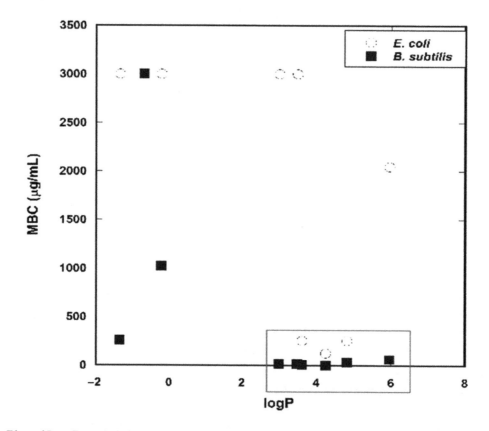

Figure 1. Plot of Log P vs. MBC. * For the sake of clarity, MBC values > 2000 µg/mL are given the value of 3000 µg/mL.

Electron microscopy is a powerful tool to further assess the effect of the imidazole derivatives and imidazolium salts on bacterial cell growth, inhibition, and death. Two compounds which showed from moderate to good antibacterial activity—the bisimidazolium salt **1c** and the monoimidazolium salt **3b**, respectively—were chosen for electron microscopy characterization. For these studies, *E. coli* and *B. subtilis* were inoculated for 20 h with each compound at their corresponding MIC (Figure 2) and $\frac{1}{2}$ MIC (Figures S1 and S2) concentrations and fixed with glutaraldehyde.

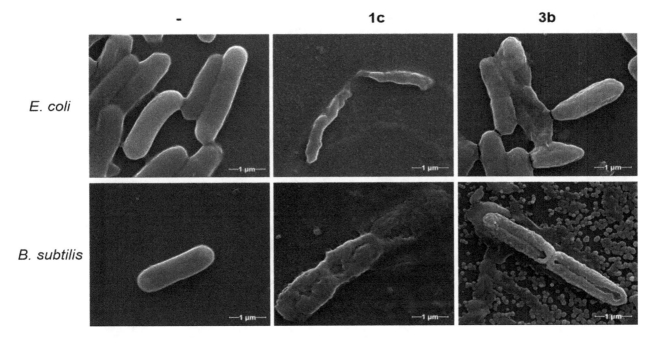

Figure 2. Scanning electron microscopy (SEM) images of *E. coli* and *B. subtilis* without treatment (-) and after incubation with compounds **1c** and **3b** at their corresponding MIC (60,000×). See Supporting Information for additional SEM images.

2.3. Aggregation Studies

The self-assembly of the compounds in aqueous medium and in the bacterial cell culture medium (LB broth) was investigated by optical and scanning electron microscopy, as well as UV-vis and fluorescence spectroscopy.

2.3.1. Fluorescence Spectroscopy

To investigate the microenvironment of the critical aggregation concentration (CAC) for self-assembly in water and in the bacterial cell culture medium by fluorescence, the intensity ratio of two of the peaks (I_1/I_3) of the pyrene fluorescence spectrum was used [43–45]. Plots of the pyrene I_1/I_3 ratio as a function of the total surfactant concentration show a typical sigmoidal decrease in the region where self-assembly takes place. At low concentrations, this ratio is larger as it corresponds to a polar environment for pyrene. When the surfactant concentration increases this ratio decreases rapidly, as the self-assembly favors the location of pyrene in a more hydrophobic environment, until reaching a roughly constant value because of the full incorporation of the probe into the hydrophobic region of the aggregates. Different approaches have been used to estimate CAC values from I_1/I_3 ratios [46]. The most common approach is the use of the break points, either directly or by extrapolating the values from the intersection of the two straight lines defined at the constant and variable regions of the I_1/I_3 sigmoidal curve [43,46–48]. As CAC represents the threshold of concentration at which self-aggregation starts, the corresponding value can be estimated from the break point at lower concentration (see Figures S9–S14) [49–52].

Fluorescence studies were carried out using MilliQ® water and 1/1 MilliQ® water/bacterial cell culture medium, because with the pure cell culture medium, a strong broad fluorescence emission band was observed precluding an accurate analysis. Furthermore, compound **3c** could not be studied due to solubility problems. The corresponding CACs obtained in water and in the 1/1 mixture of water/bacterial cell culture medium by fluorescence are shown in Table 2.

Furthermore, the MBC values of the compounds against *B. subtilis* were compared to their CAC (Figure 3). This comparison can shed light on the active form of the molecules exerting the antibacterial action, i.e., monomeric or aggregated structures.

Table 2. Estimated critical aggregation concentration (CAC) values obtained in aqueous and bacterial cell culture medium using fluorescence spectroscopy at 25 °C.

Entry	Amphiphilic Compound	CAC Fluorescence (mM) [a]		
		W [b]	CCM:W [c]	
			CAC1	CAC2
1	**1a**	0.085	0.004	0.045
2	**1b**	0.084	0.006	0.048
3	**1c**	0.010	0.016	0.21
4	**2a**	4.31	2.89	5.4
5	**2b**	4.57	3.46	8.4
6	**2c**	2.34	2.25	3.54
7	**3a**	0.033	0.018	0.325
8	**3b**	0.098	0.063	0.33
9	**3c**	nd [d]	nd [d]	

[a] CAC values from the break point. [b] In water. [c] In the 1/1 bacterial cell culture medium/water. [d] Low solubility.

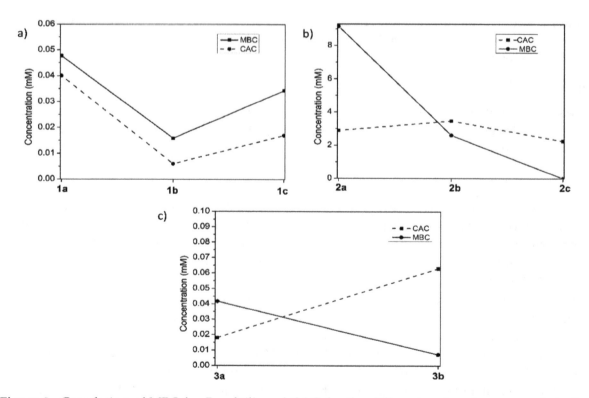

Figure 3. Correlation of MBC for *B. subtilis* and CAC for the different series of compounds in the bacterial cell culture medium: (**a**) valine derivatives with long alkyl chain; (**b**) valine derivatives with short chain; and (**c**) phenylalanine derivatives with long alkyl chain.

2.3.2. Optical Microscopy and Scanning Electron Microscopy (SEM)

The morphology of the aggregates in water, in 1/1 water/bacterial cell culture medium, and in the cell culture medium at concentrations above the CAC, were studied by optical microscopy (Figures S15–S17) and SEM (Figure 4 and Figure S18).

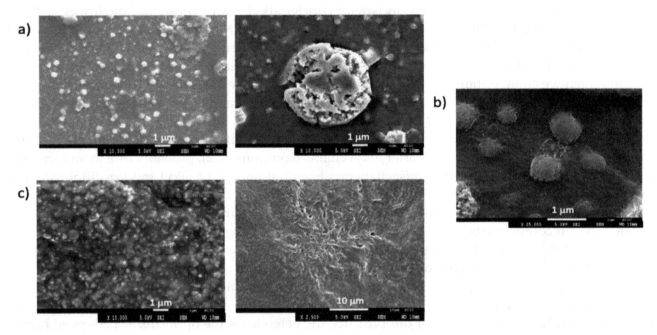

Figure 4. SEM images for **3b** (**a**) 0.5 mM in water; (**b**) 0.7 mM in 1/1 water/bacterial cell culture medium; and (**c**) 0.7 mM in the bacterial cell culture medium.

2.3.3. UV-Vis Spectroscopy

The aggregation and stability of the aggregates in the different solvents, water, 1/1 water/bacterial cell culture, and bacterial cell culture medium for **1a–c** were studied by UV-vis at 25 °C measuring the absorbance at 600 nm, for 1 mM colloidal solutions (Figure 5, Figures S19 and S20) [53,54].

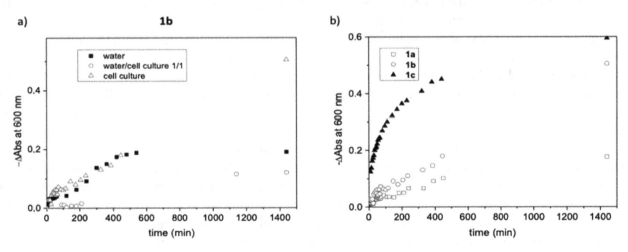

Figure 5. (**a**) Change in absorbance at 600 nm with respect to time for **1b** at 1 mM in different media. (**b**) Change in absorbance at 600 nm with respect to time for **1a–1c** at 1 mM in the bacterial cell culture medium.

3. Discussion

The Gram-positive cell wall is composed of a thick, multilayered peptidoglycan sheath outside of the cytoplasmic membrane, while the Gram-negative cell wall is composed of an outer membrane linked by lipoproteins to thin, mainly single-layered peptidoglycan. The peptidoglycan is located within the periplasmic space that is created between the outer and inner membranes [55]. It therefore follows that all the tested compounds were more active against *B. subtilis* (Gram-positive) than *E. coli* (Gram-negative) (i.e., see Table 1, entries 1 and 7). Compound **3b** (entry 8) proved to be the most active antibacterial agent possessing an MBC as low as 4 and 128 µg/mL against *B. subtilis* and *E. coli* respectively; while those compounds with shorter alkyl chains presented the lowest activity. Some of the compounds (Table 1, entries 2, 3, 6, 7, and 8) presented MIC values lower than MBC values. An antimicrobial compound is considered to be bactericidal whenever its MBC to MIC ratio is less than or equal to four. Compounds with MBC/MIC >4 are considered to be bacteriostatic [56]. In all the cases in which we could obtain exact MBC and MIC values (Table 1, entries 2, 3, 8 and 9), their ratio was equal to or minor than four. Therefore, compounds **1b**, **1c**, **3b**, and **3c** can be considered to possess true bactericidal activity.

The structural element which clearly relates to a better activity is the use of longer alkyl chains (compounds **1** and **3**) in contrast to shorter alkyl chains (compounds **2**), probably due to an increased lipophilicity. The toxicity towards miscellaneous bacterial strains of alkyl imidazolium salts has been reported to increase with the length of the alkyl chain [57]. The monoimidazolium salts with these longer alkyl chains (**1a-b** and **3a-b**) were more active against *B. subtilis* and *E. coli* than the bisimidazolium counterparts, with the monotopic salt **3b** showing the lowest MIC and MBC values (entries 2 and 8, Table 1), this indicates that the introduction of two hydrophobic alkyl chains contributes greatly to decrease the activity, opposite to the trends observed in the literature [27].

Regarding amino acid nature, the phenylalanine monotopic salt with long alkyl chain (**3b**) presented lower MIC and MBC values against *E. coli* than the analogous valine compound (**1b**) (entries 2 and 8, Table 1), however for ditopic salts, the behavior is the opposite, **3c** presented higher MIC and MBC values than **1c** (entries 3 and 9, Table 1).

Although a similar biological activity for the Gram-positive and Gram-negative organisms is preferred, it is not always the case with different strains of microorganisms. Some authors have described that Gram-positive organisms preferred a more lipophilic molecule than the Gram-negative ones [58]. This has been attributed to the difference in the cell outer membrane between bacterial types and strains: while Gram-positive bacteria have a very simple cell wall, the outer membrane of Gram-negative bacteria contains lipopolysaccharides which are cross-bridged by divalent cations, adding strength to the membrane and impermeability to lipophilic molecules. This agreed with the results obtained in Table 1 where the more lipophilic compounds showed less activity against *E. coli*.

A good correlation was obtained between the theoretical logP, calculated using the average values from VCCLab software and Molinspiration, and the retention time observed from HPLC (Figure S1). The activity observed against *B. subtilis* increases for compounds with logP > 3 with MBC ≤ 64 mg/mL. However, MBC values greater than 2000 µg/mL were obtained for both lipophilic and lipophobic compounds, with the exception of the lipophilic compounds **1b**, **1c**, and **3b** which present lower MBC values (Figure 1).

From the SEM images in Figure 2, both bacteria strains incubated with compounds **1c** and **3b** show clear signs of damage: from morphological changes to disruption of the cell membrane and leakage of cytoplasmatic material, ending with the disintegration of the bacteria into small fragments. Most images, especially of *B. subtilis*, show an "implosion" of bacteria, with a marked depression in the middle of the cell (also refer to Figures S1 and S2). In some of the images, aggregates of the compounds can be seen surrounding the bacteria, many of which are attached to the cell membrane.

Human embryonic kidney cells, HEK-293, were chosen as a cell model to evaluate the cytotoxicity of the compounds. The HEK-293 cells were incubated in the cell culture medium with varying concentrations of the examined compound and the impact of treatment was measured using the MTT cell viability assay [46]. The results indicated that compounds **1a–1c**, **3a**, and **3c** were considerably toxic with IC_{50} values lower than 36 µM (Table 1 and Table S1). Surprisingly, compound **3b** derived from phenylalanine was less toxic to the HEK-293 cell line at concentrations 15 times higher than the MIC and MBC for the *B. subtilis* strain (Table 1, entry 8) [59].

Comparing results with the commercial antibiotic alamethicin, the corresponding MIC value of **3b** against *B. subtilis* is lower than alamethicin, (Table 1, entry 10) [41], whereas the toxicity of alamethicin against MRC-5 human cells is similar to the cytotoxicity of the imidazolium salt **3b** against HEK-293 line [42].

To gain a more detailed understanding on the mechanism of cytotoxicity of these imidazole and imidazolium salts on bacteria, we studied the possible structure–activity relationship between their antibacterial activities and their aggregation behavior in bacterial cell medium [23,38].

From pyrene fluorescence studies in pure water, the plot of the I_1/I_3 ratio for the corresponding emission spectra vs. concentrations showed one single break point (Figure S9, Figure S11, and Figure S13) reaching in all cases values of $I_1/I_3 \approx 1.3$ or lower after the break point. However, in the bacterial cell culture medium, the plot of the I_1/I_3 ratios for the corresponding emission spectra vs. concentration presented two single break point and, in some cases, even three points. The two break points observed for all the compounds suggest the presence of two different processes. The first one takes place at I_1/I_3 values observed for pyrene in the absence of compounds ($I_1/I_3 = 1.16$ in water/1/1 bacterial cell culture medium) and reveals that pyrene is fully exposed to the polar solvent mixture in this first aggregation step. At the second break point, at higher concentrations, this ratio reaches lower values suggesting the formation in this region of aggregates in which the probe molecule is less solvent exposed [60]. For example, for compound **1b**, the first break point at 6 μM leads to aggregates with an appreciable solvent exposed probe ($I_1/I_3 \approx 1.1$) and the second process starts at *ca.* 48 μM affording aggregates, providing a low polarity microenvironment to pyrene, reaching I_1/I_3 values ≈ 0.8 for 1 mM concentration.

The CAC values obtained for compounds with long alkyl chain were in the μM range while for compounds **2a-c** with short alkyl chains, the CAC values obtained were in the mM range (i.e., entries 1 and 4, Table 2), where the lowest CAC values for the ditopic salts were found in water. In general, for the imidazole and monotopic salts, changing the medium from water to water/bacterial cell culture medium led to a decrease in the CAC values (i.e., Table 2, entries 1 and 2), however for ditopic salts, the CAC values did change significantly (Table 2, entries 3 and 6).

Comparing the first CAC values obtained in 1/1 water/bacterial cell culture medium and the MBC for *B. subtilis* for the different series of compounds in Figure 3, it can be observed as compounds **1a–1c** presented the CAC below the MBC, implying that these compounds exist in an aggregated form at the MBC concentration, meaning fewer imidazolium monomers will be present at these concentrations, less than is needed to produce a significant biologic effect, thus increased overall concentrations are needed to obtain the desired bactericidal effects if the monomeric form is the responsibility of the corresponding bioactivity. However, different behavior was observed for the series **3a–3b** derived from phenylalanine. Figure 3c shows how the CAC line intersects the MBC line, indicating that compound **3b** is not aggregated at the corresponding MBC value and exerts a high bactericidal effect, as observed in Table 2 (entry 8). Finally, for the **2a–2c** series, the CAC is below the MBC for **2a** but above for **2b** and **2c**, illustrating that the monomeric form is responsible for the corresponding antibacterial activity (Table 2, entry 6).

In addition to the results above, the compounds containing dodecyl chains can easily align with lipids and hence, accumulate within the bacterial cell membrane. In this regard, compounds with longer alkyl tails have CACs in the μM range in the bacterial cell culture medium and thus easily self-assemble, leading to an easy accumulation within the cell membrane. Therefore, resulting in a lower effective concentration at the site of action within the cellular cytoplasm lower. This accumulation could lead to a biocidal mechanism based on [38], as is observed in Figure 2. Furthermore, it appears that the shorter chain length results in reduced membrane interaction and an energetically unfavorable micelle formation, meaning low self-assembling capability, which leads to a lower overall bacterial cytotoxicity as seen from the corresponding MIC and MBC values (Table 1).

Consequently, by comparing the MBC for *B. subtilis* and CAC of the imidazole and imidazolium series, this study has provided a better understanding of the relationship between the biological activities of these compounds correlated with their aggregation capabilities. The results demonstrate that the compounds with longer alkyl chains provide excellent antimicrobial activity although most of them are aggregated at the antimicrobial response concentration, with only compound **3b** existing in its monomeric form at its corresponding MBC value.

Optical microscopy confirmed the formation of spherical aggregates between 0.5–20 μm diameter in size in the three different media (Figures S15–S17). Regarding the medium, in general, in the culture medium, the dispersity of the aggregates decreased for compounds with longer alkyl chains (see Figures S15 and S17). Furthermore, in the culture medium, compounds **2a–c** and **3b** were able to form worm-like aggregates at the studied concentrations (Figures S16 and S17).

SEM images for **1c** and **3b** in water, in 1/1 water/bacterial cell culture medium and in the bacterial cell culture medium revealed the formation of different aggregates morphologies. Compound **1c** produced spherical aggregates with <3 μm diameter size in all three media, with the aggregates in water being more distorted (Figure S18). Compound **3b** was able to form spherical aggregates in water and water/bacterial cell culture medium (Figure 4a,b), while in the pure culture medium, different morphologies were observed, such as spherical aggregates <1 μm in diameter coexisting with fibrillary aggregates (Figure 4c). When viewed at higher magnification, it is observed that the larger spherical aggregates consisted of several smaller aggregates or dendritic fibrillary aggregates for **3b** and **1c**, respectively (Figure 4 and Figure S18).

Regarding the stability of the aggregates formed, studies by UV-vis spectroscopy for **1a–c** are gathered in Figure 5. Figure 5a shows the change in absorbance ($-\Delta A_{600}$) of compound **1b** (1 mM) at 600 nm with respect to time in the different media. The initial rate for the change in absorbance associated to the destabilization of the aggregates is defined by the slope of the linear region of the initial $-\Delta A_{600}$ versus time plot. The slope and the total change in the absorbance was the smallest when using the water/bacterial cell culture medium, being the rate at the initial region for pure water and bacterial cell culture medium in the same ranges. However, it must be highlighted that the absorbance decreases until reaching a zero value after 500 min for pure water. A different behavior was obtained for **1a** and **1c** (see Figures S19 and S20). For compound **1a**, the absorbance at 600 nm decreased with time in the three media with similar rates, while for **1c**, the rate followed the order water > bacterial cell culture medium > 1/1 water/bacterial cell culture medium, reaching almost zero values in the tree media after 24 h.

Overall, the results obtained show that in the pure culture medium, the stability of the aggregates follows the order **1a** > **1b** > **1c** (Figure 5b), indicating that the introduction of the two headgroups and hydrophobic alkyl chains in **1c** contributes to a minor stabilization of the aggregates in this medium.

4. Materials and Methods

4.1. Materials

4.1.1. Reagents and Culture Media

Resazurin sodium salt and dimethyl sulfoxide (DMSO) were bought from Sigma-Aldrich. Luria-Bertani (LB) liquid broth (Miller's formulation) and nutrient broth (NB) were freshly prepared and sterilized by autoclave. Broth powders were bought from Scharlab. Tryptone soy agar plates were purchased from Thermo Scientific. Glutaraldehyde was purchased in solution at 25% in H_2O and Grade II from Sigma Aldrich and used as provided. Phosphate buffer was prepared from the solid salts NaH_2PO_4 and Na_2HPO_4, both purchased from Aldrich at qualities 99% and 99.5% respectively, by dissolving them in MilliQ® water and adjusting pH with NaOH and HCl solutions.

Cell culture media for cytotoxicity studies were purchased from Gibco (Grand Island, NY, USA). Fetal bovine serum (FBS) was obtained from HyClone (UT, USA). Supplements and other chemicals not listed in this section were obtained from Sigma Chemical Co. (St. Louis, MO, USA). Plastics for cell culture were supplied by Thermo Scientific BioLite (Madrid, Spain). All tested compounds were dissolved in DMSO at a concentration of 10 mM and stored at −20 °C until use. HEK-293 cell lines were maintained in Dulbecco's modified Eagle's medium (DMEM) containing glucose (1 g/L), glutamine (2 mM), penicillin (50 µg/mL), streptomycin (50 µg/mL), and amphotericin B (1.25 µg/mL) supplemented with 10% FBS.

Reagents and solvents, including NMR solvents, were purchased from commercial suppliers and were used without further purification except for pyrene, used for fluorescence studies, that was crystallized twice from methanol. Deionized water was obtained from a MilliQ® equipment (Burlington, MA, USA). Imidazoles **1a** and **2a** and imidazolium salts **1b** and **1c** were prepared as previously described [30,32].

4.1.2. Synthesis and Characterization

Imidazole **3a** and compounds **2b–c** and **3b–c** were prepared following the synthetic protocols.

General procedure for compound 3a: To a mixture of glyoxal (40% aq., 1.1 equiv, 2.6 mL) and formaldehyde (37% aq., 5.0 equiv., 7.7 mL), the (S)-2- amino-N-dodecyl-3- phenylpropanamide compound (1.0 equiv., 6.9 g, 20.8 mmol) and ammonium acetate (1.1 equiv, 1.8 g, 23.4 mmol) were dissolved previously in methanol and added. The reaction mixture was stirred at room temperature for 48 h. The solvent was evaporated under reduced pressure and the resulting crude residue was treated with saturated Na_2CO_3 solution, extracted with CH_2Cl_2 (3×), dried with anhydrous $MgSO_4$, filtered, and concentrated.

General procedure for compounds 2b–3b: To a mixture of compound **2a–3a** (1.1 equiv) and bromomethylbencene (1.0 equiv) were dissolved in acetonitrile (5 mL). The reaction was carried out under microwave irradiation using 120 W, 1.72×10^6 Pa, 150 °C, and 1 h. After solvent evaporation, the remaining solid was washed with diethyl ether (×3) to afford the desired compound.

General procedure for compounds 2c–3c: To a mixture of compound **2a–3a** (2.2 equiv) and 1, 3-(bis-bromomethyl)benzene (1.0 equiv) were dissolved in acetonitrile (5 mL). The reaction was carried out under microwave irradiation using 120 W, 1.72×10^6 Pa, 150 °C, and 1 h. After solvent evaporation, the remaining solid was washed with diethyl ether (×3) to afford the desired compound.

Compound 3a: yellow liquid (7 g, 88%), $[\alpha]^{25}_D = -7.11$ (c = 0.01, MeOH); m.p= 56.1 °C. ^{1}H NMR (400 MHz, $CDCl_3$ and CD_3OD) δ 7.26–7.07 (m, 4H), 7.00 (m, 1H), 6.97–6.89 (m, 3H), 6.48 (t, J = 5.7 Hz, NH), 4.67 (dd, J = 9.1, 6.0 Hz, 1H), 3.46 (dd, J = 14.0, 6.0 Hz, 1H), 3.19–3.00 (m, 3H), 1.30 (m, 2H), 1.26–1.04 (m, 18H), 0.85–0.77 (m, 3H). ^{13}C NMR (101 MHz, $CDCl_3$) δ 168.3, 134.0, 136.3, 129.6, 128.8, 128.7, 127.2, 118.0, 62.9, 39.8, 39.3, 31.9, 29.6, 29.6, 29.5, 29.3, 29.2, 26.8, 22.7, 14.1. MS (ESI) (m/z) calcd. for $C_{24}H_{37}N_3O$ [M+H]$^+$ = 384.3; found 383.4 (100%), 767.7 (35%, [M+M+H]$^+$). IR (ATR) = 3309, 2953, 2919, 2850, 1656, 1549, 1493, 1469, 1454 cm^{-1}. Calculated for $C_{24}H_{37}N_3O·4H_2O$: C 63.27, H 9.96, N 9.22; found C 62.97, H 9.74, N 9.58.

Compound 2b: yellow oil (150 mg, 93%); $[\alpha]^{25}_D = 41.07$ (c = 0.01, McOH); m.p. 33 °C. ^{1}H NMR (400 MHz, $CDCl_3$) δ 9.93 (s, 1H), 8.62 (t, J = 5.7 Hz, 1H), 7.75 (t, J = 1.8 Hz, 1H), 7.38–7.21 (m, 5H), 7.11 (s, 1H), 5.66 (d, J = 10.6 Hz, 1H), 5.47–5.27 (dd, J = 10.6, 2.2 Hz, 2H), 3.34–3.17 (m, 1H), 3.12–2.96 (m, 1H), 2.45–2.37 (m, 1H), 1.54–1.40 (m, 2H), 1.32–1.21 (m, 2H), 1.03 (d, J = 6.5 Hz, 3H), 0.81 (t, J = 7.3 Hz, 3H), 0.76 (d, J = 6.6 Hz, 3H). ^{13}C NMR (101 MHz, $CDCl_3$) δ 167.0, 136.1, 131.8, 130.1, 129.8, 128.6, 121.8, 120.9, 67.7, 53.9, 39.6, 31.2, 31.0, 20.2, 18.8, 18.3, 13.7. MS (ESI) (m/z) calcd. for $C_{19}H_{28}N_3O$ [M]$^+$ = 314.2; found 314.5 (100%); IR (ATR)= 3220, 3063, 2962, 2933, 2873, 1672, 1550, 1497, 1456, 1327, 1225, 1152 cm^{-1}. Calculated for $C_{19}H_{28}N_3OBr$: C 57.87, H 7.16, N 10.66; found C 57.80, H 6.98, N 11.01.

Compound 3b: yellow viscous solid (129 mg, 90%); $[\alpha]^{25}_D = -31.07$ (c = 0.01, MeOH); m.p = 16 °C. ^{1}H NMR (300 MHz, $CDCl_3$) δ 9.53 (s, 1H), 8.59 (t, J = 5.5 Hz, NH), 7.74 (s, 1H), 7.41–7.14 (m, 7H), 7.04–6.95 (m, 2H), 6.92 (s, 1H), 6.55 (m, 1H), 5.14 (q, J = 14.7 Hz, 2H), 3.51–2.95 (m, 4H), 1.83 (s, 3H), 1.44 (m, 2H), 1.17 (s, 16H), 0.92–0.70 (m, 3H). ^{13}C NMR (101 MHz, $CDCl_3$) δ 166.6, 136.1, 134.3, 131.9, 129.8, 129.7, 129.1, 129.0, 128.2, 127.5, 121.8, 120.9, 62.3, 53.6, 40.0, 39.0, 31.9, 29.7, 29.6, 29.5, 29.4,

29.2, 28.9, 27.0, 22.7, 14.1. MS (ESI) (m/z) calcd. for $C_{31}H_{44}N_3O$ $[M]^+ = 474.4$; found 474.7 (100%); IR (ATR) = 3297, 3061, 2966, 2922, 2851, 1654, 1557, 1495, 1453 cm^{-1}. Calculated for $C_{31}H_{44}N_3OBr \cdot H_2O$: C 65.02, H 8.10, N 7.34; found C 65.46, H 8.24, N 7.68.

Compound 2c: yellow oil (104 mg, 90%); $[\alpha]^{25}_D = 6.93$ (c = 0.01, MeOH); m.p.= 85 °C. ^{1}H NMR (500 MHz, CDCl$_3$) δ 10.01 (s, 2H), 8.40 (t, J = 5.6 Hz, 2H), 8.12 (s, 2H), 7.68 (d, J = 1.3 Hz, 2H), 7.47–7.36 (m, 2H), 7.34–7.23 (m, 2H), 5.73 (d, J = 14.4 Hz, 2H), 5.55–5.38 (dd, J = 10.7 Hz, J = 3.5 Hz, 4H), 3.37–3.25 (m, 2H), 3.15–3.00 (m, 2H), 2.53–2.38 (m, 2H), 1.64–1.43 (m, 4H), 1.39–1.20 (m, 4H), 1.08 (d, J = 6.6 Hz, 6H), 0.87 (t, J = 7.3 Hz, 6H), 0.82 (d, J = 6.7 Hz, 6H). 13C NMR (126 MHz, CDCl$_3$) δ 206.8, 166.7, 136.5, 134.1, 130.6, 130.5, 129.9, 122.4, 120.8, 77.3, 77.0, 76.8, 68.1, 53.2, 39.5, 31.1, 30.9, 30.9, 20.1, 18.8, 18.4, 13.6. MS (ESI) (m/z) calcd. for $C_{32}H_{50}N_6O_2$ $[M]^{2+} = 275.2$; found 275.3 (100%); IR (ATR)= 3412, 3228, 3125, 3066, 2962, 2933, 2873, 1671, 1550, 1465, 1360, 1298, 1226, 1152 cm^{-1}. Calculated for $C_{32}H_{50}N_6O_2Br_2 \cdot 2H_2O$: C 51.48, H 7.29, N 11.26; found C 50.84, H 7.32, N 11.46.

Compound 3c: yellow viscous solid (126 mg, 82%); $[\alpha]^{25}_D = 17.33$ (c = 0.01, MeOH); m.p. = 60 °C. ^{1}H NMR (300 MHz, CDCl$_3$) δ 9.47 (s, 2H), 8.21 (t, J = 5.7 Hz, NH), 7.81–7.51 (m, 6H), 7.29–7.06 (m, 16H), 6.13 (t, J = 8.0 Hz, 2H), 5.31 (s, 4H), 3.37 (dd, J = 13.6, 7.2 Hz, 2H), 3.25–3.10 (m, 4H), 3.00–2.84 (m, 2H), 1.41–1.29 (m, 4H), 1.23–1.05 (m, 32H), 0.80 (m, 6H). ^{13}C NMR (101 MHz, CDCl$_3$) δ 166.3, 136.3, 134.3, 133.6, 130.6, 130.3, 129.7, 129.2, 128.9, 127.5, 122.3, 121.0, 62.6, 53.0, 39.9, 38.9, 31.9, 29.7, 29.7, 29.6, 29.5, 29.4, 29.2, 28.9, 26.9, 22.7, 14.1. MS (ESI) (m/z) calcd. for $C_{56}H_{82}N_6O_2$ $[M]^{2+} = 435.3$; found 435.7 (100%); IR (ATR)= 3294, 3063, 2923, 2852, 1656, 1554, 1495, 1454, 1362 cm^{-1}. Calculated for $C_{56}H_{82}N_6O_2Br_2$: C 65.23, H 8.02, N 8.15; found C 65.76, H 8.57, N 8.34.

4.1.3. Microorganisms and Growth Conditions

Two bacterial strains were used in the antibacterial assays: *Escherichia coli* DH5α as a Gram-negative model and *Bacillus subtilis* 1904-E as a Gram-positive model. Both bacterial strains were donated to our laboratory and can be provided on request by contacting the corresponding authors. Both bacterial strains were incubated at 37 °C and the pre-inoculum incubation time was of 24 h. Liquid Luria-Bertani (LB) medium was used for *E. coli* DH5α and nutrient broth (NB) for *B. subtilis*.

4.2. Methods

4.2.1. Bacterial Proliferation Assay in Presence of Imidazole Derivatives

The bacteria cell bank suspensions were thawed and inoculated in the appropriate liquid broth for 24 h at 37 °C with mild agitation. A dilution from these culture solutions was used for the following tests, corresponding to an inoculum of 1×10^7 CFU/mL. Stock solutions of all the tested compounds were prepared in DMSO at a concentration of 100 mg/mL, aliquoted, and stored at −20 °C.

(A) Bacterial growth inhibition assay: Conditions here described are for testing 6 different concentrations of the compounds, with triplicates of each condition. Therefore, 4 compounds were tested per plate. An adapted version of the microdilution method was used. Firstly, the imidazole derivatives were dissolved in the corresponding broth at 2× the highest tested concentration. Then, 100 µL of the 2× solutions were added to the first (A) and second (B) row wells of a 96-well plate. In addition, 100 µL of liquid medium had been previously added to rows B to F. Subsequent dilutions at 1:2 are prepared in rows B to F, by withdrawal of 100 µL from the previous row (more concentrated) to the next row (half diluted), mixing well. Then, 100 µL were discarded from the last row (F). By now, there are 100 µL in each well, and 100 µL of bacterial suspension at 10^7 CFU/mL were added to each well. Then, the 96-well plates were incubated for 24 h at 37 °C under mild agitation. Bacterial growth was controlled both by visual observation of the turbidity in each well and by measuring the optical density (OD) at 560 nm at time 0 h and 24 h. Results are recorded as the lowest concentration of antimicrobial agent that inhibits visible growth of the bacteria, and were compared with the OD variation of a control culture containing *E. coli* or *B. subtilis* (+ control) and of solution of the tested compounds without bacteria (- control).

(B) Bacterial cell viability assay: Cell viability was analyzed using a Resazurin (7-Hydroxy-3H-phenoxazin-3-one 10-oxide) assay in a 96-well plate. Once the bacterial cultures of growth inhibition assay had been grown for a total of 24 h, 25 μL of a 0.1 mg/mL resazurin (prepared in LB or NB medium) were added to each well and incubated in the dark at 37 °C for 1 h under stirring. Resazurin has a blue color at the testing pH and turns pink when reduced by the viable bacteria to resorufin. Therefore, pink wells indicate metabolizing bacteria, while blue wells are indicative of bacteria that have lost their ability to convert resazurin to resorufin. Different controls were made in order to corroborate the MBC value obtained by the resazurin assay. The change of color was confirmed at 1, 4, and 24 h after its addition. The viability of bacteria was verified (either confirmed or rejected) by the colony plate-counting method, by seeding 10 μL from the cell culture onto tryptone soy agar plates and observing the presence or absence of bacterial growth after 24 h at 37 °C.

4.2.2. Log P Calculation and Retention Time Determination

LogP values for the different compounds were calculated using VCCLab (ALOGPS 2.1) and Molinspiration (miLogP2.2) softwares. We used LogP as the average of these values. The protonated forms for the imidazole derivatives were considered. Reverse phase HPLC (equipment: Agilent technologies 1100 series, column: Xterra MS C18 4.6×150 mm (5 μmol/L)) was also used for measuring the relative lipophilicity of these compounds, since the retention time of each molecule on the reverse phase column is related to its lipophilicity. All the products were dissolved in MeOH at 2 mmol/L concentration and eluted using 70/30 acetonitrile/water and 0.1% of formic acid for 15 min and flow rate 0.2 mL/min at 25 °C. λ used was 254, 280, and 220 nm taking the corresponding chromatogram with higher mAU (see Supporting Information).

4.2.3. H NMR Studies

NMR experiments were carried out on a Varian INOVA 500 spectrometer (500 MHz for ^{1}H and 125 MHz for ^{13}C), on a Bruker Avance III HD 400 spectrometer (400 MHz for ^{1}H and 100 MHz for ^{13}C) or on a Bruker Avance III HD 300 spectrometer (300 MHz for ^{1}H and 75 MHz for ^{13}C) at 25 °C. Chemical shifts are reported in ppm using TMS as the reference.

4.2.4. Fluorescence Spectroscopy Measurements

Pyrene was used as a fluorescence probe to determine the CAC of the compounds in water and 1/1 water/bacterial cell culture medium at 25 ± 1 °C. Fluorescence measurements were performed with a Spex Fluorolog 3-11 instrument equipped with a 450 W xenon lamp (right angle mode). Firstly, a stock pyrene solution of 1.98×10^{-4} mol/L was prepared in ultrapure methanol. Then, solutions of the imidazole and imidazolium salt compounds (ranging from 6 to 3×10^{-3} mmol/L) were prepared in different vials and 5 μL of pyrene solution was transferred into the vials, reaching a final pyrene concentration of 9.89×10^{-7} mol/L in each vial. Fluorescence spectra of pyrene were recorded from 200 to 650 nm after excitation at 337 nm, and the spectra were not corrected for the Xe lamp spectral response. The slit width was set at 5 nm for both excitation and emission. The peak intensities at 373 and 385 nm were determined as I_1 and I_3, respectively. The ratios of the peak intensities at 373 and 385 nm (I_1/I_3) for the emission spectra were recorded as a function of the logarithm of concentration. The CAC values were taken from the break point. Samples were excited with a 337 nm NanoLED.

4.2.5. Optical Images

Images were recorded with OLYMPUS COVER-018 microscopy, BX51TF model, at 25 °C. Experiments were carried out in water, 1/1 water/bacterial cell culture medium, and in bacterial cell culture medium.

4.2.6. Scanning Electron Microscopy (SEM)

SEM images of the compounds were obtained using a JEOL 7001F microscope with a digital camera; while SEM images of the incubated bacteria were obtained using an Inspect F50 microscope, at 10 kV and spot size of 3.0, with a digital camera. Bacteria solutions at ca. 0.5×10^7 CFU/mL were incubated overnight without and with compounds **1c** and **3b** at their $\frac{1}{2}$ MIC and MIC. After this, bacteria were washed with sterile PBS and fixed by incubation for 2 h in a 2.5% glutaraldehyde solution in phosphate buffer 10 mmol/L at pH 7.2. The fixed bacteria were subsequently washed once with phosphate buffer saline solution and four times with MilliQ water to remove any residual salts and glutaraldehyde. Finally, bacteria were resuspended in MilliQ water and 10 μL of these solutions were placed on silicon wafers and allowed to dry by evaporation overnight. Samples were coated with platinum using the sputtering technique in which microscopic particles of platinum are rejected from the surface after the material is itself bombarded by energetic particles of a plasma or gas. Experiments were carried out in water, 1/1 water/bacterial cell culture medium, and in bacterial cell culture medium.

4.2.7. UV-Vis Spectroscopy

UV-Vis absorption spectra of the colloidal solutions were recorded on a Hewlett-Packard 8453 spectrophotometer at 25 °C. Experiments were carried out in water, 1/1 water/bacterial cell culture medium, and in bacterial cell culture medium.

4.2.8. Cell Proliferation Assay for Cytotoxicity Studies

In 96-well plates, 3×10^3 HEK-293 cells per well were seeded and incubated with serial dilutions of the tested compounds (from 200 to 0.2 μM) to a total volume of 100 μL of their growth media. The 3-(4,5-dimethylthiazol-2-yl)-2,5-diphenyltetrazolium bromide (MTT; Sigma Chemical Co.) dye reduction assay in 96-well microplates was used, as previously described [18]. After 2 days of incubation (37 °C, 5% CO_2 in a humid atmosphere), 10 μL of MTT (5 mg/mL in phosphate-buffered saline, PBS) was added to each well, and the plate was incubated for a further 3 h (37 °C). The supernatant was discarded and replaced by 100 μL of DMSO to dissolve formazan crystals. The absorbance was then read at 540 nm by Multiskan^{TM} FC microplate reader. For all concentrations of compound, cell viability was expressed as the percentage of the ratio between the mean absorbance of treated cells and the mean absorbance of untreated cells. Three independent experiments were performed, and the IC_{50} values (i.e., concentration half inhibiting cell proliferation) were graphically determined using GraphPad Prism 4 software.

Statistical analysis: GraphPad Prism v4.0 software (GraphPad Software Inc., La Jolla, CA, USA) was used for statistical analysis. For all experiments, the obtained results of the triplicates were represented as means with standard deviation (SD).

5. Conclusions

A series of novel imidazole and imidazolium salts derived from *L*-valine and *L*-phenylalanine containing different hydrophobic groups have been synthesized and their antibacterial activity studied against *E. coli* and *B. subtilis*. The results demonstrate that an optimum lipophilicity of the alkyl chain and the amino acid side chain is needed to achieve antibacterial activity. The compounds presented better antibacterial activity against *B. subtilis* than *E. coli*, where compound **1a–1b** and **3a–3b** were the most active against *B. subtilis*, showing MBC values corresponding to 16 μg/mL or lower. Monotopic compound **3b** was 15 times less active against human embryonic kidney cells HEK-293 than toward *B. subtilis*, thus demonstrating its potential as an effective antibacterial agent with good biocompatibility. Aqueous aggregation studies revealed CAC values for compounds **1a–1c** and **3a–3c** in the μM range in water alone, however these CAC values decreased for imidazole and monotopic species when water was replaced with bacterial cell culture medium. Optical microscopy and SEM images confirmed the formation of these spherical aggregates. It is important to note that most of the bioactive compounds were aggregated to some extent at their MIC/MBC concentrations, however the monotopic compound **3b** was not aggregated at its corresponding MBC, suggesting that the monomeric species was responsible for the observed antibacterial activity.

Author Contributions: Conceptualization, B.A. and S.G.M.; methodology, B.A. and S.G.M.; software, A.V. and J.J.A.; validation, B.A., S.G.M. and E.A.-B.; formal analysis, B.A.; investigation, A.V., J.J.A., E.A.-B., and E.F.; resources, B.A.; data curation, S.G.M.; writing—original draft preparation, B.A.; writing—review and editing, B.A., S.G.M. and E.A.-B.; supervision, B.A., S.G.M. and S.V.L.; funding acquisition, S.V.L., E.A.-B., and S.G.M.

Acknowledgments: The electron microscopy characterization was conducted at the Laboratorio de Microscopias Avanzadas (LMA) at Universidad de Zaragoza. Authors acknowledge the LMA for offering access to their instruments and expertise. Technical support from the SECIC of the UJI is acknowledged.

References

1. Rani, N.; Sharma, A.; Singh, R. Imidazoles as Promising Scaffolds for Antibacterial Activity: A Review. *Mini-Rev. Med. Chem.* **2013**, *13*, 1812–1835. [CrossRef] [PubMed]
2. Duan, Y.T.; Wang, Z.C.; Sang, Y.L.; Tao, X.X.; Zhu, H.L. Exploration of Structure-Based on Imidazole Core as Antibacterial Agents. *Curr. Top. Med. Chem.* **2013**, *13*, 3118–3130. [CrossRef] [PubMed]
3. Li, W.J.; Li, Q.; Liu, D.; Ding, M.W. Synthesis, Fungicidal Activity, and Sterol 14α-Demethylase Binding Interaction of 2-Azolyl-3,4-dihydroquinazolines on Penicillium digitatum. *J. Agric. Food Chem.* **2013**, *61*, 1419–1426. [CrossRef] [PubMed]
4. Chen, L.; Zhao, B.; Fan, Z.J.; Liu, X.M.; Wu, Q.F.; Li, H.P.; Wang, H.X. Synthesis of Novel 3,4-Chloroisothiazole-Based Imidazoles as Fungicides and Evaluation of Their Mode of Action. *J. Agric. Food Chem.* **2018**, *66*, 7319–7327. [CrossRef]
5. Hu, Y.; Shen, Y.F.; Wu, X.H.; Tu, X.; Wang, G.X. Synthesis and biological evaluation of coumarin derivatives containing imidazole skeleton as potential antibacterial agents. *Eur. J. Med. Chem.* **2018**, *143*, 958–969. [CrossRef]
6. Wang, P.-Y.; Wang, M.-W.; Zeng, D.; Xiang, M.; Rao, J.-R.; Liu, Q.-Q.; Liu, L.-W.; Wu, Z.-B.; Li, Z.; Song, B.A.; et al. Rational Optimization and Action Mechanism of Novel Imidazole (or Imidazolium)-Labeled 1,3,4 Oxadiazole Thioethers as Promising Antibacterial Agents against Plant Bacterial Diseases. *J. Agric. Food Chem.* **2019**, *67*, 3535–3545. [CrossRef]
7. Rossi, R.; Ciofalo, M. An Updated Review on the Synthesis and Antibacterial Activity of Molecular Hybrids and Conjugates Bearing Imidazole Moiety. *Molecules* **2020**, *25*, 5133. [CrossRef]
8. Shamshina, J.L.; Kelley, S.P.; Gurau, G.; Rogers, R.D. Chemistry: Develop ionic liquid drugs. *Nature* **2015**, *528*, 188–189. [CrossRef]
9. Hauss, D. Oral lipid-based formulations. *J. Adv. Drug Deliv. Rev.* **2007**, *59*, 667–676. [CrossRef]
10. Guillory, J.K. *Pharmaceutical Salts: Properties, Selection, and Use*, 2nd ed.; Stahl, P.H., Wermuth, C.G., Eds.; Wiley-VCH: Weinheim, Germany, 2002. [CrossRef]
11. Becerril, R.; Nerín, C.; Silva, F. Encapsulation Systems for Antimicrobial Food Packaging Components: An Update. *Molecules* **2020**, *25*, 1134. [CrossRef]
12. Stoimenovski, J.; MacFarlane, D.R.; Bica, K.; Rogers, R.D. Crystalline vs. Ionic Liquid Salt Forms of Active Pharmaceutical Ingredients: A Position Paper. *Pharm. Res.* **2010**, *27*, 521–526. [CrossRef] [PubMed]
13. Shadid, M.; Gurau, G.; Shamshina, J.L.; Chuang, B.-C.; Hailu, S.; Guan, E.; Chowdhury, S.K.; Wu, J.T.; Rizvi, S.A.A.; Griffin, R.J.; et al. Sulfasalazine in ionic liquid form with improved solubility and exposure. *Med. Chem. Comm.* **2015**, *6*, 1837–1841. [CrossRef]
14. Egorova, K.S.; Gordeev, E.G.; Ananikov, V.P. Biological activity of ionic liquids and their application in pharmaceutics and medicine. *Chem. Rev.* **2017**, *117*, 7132–7189. [CrossRef]
15. Ferraz, R.; Branco, L.C.; Prudencio, C.; Noronha, J.P.; Petrovski, Z. Ionic liquids as active pharmaceutical ingredients. *ChemMedChem* **2011**, *6*, 975–985. [CrossRef]
16. Miskiewicz, A.; Ceranowicz, P.; Szymczak, M.; Bartus, K.; Kowalczyk, P. The Use of Liquids Ionic Fluids as Pharmaceutically Active Substances Helpful in Combating Nosocomial Infections Induced by Klebsiella Pneumoniae New Delhi Strain, Acinetobacter Baumannii and Enterococcus Species. *Int. J. Mol. Sci.* **2018**, *19*, 2779. [CrossRef]

17. Cuervo-Rodríguez, R.; Muñoz-Bonilla, A.; López-Fabal, F.; Fernández-García, M. Hemolytic and Antimicrobial Activities of a Series of Cationic Amphiphilic Copolymers Comprised of Same Centered Comonomers with Thiazole Moieties and Polyethylene Glycol Derivatives. *Polymers* **2020**, *12*, 972. [CrossRef]

18. Messali, M.; Moussa, Z.; Alzahrani, A.Y.; El-Naggar, M.Y.; ElDouhaibi, A.S.; Judeh, Z.M.A.; Hammouti, B. Synthesis, characterization and the antimicrobial activity of new eco-friendly ionic liquids. *Chemosphere* **2013**, *91*, 1627–1634. [CrossRef]

19. Wang, D.; Richter, C.; Rühling, A.; Drücker, P.; Siegmund, D.; Metzler-Nolte, N.; Glorius, F.; Galla, H.-J. A Remarkably Simple Class of Imidazolium-Based Lipids and Their Biological Properties. *Chem. Eur. J.* **2015**, *21*, 15123–15126. [CrossRef]

20. Chen, H.-L.; Kao, H.-F.; Wang, J.-Y.; Wei, G.-T. Cytotoxicity of Imidazole Ionic Liquids in Human Lung Carcinoma A549 Cell Line. *J. Chin. Chem. Soc.* **2014**, *61*, 763–769. [CrossRef]

21. Malhotra, S.V.; Kumar, V.; Velez, C.; Zayas, B. Imidazolium-Derived Ionic Salts Induce Inhibition of Cancerous Cell Growth through Apoptosis. *MedChemComm* **2014**, *5*, 1404–1409. [CrossRef]

22. Pernak, J.; Sobaszkiewicz, K.; Mirska, I. Anti-microbial activities of ionic liquids. *Green Chem.* **2003**, *5*, 52–56. [CrossRef]

23. Kuznetsova, D.A.; Gabdrakhmanov, D.R.; Lukashenko, S.S.; Voloshina, A.D.; Sapunova, A.S.; Kulik, N.V.; Nizameev, I.R.; Kadirov, M.K.; Kashapov, R.R.; Zakharova, Y.L. Supramolecular systems based on cationic imidazole-containing amphiphiles bearing hydroxyethyl fragment: Aggregation properties and functional activity. *J. Mol. Liq.* **2019**, *289*, 111058. [CrossRef]

24. Garcia, M.T.; Ribosa, I.; Perez, L.; Manresa, A. Micellization and antimicrobial properties of surface-active ionic liquids containing cleavable carbonate linkages. *Langmuir* **2017**, *33*, 6511–6520. [CrossRef]

25. Gindri, I.M.; Siddiqui, D.A.; Bhardwaj, P.; Rodriguez, L.C.; Palmer, K.L.; Frizzo, C.P.; Martinsc, M.A.P.; Rodrigues, D.C. Dicationic imidazolium-based ionic liquids: A new strategy for non-toxic and antimicrobial materials. *RSC Adv.* **2014**, *4*, 62594–62602. [CrossRef]

26. Pałkowski, Ł.; Błaszczyński, J.; Skrzypczak, A.; Błaszczak, J.; Kozakowska, K.; Wróblewska, J.; Kożuszko, S.; Gospodarek, E.; Krysiński, J.; Słowiński, R. Antimicrobial activity and SAR study of new gemini imidazolium-based chlorides. *J. Chem. Biol. Drug Des.* **2014**, *83*, 278–288. [CrossRef]

27. Voloshina, A.D.; Gumerova, S.K.; Sapunova, A.S.; Kulik, N.V.; Mirgorodskaya, A.B.; Kotenko, A.A.; Prokopyeva, T.M.; Mikhailov, V.A.; Zakharova, L.Y.; Sinyashin, O.G. The structure—Activity correlation in the family of dicationic imidazolium surfactants: Antimicrobial properties and cytotoxic effect. *BBA Gen. Subj.* **2020**, *1864*, 129728. [CrossRef] [PubMed]

28. Wang, L.; Qin, H.; Ding, L.; Huo, S.; Deng, Q.; Zhao, B.; Meng, L.; Yan, T. Preparation of a novel class of cationic gemini imidazolium surfactants containing amide groups as the spacer: Their surface properties and antimicrobial activity. *J. Surfactant Deterg.* **2014**, *17*, 1099–1106. [CrossRef]

29. Kapitanov, I.V.; Jordan, A.; Karpichev, Y.; Spulak, M.; Perez, L.; Kellett, A.; Kümmerer, K.; Gathergood, N. Synthesis, self-assembly, bacterial and fungal toxicity, and preliminary biodegradation studies of a series of L-phenylalanine-derived surface-active ionic liquids. *Green Chem.* **2019**, *21*, 1777–1794. [CrossRef]

30. González, L.; Escorihuela, J.; Altava, B.; Burguete, M.I.; Luis, S.V. Chiral Room Temperature Ionic Liquids as Enantioselective Promoters for the Asymmetric Aldol Reaction. *Eur. J. Org. Chem.* **2014**, *2014*, 5356–5363. [CrossRef]

31. González, L.; Altava, B.; Bolte, M.; Burguete, M.I.; García-Verdugo, E.; Luis, S.V. Synthesis of Chiral Room Temperature Ionic Liquids from Amino Acids–Application in Chiral Molecular Recognition. *Eur. J. Org. Chem.* **2012**, *2012*, 4996–5009. [CrossRef]

32. González-Mendoza, L.; Escorihuela, J.; Altava, B.; Burguete, M.I.; Luis, S.V. Application of optically active chiral bis(imidazolium) salts as potential receptors of chiral dicarboxylate salts of biological relevance. *Org. Biomol. Chem.* **2015**, *13*, 5450–5459. [CrossRef] [PubMed]

33. González-Mendoza, L.; Escorihuela, J.; Altava, B.; Burguete, M.I.; Hernando, E.; Luis, S.V.; Quesada, R.; Vicent, C. Bis(imidazolium) salts derived from amino acids as receptors and transport agents for chloride anions. *RSC Adv.* **2015**, *5*, 34415–34423. [CrossRef]

34. Baltazar, Q.Q.; Chandawalla, J.; Sawyer, K.; Anderson, J.L. Interfacial and micellar properties of imidazolium-based monocationic and dicationic ionic liquids. *Colloids Surf. A* **2007**, *302*, 150–156. [CrossRef]

35. Kamboj, R.; Singh, S.; Bhadani, A.; Kataria, H.; Kaur, G. Gemini Imidazolium Surfactants: Synthesis and Their Biophysiochemical Study. *Langmuir* **2012**, *28*, 11969–11978. [CrossRef]

36. Zhuang, L.-H. Synthesis and properties of novel ester-containing gemini imidazolium surfactants. *J. Colloid*

Interface Sci. **2013**, *408*, 94–100. [CrossRef] [PubMed]

37. Bhadani, A.; Singh, T.M.S.; Sakai, K.; Sakai, H.; Abe, M. Structural diversity, physicochemical properties and application of imidazolium surfactants: Recent advances. *Adv. Colloid Interface Sci.* **2016**, *231*, 36–58. [CrossRef] [PubMed]

38. Wang, D.; Galla, H.-J.; Drücker, P. Membrane interactions of ionic liquids and imidazolium salts. *Biophys. Rev.* **2018**, *10*, 735–746. [CrossRef]

39. Knight, N.J.; Hernando, E.; Haynes, C.J.E.; Busschaert, M.; Clarke, H.J.; Takimoto, K.; García-Valverde, M.; Frey, J.G.; Quesada, R.; Gale, P.A. QSAR analysis of substituent effects on tambjamine anion transporters. *Chem. Sci.* **2016**, *7*, 1600–1608. [CrossRef]

40. Gorczyca, M.; Korchowiec, B.; Korchowiec, J.; Trojan, S.; Rubio-Magnieto, J.; Luis, S.V.; Rogalska, E. A Study of the Interaction between a Family of Gemini Amphiphilic Pseudopeptides and Model Monomolecular Film Membranes Formed with a Cardiolipin. *J. Phys. Chem. B* **2015**, *119*, 6668–6679. [CrossRef]

41. Barns, K.J.; Weisshaar, J.C. Single-cell, time-resolved study of the effects of the antimicrobial peptide alamethicin on Bacillus subtilis. *Biochim. Biophys. Acta* **2016**, *1858*, 725–732. [CrossRef]

42. Ishiyama, A.; Otoguro, K.; Iwatsuki, M.; Namatame, M.; Nishihara, A.; Nonaka, K.; Kinoshita, Y.; Takahashi, Y.; Masuma, R.; Shiomi, K.; et al. In vitro and in vivo antitrypanosomal activities of three peptide antibiotics: Leucinostatin A and B, alamethicin I and tsushimycin. *J. Antibiot.* **2009**, *62*, 303–308. [CrossRef] [PubMed]

43. Kalyanasundaram, K.; Thomas, J.K. Environmental effects on vibronic band intensities in pyrene monomer fluorescence and their application in studies of micellar Systems. *J. Am. Chem. Soc.* **1977**, *99*, 2039–2044. [CrossRef]

44. Kalyanasundaram, K. *Photochemistry in Microheterogeneous Systems*, 1st ed.; Academic Press: New York, NY, USA, 1987.

45. Aguiar, J.; Carpena, P.; Molina-Bolívar, J.A.; Carnero Ruiz, C. On the determination of the critical micelle concentrationby the pyrene 1:3 ratio method. *J. Colloid Interface Sci.* **2003**, *258*, 116–122. [CrossRef]

46. Stockert, J.C.; Horobin, R.W.; Colombo, L.L.; Blázquez-Castro, A. Tetrazolium salts and formazan products in Cell Biology: Viability assessment, fluorescence imaging, and labeling perspectives. *Acta Histochem.* **2018**, *120*, 159–167. [CrossRef] [PubMed]

47. Frindi, M.; Michels, B.; Zana, R. Ultrasonic Absorption Studies of Surfactant Exchange between Micelles and Bulk Phase In Aqueous Micellar Solutions of Nonionic Surfactants with Short Alkyl Chains. 1,2-Hexanedlol and 1,2,3-Octanetrlol. *J. Phys. Chem.* **1991**, *95*, 4832–4837. [CrossRef]

48. Regev, O.; Zana, R. Aggregation Behavior of Tyloxapol, a Nonionic Surfactant Oligomer, in Aqueous Solution. *J. Colloid Interface Sci.* **1999**, *210*, 8–17. [CrossRef]

49. Ananthapadmanabhan, K.P.; Goddard, E.D.; Turro, N.J.; Kuo, P.L. Fluorescence Probes for Critical Micelle Concentration. *Langmuir* **1985**, *2*, 352–355. [CrossRef]

50. Liu, C.G.; Desai, K.G.H.; Chen, X.G.; Park, H.J. Linolenic acid-modified chitosan for formation of selfassembled nanoparticles. *J. Agric. Food Chem.* **2005**, *53*, 437–441. [CrossRef]

51. Dong, X.; Liu, C. Preparation and Characterization of Self-Assembled Nanoparticles of Hyaluronic Acid-Deoxycholic Acid Conjugates. *J. Nanomat.* **2010**, *2010*, 1–9. [CrossRef]

52. Yoshimura, T.; Ichinokawa, T.; Kaji, M.; Esumi, K. Synthesis and surface-active properties of sulfobetaine-type zwitterionic gemini surfactants. *Colloids Surf. A Physicochem. Eng. Asp.* **2006**, *273*, 208–212. [CrossRef]

53. Gregory, J. Monitoring particle aggregation processes. *Adv. Colloid Interface Sci.* **2009**, *147–148*, 109–123. [CrossRef] [PubMed]

54. Aslan, K.; Luhrs, C.C.; Pérez-Luna, V.H. Controlled and Reversible Aggregation of Biotinylated Gold Nanoparticles with Streptavidin. *J. Phys. Chem. B* **2004**, *108*, 15631–15639. [CrossRef]

55. Brown, L.; Wolf, J.M.; Prados-Rosales, R.; Casadevall, A. Through the wall: Extracellular vesicles in gram-positive bacteria, mycobacteria and fungi. *Nat. Rev. Microbiol.* **2015**, *13*, 620–630. [CrossRef] [PubMed]

56. Bury-Moné, S. Antibacterial Therapeutic Agents: Antibiotics and Bacteriophages. In *Reference Module in Biomedical Sciences*, 3rd ed.; Elsevier: Amsterdam, The Netherlands, 2014; pp. 1–13. ISBN 9780128012383.

57. Ghanema, O.B.; Mutaliba, M.J.A.; El-Harbawi, M.; Gonfaa, G.; Kait, C.F.; Alitheend, N.B.M.; Leveque, J.M. Effect of imidazolium-based ionic liquids on bacterial growth inhibition investigated via experimental and QSAR modelling studies. *J. Hazard. Mater.* **2015**, *297*, 198–206. [CrossRef] [PubMed]

58. Lien, E.; Hansch, C.; Anderson, S. Structure-activity correlations for antibacterial agents on gram-positive and gram-negative cells. *J. Med. Chem.* **1968**, *11*, 430–441. [CrossRef] [PubMed]

59.   Coleman, D.; Špulák, S.; Garcia, M.T.; Gathergood, N. Antimicrobial toxicity studies of ionic liquids leading to a 'hit' MRSA selective antibacterial imidazolium salt. *Green Chem.* **2012**, *14*, 1350–1356. [CrossRef]

60.   Roy, S.; Dey, J. Spontaneously Formed Vesicles of Sodium N-(11-Acrylamidoundecanoyl)-glycinate and l-Alaninate in Water. *Langmuir* **2005**, *21*, 10362–10369. [CrossRef]

6

In Vitro Assessment of Antimicrobial, Antioxidant, and Cytotoxic Properties of Saccharin–Tetrazolyl and –Thiadiazolyl Derivatives: The Simple Dependence of the pH Value on Antimicrobial Activity

Luís M. T. Frija [1,*], Epole Ntungwe [2]⬤, Przemysław Sitarek [3], Joana M. Andrade [2], Monika Toma [4], Tomasz Śliwiński [4]⬤, Lília Cabral [5], M. Lurdes S. Cristiano [5], Patrícia Rijo [2,6,*]⬤ and Armando J. L. Pombeiro [1]

[1]   Centro de Química Estrutural (CQE), Instituto Superior Técnico, Universidade de Lisboa, Av. Rovisco Pais, 1049-001 Lisboa, Portugal; pombeiro@ist.utl.pt
[2]   CBIOS—Research Center for Health Sciences & Technologies, ULusófona de Humanidades e Tecnologias, Campo Grande 376, 1749-024 Lisboa, Portugal; ntungweepolengolle@yahoo.com (E.N.); p5319@ulusofona.pt (J.M.A.)
[3]   Department of Biology and Pharmaceutical Botany, Medical University of Lodz, Muszyńskiego Street 1, 90-151 Łódź, Poland; przemyslaw.sitarek@umed.lodz.pl
[4]   Laboratory of Medical Genetics, Faculty of Biology and Environmental Protection, University of Lodz, 90-151 Lodz, Poland; monika.toma@biol.uni.lodz.pl (M.T.); tomasz.sliwinski@biol.uni.lodz.pl (T.Ś.)
[5]   Department of Chemistry and Pharmacy (FCT) and Center of Marine Sciences (CCMar), Universidade do Algarve, P-8005-039 Faro, Portugal; liliacabral80@gmail.com (L.C.); mcristi@ualg.pt (M.L.S.C.)
[6]   iMed.ULisboa - Research Institute for Medicines, Faculdade de Farmácia, Universidade de Lisboa, Av. Prof. Gama Pinto, 1649-003 Lisboa, Portugal
*   Correspondence: luisfrija@tecnico.ulisboa.pt (L.M.T.F.); patricia.rijo@ulusofona.pt (P.R.)

Abstract: The antimicrobial, antioxidant, and cytotoxic activities of a series of saccharin–tetrazolyl and –thiadiazolyl analogs were examined. The assessment of the antimicrobial properties of the referred-to molecules was completed through an evaluation of minimum inhibitory concentration (MIC) and minimum bactericidal concentration (MBC) values against Gram-positive and Gram-negative bacteria and yeasts. Scrutiny of the MIC and MBC values of the compounds at pH 4.0, 7.0, and 9.0 against four Gram-positive strains revealed high values for both the MIC and MBC at pH 4.0 (ranging from 0.98 to 125 µg/mL) and moderate values at pH 7.0 and 9.0, exposing strong antimicrobial activities in an acidic medium. An antioxidant activity analysis of the molecules was performed by using the DPPH (2,2-diphenyl-1-picrylhydrazyl) method, which showed high activity for the TSMT (N-(1-methyl-2H-tetrazol-5-yl)-N-(1,1-dioxo-1,2-benzisothiazol-3-yl) amine, **7**) derivative (90.29% compared to a butylated hydroxytoluene positive control of 61.96%). Besides, the general toxicity of the saccharin analogs was evaluated in an *Artemia salina* model, which displayed insignificant toxicity values. In turn, upon an assessment of cell viability, all of the compounds were found to be nontoxic in range concentrations of 0–100 µg/mL in H7PX glioma cells. The tested molecules have inspiring antimicrobial and antioxidant properties that represent potential core structures in the design of new drugs for the treatment of infectious diseases.

Keywords: saccharin; tetrazole; 1,3,4-thiadiazole; H7PX glioma cells; antimicrobial screening; antioxidant capacity

1. Introduction

In 1878, 1,2-benzisothiazole-3-one 1,1-dioxide (**1**, Figure 1), commercially known as saccharin, was discovered accidentally by Fahlberg during an investigation of the oxidation of o-toluenesulfonamide [1,2]: it was published by Remsen and Fahlberg one year later [3]. For more than a century, saccharin has been commonly used as a noncaloric artificial sweetener in the form of its water-soluble salts (mainly sodium, ammonium, and calcium), and it is the principal sweetening component of diabetic diets. For about three decades (since reports on carcinogenicity in laboratory animals were published), the debate on its toxicity to humans has not reached a consensus [4–6]. Numerous N-substituted derivatives of saccharin have been assessed for in vitro biological activity [7–10]. For example, first-row transition metal saccharinates as well as dioxovanadium(VI), dioxouranium(VI), and cerium(IV) saccharinates have been classified as protease inhibitors, and several metal(II) saccharinates have displayed superoxide dismutase-like activity [11]. Besides, structure–activity relationship studies have shown that the saccharin scaffold is an effective element for the development of inhibitors of human leukocyte clastase (HLE), cathepsin G (Cat G), and proteinase 3 (PR3), as well as antimycobacterium and central nervous system agents [9,12–14]. Recently, different saccharin-based antagonists have been recognized for their interferon-signaling pathways, showing antitumor activity through the inhibition of cancer-related isoforms in humans [15]. It should also be noted that the first non-benzoannelated 4-amino-2,3-dihydroisothiazole 1,1-dioxide, which lacks a 3-oxo group, has been described and shows anti-HIV-1 activity. Additionally, saccharin and isothiazolyl derivatives have been used in agriculture as herbicides, fungicides, and pesticides [16].

Azole-type heterocyclic cores on the genesis
of the molecules tested in this study:

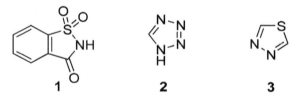

Figure 1. Structures of 1,2-benzisothiazole-3-one 1,1-dioxide (**1**, saccharin), 1H-tetrazole (**2**), and 1,3,4-thiadiazole (**3**).

Tetrazole (CN_4H_2) and its derivatives have attracted much attention as well due to their practical applications. The tetrazolic acid fragment $-CN_4H$ has acidity similar to the carboxylic acid group $-CO_2H$ and is almost allosteric with it, but it is metabolically more stable at the physiologic pH [17]. Hence, synthetic methodologies leading to the replacement of $-CO_2H$ groups by $-CN_4H$ groups in biologically active molecules are of major relevance [18]. Indeed, the number of patent claims and publications related to medicinal uses of tetrazolyl derivatives continues to grow rapidly and cover a wide range of applications: tetrazoles have been found, for instance, in compounds with antihypertensive, antiasthmatic, antitubercular, antimalarial, and antibiotic activity [19–22]. Several tetrazole derivatives have shown potential as anticonvulsants and anticancer and anti-HIV-1 drugs [23–25]. Tetrazoles have also had important applications in agriculture as plant growth regulators, herbicides, fungicides [26], and stabilizers in photography and photoimaging [27]. Due to the high enthalpy of formation, tetrazole decomposition results in the liberation of two nitrogen molecules and a significant amount of energy. Therefore, several tetrazole derivatives have been explored as explosives, propellant components for missiles, and gas generators for airbags (applicable to the automobile industry) [28]. In addition, various tetrazole-based compounds have good coordination properties and are able to form stable complexes with several metal ions. This ability is successfully used in analytical chemistry for the removal of heavy metal ions from liquids and in chemical systems formulated for metal protection against corrosion [29]. Many physical, chemical, physicochemical, and biological properties of tetrazoles are closely related to their ability to behave as acids and bases. In the tetrazole ring, the four nitrogen atoms connected in succession are able to be involved in proteolytic processes. This heterocyclic system is unusual in structure and unique in terms of acid–base characteristics.

In line with what is mentioned above for saccharin and tetrazole derivatives, the 1,3,4-thiadiazole scaffold represents an important class of core structures that are of great interest mainly because of their various biological activities and respective therapeutic applications. The 1,3,4-thiadiazole ring is a very weak base, possesses relatively high aromaticity, and is moderately stable in aqueous acid solutions although it is vulnerable to ring cleavage with an aqueous base [30]. Besides, this heterocyclic ring is very electron-deficient due to the electron-withdrawing effect of the nitrogen atoms and is relatively inert toward electrophilic substitution but susceptible to nucleophilic attack, whereas when substitutions are introduced into the 2' or 5' position of this ring, it is highly activated and readily reacts to produce varied derivatives [31]. To some extent, these specific properties lead to the application of 1,3,4-thiadiazole derivatives in pharmaceutical, agricultural, and material chemistry. Therefore, several 1,3,4-thiadiazole-based compounds display a broad spectrum of biological activities, such as antimicrobial [32], antituberculosis [33], antioxidant [34], anti-inflammatory [35], anticonvulsant [36], antidepressant, anxiolytic [37], antihypertensive [38], anticancer [39], and antifungal activity [40]. The most prominent thiadiazole derivative is possibly the acetazolamide [*N*-(5-sulfamoyl-1,3,4-thiadiazol-2-yl)acetamide], a very well-known carbonic anhydrase inhibitor that is used in the treatment of glaucoma [41], high-altitude illness [42], epileptic seizures [43], idiopathic intracranial hypertension [44], hemiplegic migraine [45], cystinuria [46], obstructive sleep apnea [47], and congenital myasthenic syndromes [48].

The search for new molecular entities, whether natural or synthetic, with relevant pharmacological activities for effective applications in medical practices continues to be a hot topic in health science as well as in science as a whole. This permanent search is well documented in the immense scientific literature and is mainly supported by the fact that many pathogenic organisms are able to develop mechanisms of resistance to high-activity medicines in their early lives [49–54]. In this context, and given our prior interest in the synthesis, reactivity, and bioactivity of tetrazole and thiazole derivatives, our collaborative interest was piqued by the great potential of these heterocycles for medical applications. Herein, we report on the antimicrobial, antioxidant, and cytotoxic activities of four mixed-azole compounds of benzisothiazole–tetrazolyl and benzisothiazole–thiadiazolyl.

2. Results and Discussion

2.1. Chemistry

The 3-chloro-1,2-benzisothiazole 1,1-dioxide (**2**), one of the strategic building blocks for the synthesis of the studied molecules, was first prepared through the halogenation of saccharin (**1**), as previously described (Scheme 1 (A)) [55]. The three saccharin–tetrazolyl analogs (TS (**5**), 2MTS (**6**), and TSMT (**7**)) were synthetized through a combination of the amino-tetrazoles **3**, **4a**, and **4b** with **2**, following a nucleophilic substitution reaction of the chloride anion by the amine functionality (Scheme 1 (B)). Similarly, compound **9** (MTSB) was prepared by coupling **2** and 5-methyl-1,3,4-thiadiazole-2-thiol (**8**) (Scheme 1 (C)). All of the reactions proceeded smoothly under experimental protocols originally developed by us [56–59], affording crystalline products in reasonable to very good yields.

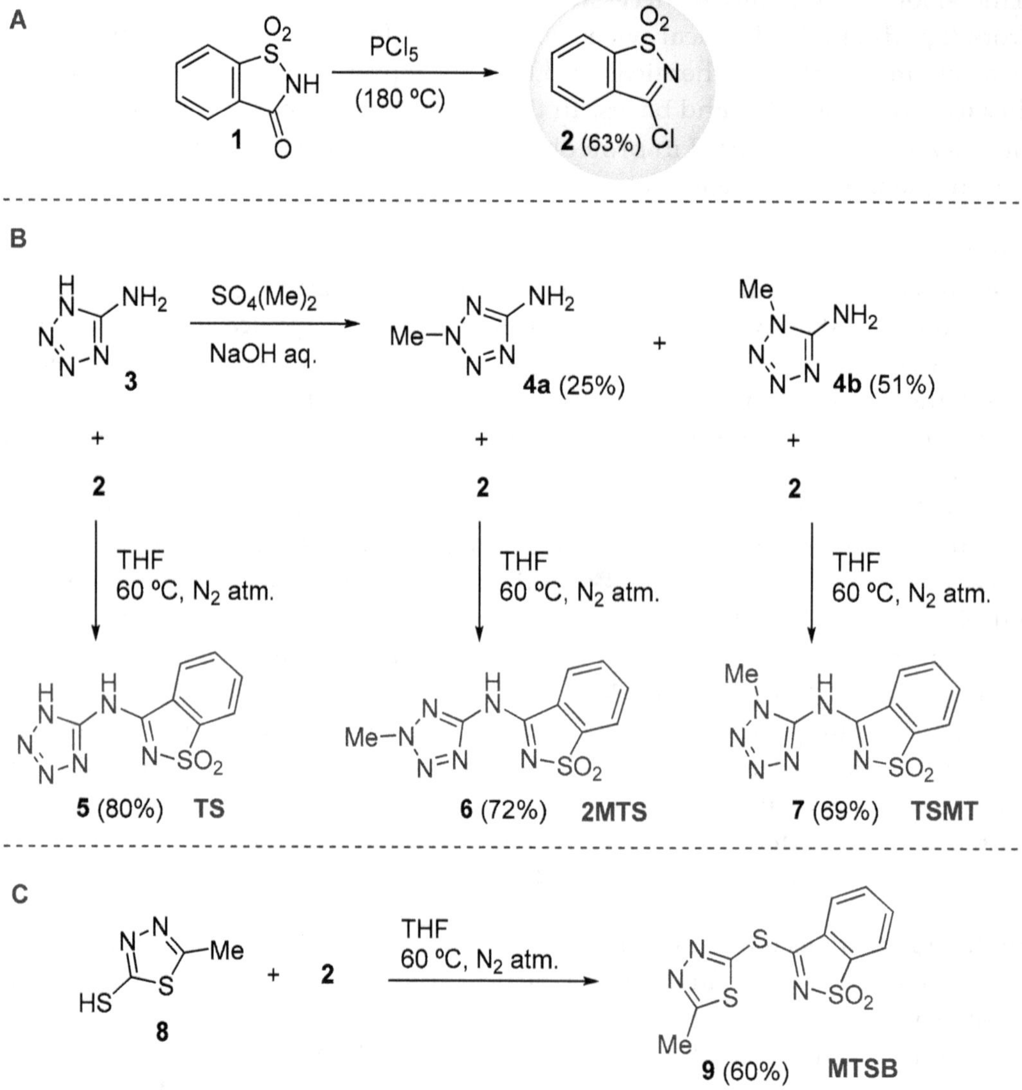

Scheme 1. Synthesis of saccharin–tetrazolyl (TS, 2MTS, and TSMT) and saccharin–thiadiazolyl (MTSB) derivatives.

2.2. Biological Assays

2.2.1. Antimicrobial Activity

The assessment of the antibacterial properties of compounds TSMT, MTSB, TS, and 2MTS was determined through minimum inhibitory concentration (MIC) and minimum bactericidal concentration (MBC) values against Gram-positive (*Staphylococcus aureus* and *Enterococcus faecalis*), Gram-negative (*Pseudomonas aeruginosa* and *Escherichia coli*), and yeast (*Saccharomyces cerevisiae* and *Candida albicans*) strains obtained from the American Type Culture Collection (ATCC) (Table 1). The MIC value corresponding to the lowest concentration at which no visible growth was observed was assessed by the microdilution method [60]. For MBC evaluation, the bacterial suspension in the wells was homogenized, serially diluted, spread in triplicate on appropriate medium, and incubated at 37 °C. All compounds and respective positive controls were tested at the same concentration of 500 µg/mL.

Table 1. Minimum inhibitory concentration (MIC) and minimum bactericidal concentration (MBC) values of TSMT, MTSB, TS, and 2MTS (obtained through the microdilution method against Gram-positive bacteria, Gram-negative bacteria, and yeast strains (in μM)).

Sample	E. faecalis		S. aureus		P. aeruginosa		E. coli		S. cerevisiae		C. albicans	
	MIC	MBC	MIC	MBC	MIC	MBC	MIC	MBC	MIC	MBC	MIC	MBC
TSMT	236.5	1892.1	118.3	1892.1	118.3	946.0	236.5	473.0	473.0	946.0	236.5	1892.1
MTSB	219.0	1752.1	109.5	1752.1	109.5	876.1	219.0	438.0	438.0	876.1	219.0	1752.1
TS	249.8	1998.1	124.9	1998.1	124.9	999.0	249.8	499.5	499.5	999.0	249.8	1998.1
2MTS	236.5	1892.1	118.3	1892.1	118.3	946.0	236.5	473.0	473.0	946.0	236.5	1892.1
Positivecontrol	1.95	nt	1.95	nt	0.977	nt	0.488	nt	15.6	nt	7.81	nt
	VAN		VAN		NOR		NOR		NYS		NYS	

VAN: vancomycin; NOR: norfloxacin; NYS: nystatin; nt: not tested. Data are the median values of at least three replicates.

The results of the antimicrobial assay showed that the compounds tested were bacteriostatic. This was concluded because the MBC values were much higher than the MIC values (see Table 1). The compounds were more active against the Gram-negative *P. aeruginosa* and the Gram-positive *S. aureus* bacteria. However, it seemed that the MIC and MBC values were more similar against *E. coli*. Additionally, antimicrobial tests were performed at different pH values (pH 4.0, 7.0, and 9.0), also using the microdilution method (see Tables 2–4). The microorganisms used in these tests were chosen based on the initial results from the antimicrobial screening of Gram-positive bacteria and comprised four Gram-positive strains, namely *S. aureus* CIP6538, *E. faecalis* ATCC 29212, methicillin-resistant *S. aureus* CIP106760 (MRSA), and vancomycin-resistant *E. faecalis* ATCC51299 (VRE).

Table 2. MIC and MBC values of TSMT, MTSB, TS, and 2MTS (obtained through the microdilution method against Gram-positive bacteria at pH 4.0).

Sample	S. aureus CIP6538		E. faecalis ATCC51299 (VRE)		S. aureus CIP106760 (MRSA)		E. faecalis 29212	
	MIC	MBC	MIC	MBC	MIC	MBC	MIC	MBC
TSMT	473.0	1892.1	236.5	1892.1	236.5	473.0	236.5	1892.1
MTSB	13.7	109.5	13.7	109.5	3.42	1.71	3.42	27.4
TS	62.5	499.5	31.2	249.8	3.90	1.95	7.80	62.5
2MTS	29.6	236.5	14.8	118.3	3.70	1.85	473.0	1892.1
Positive control	1.95	nt	1.95	nt	0.977	nt	0.488	nt
	VAN		VAN		NOR		NOR	

VAN: vancomycin; NOR: norfloxacin; NYS: nystatin; nt: not tested. Data are the median values of at least three replicates.

Table 3. MIC and MBC values of TSMT, MTSB, TS, and 2MTS (obtained through the microdilution method against Gram-positive bacteria at pH 7.0).

Sample	S. aureus CIP6538		E. faecalis ATCC51299 (VRE)		S. aureus CIP106760 (MRSA)		E. faecalis 29212	
	MIC	MBC	MIC	MBC	MIC	MBC	MIC	MBC
TSMT	473.0	1892.1	236.5	1892.1	473.0	1892.1	946.0	1892.1
MTSB	438.0	1752.1	219.0	1752.1	438.0	1752.1	876.1	1752.1
TS	499.5	1998.1	249.8	1998.1	499.5	1998.1	999.0	1998.1
2MTS	473.0	1892.1	236.5	1892.1	473.0	1892.1	946.0	1892.1
Positive control	1.95	nt	1.95	nt	0.977	nt	0.488	nt
	VAN		VAN		NOR		NOR	

VAN: vancomycin; NOR: norfloxacin; NYS: nystatin; nt: not tested. Data are the median values of at least three replicates.

Table 4. MIC and MBC values of TSMT, MTSB, TS, and 2MTS (obtained through the microdilution method against Gram-positive bacteria at pH 9.0).

Sample	S. aureus CIP6538		E. faecalis ATCC51299 (VRE)		S. aureus CIP106760 (MRSA)		E. faecalis 29212	
	MIC	MBC	MIC	MBC	MIC	MBC	MIC	MBC
TSMT	946.0	1892.1	473.0	1892.1	473.0	1892.1	473.0	1892.1
MTSB	438.0	1752.1	219.0	1752.1	438.0	1752.1	438.0	1752.1
TS	499.5	1998.1	499.5	1998.1	999.0	1998.1	499.5	1998.1
2MTS	473.0	1892.1	473.0	1892.1	473.0	1892.1	473.0	1892.1
Positive control	1.95	nt	1.95	nt	0.977	nt	0.488	nt
	VAN		VAN		NOR		NOR	

VAN: vancomycin; NOR: norfloxacin; NYS: nystatin; nt: not tested. Data are the median values of at least three replicates.

The results of the antimicrobial assays at the different pH values showed that lowering the medium pH to 4.0 had a positive effect on the compounds MTSB, TS, and 2MTS against the methicillin-resistant *S. aureus* CIP106760 (MRSA). Overall, it was attested that MTSB at pH 4.0 was the most active derivative against all Gram-positive strains. It should be noted that MTSB was the sole compound comprising the thiadiazole function, and presumably, the different activity must be correlated with the type of heterocycle ring. The results for pH 7.0 and 9.0 did not provide better results than those previously obtained.

In terms of pH-dependent antimicrobial mechanisms, it should be emphasized that several antimicrobial peptides (AMPs) have increasingly been reported as potent antibiotics that utilize pH-dependent antimicrobial mechanisms [61]. Some of these antibiotics display high pH optima related to their antimicrobial activity and show activity against microbes that present low pH optima, which reflects the acidic pH generally found at their sites of action, namely the skin. This effect should be comparable to our compounds and could be the explanation for the high antimicrobial activity of our compounds at low pH. Several pH-dependent AMPs and other antimicrobial proteins have been developed for medical purposes and have successfully gone through clinical trials, namely kappacins, LL-37, histatins, lactoferrin, and their derivatives. The major examples of the therapeutic applications of these antimicrobial compounds include wound healing as well as the treatment of multiple infections. Generally, such applications involve topical administration, a source of novel biologically active agents that could aid in the fulfilment of the urgent need for alternatives to conventional antibiotics, helping to avert a return to the pre-antibiotic era: our compounds could be a key development.

2.2.2. Antioxidant Activity

The antioxidant activity of the studied compounds was evaluated using a DPPH assay, which evaluates the potential of test samples to quench DPPH radicals via hydrogen-donating ability. The antioxidant agents convert DPPH into a stable diamagnetic molecule, 1-1diphenyl-2-picryl hydrazine, through electron or hydrogen transfers. A color change from purple to yellow indicates the increasing radical scavenging activity of the test compounds. Herein, it was observed that TSMT and MTSB derivatives possessed a high free radical scavenging ability (see Figure 2). These two molecules had the highest reducing power, indicating that they were good electron/hydrogen donors and could prevent oxidative stress.

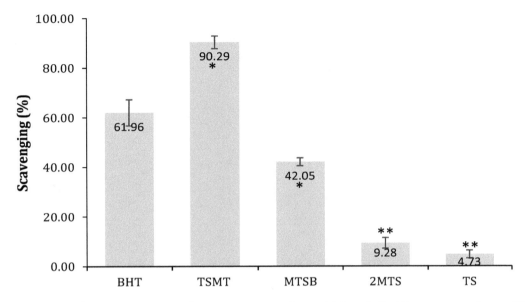

Figure 2. Antioxidant activity tested at a concentration of 10 μg/mL. The mean value ± SD was calculated from three independent experiments and compared to butylated hydroxytoluene (BHT) (∗ $p < 0.05$; ∗∗ $p < 0.001$).

2.2.3. Brine Shrimp Lethality Bioassay (General Toxicity)

The *Artemia salina* test is a known, simple, fast, and low-cost test and was used in this investigation to check the general toxicity of the compounds. As a general rule, it was observed that all of the compounds exhibited low toxicity in the *Artemia salina* model (Figure 3). Nevertheless, it should be emphasized that the MTSB and TSMT derivatives presented with higher toxicity, making them potential lead therapeutic agents, and thus they must further be tested using different cell- and microorganism-based assays.

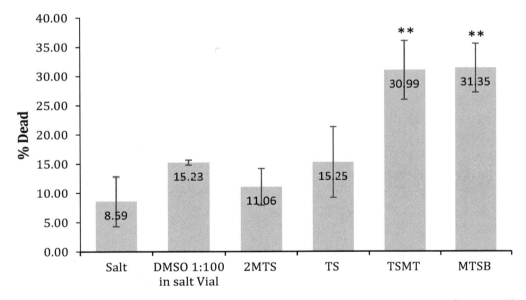

Figure 3. General toxicity screening at a concentration of 10 ppm using the *Artemia salina* test. The mean value ± SD was calculated from three independent experiments and compared to salt (∗∗ $p < 0.001$).

2.2.4. Cell Viability after Treatment with MTSB, TS, TSMS, and 2MTS in H7PX Glioma Cells (IV Grade)

In the course of this study, H7PX cells were treated with a concentration range of 0–100 μg/mL of the four compounds (MTSB, TS, TSMS, and 2MTS) over 24 h, after which the percentage of cell viability was determined by an MTT assay. It was demonstrated that none of the tested compounds reduced the viability of human H7PX cells in the stated range of concentration (0–100 μg/mL) after 24 h (Figure 4). None of the compounds' IC_{50} values were reached. Similar effects were observed with 48 h of incubation (data not shown).

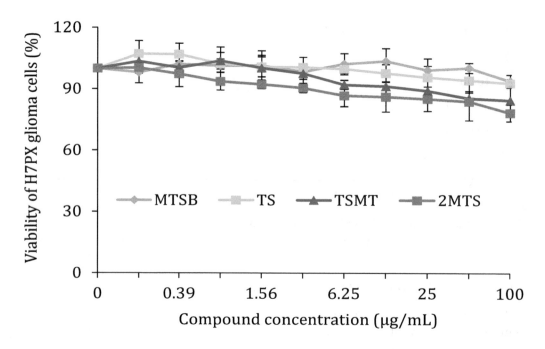

Figure 4. Effect of MTSB, TS, TSMT, and 2MTS treatment on the viability of H7PX glioma cells after 24 h of incubation (data are reported as means ± SD of three determinations).

3. Experimental Section

3.1. Chemistry

3.1.1. General

Unless indicated otherwise, solvents and starting materials were obtained from Sigma. All chemicals used were of reagent grade without further purification before use. Column chromatography was performed using silica gel 60 MN, and aluminum-backed silica gel Merck 60 F254 plates were used for analytical thin-layer chromatography (TLC). Melting points were recorded and are uncorrected. ^{1}H and ^{13}C NMR spectra were recorded at room temperature on a Bruker Avance II 400 (UltraShield™ Magnet, Billerica, MA, USA) spectrometer operating at 400 MHz (^{1}H) and 101 MHz (^{13}C). The chemical shifts are reported in ppm using TMS (tetramethylsilane) as an internal standard. Carbon, hydrogen, and nitrogen elemental analyses were carried out by the Microanalytical Service of the Instituto Superior Técnico—University of Lisbon. FT-IR spectra (4000–400 cm^{-1}) were recorded on a VERTEX 70 (Bruker, Billerica, MA, USA) spectrometer using KBr pellets. Mass spectra were obtained on a VG 7070E mass spectrometer through electron ionization (EI) at 70 eV.

3.1.2. Synthetic Protocols

The synthesis of 3-chloro-1,2-benzisothiazole-1,1-dioxide (**2**), 2-methyl-(2*H*)-tetrazole-5-amine (**4a**), 1-methyl-(1*H*)-tetrazole-5-amine (**4b**), *N*-(1*H*-tetrazol-5-yl)-*N*-(1,1-dioxo-1,2-benzisothiazol-3-yl) amine (**5**) (TS), *N*-(2-methyl-2*H*-tetrazol-5-yl)-*N*-(1,1-dioxo-1,2-benzisothiazol-3-yl) amine (**6**) (2MTS), *N*-(1-methyl-2*H*-tetrazol-5-yl)-*N*-(1,1-dioxo-1,2-benzisothiazol-3-yl) amine (**7**) (TSMT), and 3-[(5-methyl-1,3,4-thiadiazol-2-yl)sulfanyl]-1,2-benzisothiazole 1,1-dioxide (**9**) (MTSB) was carried out as previously described [55,56,58,59].

3.2. Biologic Activities

3.2.1. Antioxidant Activity (DPPH Method)

The antioxidant activity of all the compounds was measured by the DPPH method, as described by Rijo et al. [62]. Accordingly, a mixture containing 10 μL of sample and 990 μL of DPPH solution (0.002% in methanol) was incubated for 30 min at room temperature followed by absorbance measurements at 517 nm against the corresponding blank sample. The antioxidant activity of each compound was calculated using Equation (1). AA denotes the antioxidant activity, A_{DPPH} is the absorption of DPPH against the blank, and A_{sample} represents the absorption of the compound or control against the blank. All tests were carried out in triplicate at a sample concentration of 10 μg/mL. The reference standard used for this procedure was butylated hydroxytoluene (BHT) in the same conditions as the samples:

$$AA = \frac{A_{DPPH} - A_{Sample}}{A_{DPPH}} \times 100\%,$$ (1)

3.2.2. Brine Shrimp Lethality Bioassay (General Toxicity)

The general toxicity of the compounds was evaluated by the use of a test of lethality to *Artemia salina* (brine shrimp) [63]. Concentrations of 10 ppm of each sample were tested. The number of dead larvae was recorded after 24 h and was used to calculate the lethal concentration (%) according to Equation (2) (where $Total_{A.\ salina}$ = the total number of larvae in the assay and $Alive_{A.\ salina}$ = the number of alive *A. salina* larvae in the assay):

$$\text{Letal concentration} = \frac{Total_{A.\ salina} - Alive_{A.\ salina}}{Total_{A.\ salina}} \times 100\%,$$ (2)

3.2.3. Cell Culture

An H7PX primary glioblastoma cell line was cultivated in DMEM (Biowest, Nuaollé, France) supplemented with 10% FBS (Euroclone, Pero, Italy), 100 IU/mL penicillin (Sigma-Aldrich, Saint Louis, MO, USA), 100 μg/mL streptomycin (Sigma-Aldrich, Saint Louis, MO, USA) and 50 μg/mL gentamicin (Biowest, Nuaollé, France) in a humidified atmosphere (5% CO_2, 37 °C).

3.2.4. In Vitro Cell Viability by MTT Assay

An MTT (3-(4,5-dimethylthiazol-2-yl)-2,5-diphenyl tetrazolium bromide) assay was employed to measure the viability of H7PX cells (glioma cells in IV grade derived from patient) treated with different concentrations of TS (**5**), 2MTS (**6**), TSMT (**7**), or MTSB (**9**). Cells were seeded at 1×10^4 cells per well in 96-well culture plates and were left overnight before treatments for attachment. Subsequently, the cells were incubated for 24 h with all compounds over a range of concentrations: 0.0 (control), 0.39, 0.78, 1.56, 3.13, 6.25, 12.5, 25, 50, and 100 μg/mL. Following this, the cells were incubated with 0.5 mg/mL of MTT at 37 °C for 1.5 h. After that, the MTT was carefully removed, and DMSO (100 μL) was added to each well and vortexed at low speed for 5 min to fully dissolve the formazan crystals. Absorbance was measured at 570 nm with a reference at 630 nm using a Bio-Tek Synergy HT Microplate Reader (Bio-Tek Instruments, Winooski, VT, USA). All experiments were repeated in triplicate. Cell viability was expressed as a percentage relative to the untreated cells, which was defined as 100%. The study was approved by the Ethical Commission of the Medical University of Lodz, and informed consent was obtained from the patients (Nr. RNN/194/12/KE).

3.2.5. Antimicrobial Activity

Microorganisms and growth conditions: The strains used in this study comprised *Staphylococcus aureus* (ATCC 25,923 and CIP 106760), *Enterococcus faecalis* (ATCC 51,299 and ATCC29212), *Escherichia coli* ATCC 25922, *Pseudomonas aeruginosa* ATCC 27,853, and the yeasts *Candida albicans* ATCC 10,231 and *Saccharomyces cerevisiae* ATCC 2601. All bacteria were grown at 37 °C in Mueller–Hinton broth (Biokar Diagnostics, Beauvais, France), and the yeasts were grown in Sabouraud dextrose agar (Biokar Diagnostics, Allone, France).

Microdilution method (MIC determination): The minimum inhibitory concentrations (MICs) of the compounds (dissolved in the respective pH aqueous solutions) were evaluated using a twofold serial broth microdilution assay (CLSI, 2011) in Mueller–Hinton broth (MHB, Biokar Diagnostics, Beauvais, France). Overnight cultures were diluted in MHB with increasing concentrations of each compound (in µM). Vancomycin (VAN), norfloxacin (NOR), and nystatin (NYS) were used as positive controls for Gram-positive bacteria, Gram-negative bacteria, and yeasts, respectively. The negative control for the aqueous solutions at different pH values showed no inhibition growth. The cultures were incubated for 24 h at 37 °C, and Optical Density at 620 nm was measured using a Microplate Reader (Thermo Scientific Multiskan FC, Loughborough, UK). Assays were carried out in triplicate for each tested microorganism.

Minimum bactericidal concentration (MBC) assessment: To define the minimum bactericidal concentration (MBC) for each set of wells in the MIC determination, a loopful of agar was collected from the wells without any growth and inoculated on sterile Mueller–Hilton medium broth (for bacteria) through streaking. Plates inoculated with bacteria were incubated at 37 °C for 24 h. After incubation, the lowest concentration was noted as the MBC (for bacteria) at which no visible growth was observed.

3.2.6. Statistical Analysis

The values in this study are expressed as means ± SD. The Shapiro–Wilk test was used for verification of the normality of the data. Statistical differences were determined by one-way ANOVA. The results were analyzed using STATISTICA 12.0 software (StatSoft, Tulsa, OK, USA). Differences of $p < 0.05$ were considered statistically significant.

4. Conclusions

The antimicrobial, antioxidant, and cytotoxic activities of three saccharin–tetrazolyl (TS, TSMT, and 2MTS) derivatives and one saccharin–thiadiazolyl (MTSB) derivative were addressed throughout this investigation. The antimicrobial activity of the synthesized compounds was evaluated against a series of Gram-positive and Gram-negative bacteria and yeast strains. An evaluation of the MIC and MBC values of the four derivatives was completed at pH 4.0, 7.0, and 9.0 against four Gram-positive strains (*S. aureus*, *E. faecalis*, *S. aureus* (MRSA), and *E. faecalis* (VRE)), showing high values for the MIC and MBC at pH 4.0 (ranging from 3.42 to 473.0 µM). It was attested that the derivative MTSB, the sole compound comprising the thiadiazole function, was the most active against all of the considered Gram-positive strains at pH 4.0.

In addition, the antioxidant activity of the compounds (calculated by using the DPPH method) was the highest value for TSMT (90.29% compared to the BHT positive control of 61.96%). Finally, we demonstrated for the first time that the TS, TSMT, 2MTS, and MTSB compounds did not show in vitro cytotoxic effects on H7PX glioma cells.

The present study exposed the influence of the pH of the medium on the antimicrobial activity of the TS, TSMT, 2MTS, and MTSB compounds, which is similar to well-described antimicrobial peptide antibiotics. Therefore, the use of these kinds of molecules to produce new antibiotics should be considered in the future, although further studies are needed to confirm this hypothesis.

Author Contributions: L.M.T.F. and P.R. designed the study, analyzed the data, and wrote the paper; E.N., P.S., J.M.A., M.T., and T.Ś. performed the biological assays; L.M.T.F. and L.C. performed the synthesis and characterization of the compounds; M.L.S.C. and A.J.L.P. were responsible for supervision and reviewing the draft.

References

1. Schulze, B.; Illgen, K. Isothiazol-1,1-dioxide—Vom Süßstoff zum chiralen Auxiliar in der stereoselektiven Synthese. *J. Prakt. Chem.* **1997**, *339*, 1–14. [CrossRef]
2. Ellis, J.W.J. Overview of sweeteners. *Chem. Educ.* **1995**, *72*, 671–675. [CrossRef]
3. Remsen, I.; Fahlberg, C. On the oxidation of substitution products of aromatic hydrocarbons. IV. On the oxidation of orthotoluenesulphonamide. *J. Am. Chem. Soc.* **1879**, *1*, 426–438. [CrossRef]
4. Price, M.J.; Biava, G.C.; Oser, L.B.; Vogin, E.E.; Steinfeld, J.; Ley, L.H. Bladder tumors in rats fed cyclohexylamine or high doses of a mixture of cyclamate and saccharin. *Science* **1970**, *167*, 1131–1132. [CrossRef] [PubMed]
5. Masui, T.; Mann, M.A.; Borgeson, D.C.; Garland, M.E.; Okamura, T.; Fujii, H.; Pelling, C.J.; Cohen, M.S. Sequencing analysis of HA-RAS, KI-RAS, and N-RAS genes in rat urinary-bladder tumors induced by N-[4-(5-Nitro-2-furyl)-2-thiazolyl]formamide (FANFT) and sodium saccharin. *Terat. Carcin. Mutagen.* **1993**, *13*, 225–233. [CrossRef] [PubMed]
6. Garland, M.E.; Sakata, T.; Fisher, M.J.; Masui, T.; Cohen, M.S. Influences of Diet and Strain on the Proliferative Effect on the Rat Urinary Bladder Induced by Sodium Saccharin. *Cancer Res.* **1989**, *49*, 3789–3794. [PubMed]
7. Groutas, W.C.; Houser-Archield, N.; Chong, L.S.; Venkataraman, R.; Epp, J.B.; Huang, H.; McClenahan, J.J. Efficient inhibition of human-leukocyte elastase and cathepsin-G by saccharin derivatives. *J. Med. Chem.* **1993**, *36*, 3178–3181. [CrossRef] [PubMed]
8. Groutas, W.C.; Chong, L.S.; Venkataraman, R.; Kuang, R.; Epp, J.B.; Houser-Archield, N.; Huang, H.; Hoydal, R.J. Amino acid-derivative phthalimide and saccharin derivatives as inhibitors of human leukocyte elastase, cathepsin G, and proteinase 3. *Arch. Biochem. Biophys.* **1996**, *332*, 335–340. [CrossRef] [PubMed]
9. Groutas, W.C.; Epp, J.B.; Venkataraman, R.; Kuang, R.; Truong, T.M.; McClenahan, J.J.; Prakash, O. Design, synthesis, and in vitro inhibitory activity toward human leukocyte elastase, cathepsin G, and proteinase 3 of saccharin-derived sulfones and congeners. *Bioorg. Med. Chem.* **1996**, *4*, 1393–1400. [CrossRef]
10. Elghamry, I.; Youssef, M.M.; Al-Omair, M.A.; Elsawy, H. Synthesis, antimicrobial, DNA cleavage and antioxidant activities of tricyclic sultams derived from saccharin. *Eur. J. Med. Chem.* **2017**, *139*, 107–113. [CrossRef] [PubMed]
11. Apella, M.C.; Totaro, R.; Baran, E.J. Determination of superoxide dismutase-like activity in some divalent metal saccharinates. *Biol. Trace Elem. Res.* **1993**, *37*, 293–299. [CrossRef] [PubMed]
12. Guenther, U.; Wrigge, H.; Theuerkauf, N.; Boettcher, M.F.; Wensing, G.; Zinserling, J.; Putensen, C.; Hoeft, A. Repinotan, a selective 5-HT1A-R-agonist, antagonizes morphine-induced ventilator depression in anesthetized rats. *Anesth. Analg.* **2010**, *111*, 901–907. [PubMed]
13. Malinka, W.; Ryng, S.; Sieklucka-Dziuba, M.; Rajtar, G.; Gownial, A.; Kleinrok, Z. 2-Substituted-3-oxoisothiazolo[5,4-b]pyridines as potential central nervous system and antimycobacterial agents. *Farmaco* **1998**, *53*, 504–512. [CrossRef]
14. Malinka, W.; Ryng, S.; Sieklucka-Dziuba, M.; Rajtar, G.; Gownial, A.; Kleinrok, Z. Synthesis and preliminary screening of derivatives of 2-(4-arylpiperazine-1-ylalkyl)-3-oxoisothiazolo[5,4,b]pyridines as CNS and antimycobacterial agents. *Pharmazie* **2000**, *55*, 416–425. [PubMed]
15. Csakai, A.; Smith, C.; Davis, E.; Martinko, A.; Coulp, S.; Yin, H. Saccharin derivatives as inhibitors of interferon-mediated inflammation. *J. Med. Chem.* **2014**, *57*, 5348–5355. [CrossRef] [PubMed]
16. Fischer, R.; Kretschik, O.; Schenke, T.; Schenkel, R.; Wiedemann, J.; Erdelen, C.; Loesel, P.; Drewes, M.W.; Feucht, D.; Andersch, W.W. *Ger. Offen.* DE 1999244668. 1999. *Chem. Abstr.* **2001**, *134*, 4932.
17. Singh, H.; Chawla, A.S.; Kapoor, V.K.; Paul, D.; Malhotra, R.K. Medicinal chemistry of tetrazoles. *Prog. Med. Chem.* **1980**, *17*, 151–183. [PubMed]
18. Noda, K.; Saad, Y.; Kinoshita, A.; Boyle, T.P.; Graham, R.M.; Husain, A.; Karnik, S.S. Tetrazole and carboxylate receptor antagonists bind to the same subsite by different mechanisms. *J. Biol. Chem.* **1995**, *270*, 2284–2289. [CrossRef] [PubMed]
19. Mavromoustakos, T.; Kolocouris, A.; Zervou, M.; Roumelioti, P.; Matsoukas, J.; Weisemann, R. An effort to understand the molecular basis of hypertension through the study of conformational analysis of Losartan and Sarmesin using a combination of nuclear magnetic resonance spectroscopy and theoretical calculations. *J. Med. Chem.* **1999**, *42*, 1714–1722. [CrossRef] [PubMed]

20. Toney, J.H.; Fitzgerald, P.M.D.; Grover-Sharma, N.; Olson, S.H.; May, W.J.; Sundelof, J.G.; Vanderwall, D.E.; Cleary, K.A.; Grant, S.K.; Wu, J.K.; et al. Antibiotic sensitization using biphenyl tetrazoles as potent inhibitors of *Bacteroides fragilis* metallo-β-lactamase. *Chem. Biol.* **1998**, *5*, 185–196. [CrossRef]

21. Gao, C.; Chang, L.; Xu, Z.; Yan, X.-F.; Ding, C.; Zhao, F.; Wu, X.; Feng, L.-S. Recent advances of tetrazole derivatives as potential anti-tubercular and anti-malarial agents. *Eur. J. Med. Chem.* **2019**, *163*, 404. [CrossRef] [PubMed]

22. Hashimoto, Y.; Ohashi, R.; Kurosawa, Y.; Minami, K.; Kaji, H.; Hayashida, K.; Narita, H.; Murata, S. Pharmacologic Profile of TA-606, a Novel Angiotensin II-Receptor Antagonist in the Rat. *J. Cardiovasc. Pharmacol.* **1998**, *31*, 568–575. [CrossRef] [PubMed]

23. Desarro, A.; Ammendola, D.; Zappala, M.; Grasso, S.; Desarro, G.B. Relationship between Structure and Convulsant Properties of Some b-Lactam Antibiotics following Intracerebroventricular Microinjection in Rats. *Antimicrob. Agents Chemother.* **1995**, *39*, 232–237. [CrossRef] [PubMed]

24. Tamura, Y.; Watanabe, F.; Nakatani, T.; Yasui, K.; Fuji, M.; Komurasaki, T.; Tsuzuki, H.; Maekawa, R.; Yoshioka, T.; Kawada, K.; et al. Highly Selective and Orally Active Inhibitors of Type IV Collagenase (MMP-9 and MMP-2): N-Sulfonylamino Acid Derivatives. *J. Med. Chem.* **1998**, *41*, 640–649. [CrossRef] [PubMed]

25. Abell, A.D.; Foulds, G.J. Synthesis of a cis-conformationally restricted peptide bond isostere and its application to the inhibition of the HIV-1 protease. *J. Chem. Soc. Perkin Trans.* **1997**, *1*, 2475–2482. [CrossRef]

26. Sandmann, G.; Schneider, C.; Boger, P. A New Non-Radioactive Assay of Phytoene Desaturase to Evaluate Bleaching Herbicides. *Z. Naturforsch. C* **1996**, *51*, 534–538. [CrossRef] [PubMed]

27. Koldobskii, G.I.; Ostrovskii, V.A.; Poplavskii, V.S. Advances in tetrazole chemistry. *Khim. Geterotsikl. Soedin.* **1981**, *10*, 1299.

28. Ostrovskii, V.A.; Pevzner, M.S.; Kofman, T.P.; Shcherbinin, M.B.; Tselinskii, I.V. *Targets in Heterocyclic Systems. Chemistry and Properties*; Attanasi, O.A., Spinelli, D., Eds.; Societa Chimica Italiana: Rome, Italy, 1999; Volume 3, p. 467.

29. Moore, D.S.; Robinson, S.D. Catenated Nitrogen Ligands Part II. Transition Metal Derivatives of Triazoles, Tetrazoles, Pentazoles, and Hexazine. *Adv. Inorg. Chem.* **1988**, *32*, 171–239.

30. Balaban, A.T.; Oniciu, D.C.; Katritzky, A.R. Aromaticity as a cornerstone of heterocyclic chemistry. *Chem. Rev.* **2004**, *104*, 2777–2812. [CrossRef] [PubMed]

31. Hu, Y.; Li, C.-Y.; Wang, X.-M.; Yang, Y.-H.; Zhu, H.-L. 1,3,4-Thiadiazole: Synthesis, reactions, and applications in medicinal, agricultural, and materials chemistry. *Chem. Rev.* **2014**, *114*, 5572–5610. [CrossRef] [PubMed]

32. Almajan, G.L.; Barbuceanu, S.F.; Bancescu, G.; Saramet, I.; Saramet, G.; Draghici, C. Synthesis and antimicrobial evaluation of some fused heterocyclic [1,2,4]triazolo[3,4-b][1,3,4]thiadiazole derivatives. *Eur. J. Med. Chem.* **2010**, *45*, 6139–6146. [CrossRef] [PubMed]

33. Kolavi, G.; Hegde, V.; Khazi, I.; Gadad, P. Synthesis and evaluation of antitubercular activity of imidazo[2,1-b][1,3,4]thiadiazole derivatives. *Bioorg. Med. Chem.* **2006**, *14*, 3069–3080. [CrossRef] [PubMed]

34. Khan, I.; Ali, S.; Hameed, S.; Rama, N.H.; Hussain, M.T.; Wadood, A.; Uddin, R.; Ul-Haq, Z.; Khan, A.; Ali, S.; et al. Synthesis, antioxidant activities and urease inhibition of some new 1,2,4-triazole and 1,3,4-thiadiazole derivatives. *Eur. J. Med. Chem.* **2010**, *45*, 5200–5207. [CrossRef] [PubMed]

35. Hafez, H.N.; Hegab, M.I.; Ahmed-Farag, I.S.; El-Gazzar, A.B.A. A facile regioselective synthesis of novel *spiro*-thioxanthene and *spiro*-xanthene-9',2-[1,3,4]thiadiazole derivatives as potential analgesic and anti-inflammatory agents. *Bioorg. Med. Chem. Lett.* **2008**, *18*, 4538–4543. [CrossRef] [PubMed]

36. Jatav, V.; Mishra, P.; Kashaw, S.; Stables, J.P. CNS depressant and anticonvulsant activities of some novel 3-[5-substituted 1,3,4-thiadiazole-2-yl]-2-styryl quinazoline-4(3H)-ones. *Eur. J. Med. Chem.* **2008**, *43*, 1945–1954. [CrossRef] [PubMed]

37. Clerici, F.; Pocar, D.; Guido, M.; Loche, A.; Perlini, V.; Brufani, M. Synthesis of 2-amino-5-sulfanyl-1,3,4-thiadiazole derivatives and evaluation of their antidepressant and anxiolytic activity. *J. Med. Chem.* **2001**, *44*, 931–936. [CrossRef] [PubMed]

38. Hasui, T.; Matsunaga, N.; Ora, T.; Ohyabu, N.; Nishigaki, N.; Imura, Y.; Igata, Y.; Matsui, H.; Motoyaji, T.; Tanaka, T.; et al. Identification of benzoxazin-3-one derivatives as novel, potent, and selective nonsteroidal mineralocorticoid receptor antagonists. *J. Med. Chem.* **2011**, *54*, 8616–8631. [CrossRef] [PubMed]

39. Noolvi, M.N.; Patel, H.M.; Singh, N.; Gadad, A.K.; Cameotra, S.S.; Badiger, A. Synthesis and anticancer evaluation of novel 2-cyclopropylimidazo[2,1-b][1,3,4]-thiadiazole derivatives. *Eur. J. Med. Chem.* **2011**, *46*, 4411–4418. [CrossRef] [PubMed]

40. Liu, X.H.; Shi, Y.X.; Ma, Y.; Zhang, C.Y.; Dong, W.L.; Pan, L.; Wang, B.L.; Li, B.J.; Li, Z.M. Synthesis, antifungal activities and 3D-QSAR study of N-(5-substituted-1,3,4-thiadiazol-2-yl)cyclopropanecarboxamides. *Eur. J. Med. Chem.* **2009**, *44*, 2782–2786. [CrossRef] [PubMed]

41. Kaur, I.P.; Smitha, R.; Aggarwal, D.; Kapil, M. Acetazolamide: Future perspective in topical glaucoma therapeutics. *Int. J. Pharm.* **2002**, *248*, 1–14. [CrossRef]

42. Luks, A.M.; McIntosh, S.E.; Grissom, C.K.; Auerbach, P.S.; Rodway, G.W.; Schoene, R.B.; Zafren, K.; Hackett, P.H. Wilderness Medical Society consensus guidelines for the prevention and treatment of acute altitude illness. *Wilderness Environ. Med.* **2010**, *21*, 146–155. [CrossRef] [PubMed]

43. Wolf, P. Acute drug administration in epilepsy: A review. *CNS Neurosci. Ther.* **2011**, *17*, 442–448. [CrossRef] [PubMed]

44. Rangwala, L.M.; Liu, G.T. Pediatric idiopathic intracranial hypertension. *Surv. Ophthalmol.* **2007**, *52*, 597–617. [CrossRef] [PubMed]

45. Russell, M.B.; Ducros, A. Sporadic and familial hemiplegic migraine: Pathophysiological mechanisms, clinical characteristics, diagnosis, and management. *Lancet Neurol.* **2011**, *10*, 457–470. [CrossRef]

46. Tiselius, H.G. New horizons in the management of patients with cystinuria. *Curr. Opin. Urol.* **2010**, *20*, 169–173. [CrossRef] [PubMed]

47. Jalandhara, N.B.; Patel, A.; Arora, R.R.; Jalandhara, P. Obstructive sleep apnea: A cardiopulmonary perspective and medical therapeutics. *Am. J. Ther.* **2009**, *16*, 257–263. [CrossRef] [PubMed]

48. Schara, U.; Lochmuller, H. Therapeutic strategies in congenital myasthenic syndromes. *Neurotherapeutics* **2008**, *5*, 542–547. [CrossRef] [PubMed]

49. Superti-Furga, G.; Cochran, J.; Crews, C.M.; Frye, S.; Neubauer, G.; Prinjha, R.; Shokat, K. Where is the Future of Drug Discovery for Cancer? *Cell* **2017**, *168*, 564–565.

50. Gulçin, I. Antioxidant activity of food constituents: An overview. *Arch. Toxicol.* **2012**, *86*, 345–391. [CrossRef] [PubMed]

51. Walker, B.; Barrett, S.; Polasky, S.; Galaz, V.; Folke, C.; Engstrom, G.; Ackerman, F.; Arrow, K.; Carpenter, S.; Chopra, K.; et al. Environment. Looming global-scale failures and missing institutions. *Science* **2009**, *325*, 1345–1346. [CrossRef] [PubMed]

52. D'Costa, V.M.; King, C.E.; Kalan, L.; Morar, M.; Sung, W.W.; Schwarz, C.; Froese, D.; Zazula, G.; Calmels, F.; Debruyne, R.; et al. Antibiotic resistance is ancient. *Nature* **2011**, *477*, 457. [CrossRef] [PubMed]

53. Andersson, D.I.; Hughes, D. Antibiotic resistance and its cost: Is it possible to reverse resistance? *Nat. Rev. Microbiol.* **2010**, *8*, 260. [CrossRef] [PubMed]

54. Cassir, N.; Rolain, J.M.; Brouqui, P. A new strategy to fight antimicrobial resistance: The revival of old antibiotics. *Front. Microbiol.* **2014**, *5*, 551. [CrossRef] [PubMed]

55. Brigas, A.F.; Fonseca, C.S.C.; Johnstone, R.A.W. Preparation of 3-Chloro-1,2-Benzisothiazole 1,1-Dioxide (Pseudo-Saccharyl Chloride). *J. Chem. Res.* **2002**, *6*, 299–300. [CrossRef]

56. Frija, L.M.T.; Alegria, E.C.B.A.; Sutradhar, M.; Cristiano, M.L.S.; Ismael, A.; Kopylovich, M.N.; Pombeiro, A.J.L. Copper(II) and cobalt(II) tetrazole-saccharinate complexes as effective catalysts for oxidation of secondary alcohols. *J. Mol. Catal. A Chem.* **2016**, *425*, 283–290. [CrossRef]

57. Frija, L.M.T.; Fausto, R.; Loureiro, R.M.S.S.; Cristiano, M.L.S. Synthesis and structure of novel benzisothiazole-tetrazolyl derivatives for potential application as nitrogen ligands. *J. Mol. Catal. A Chem.* **2009**, *305*, 142–146. [CrossRef]

58. Ismael, A.; Paixão, J.A.; Fausto, R.; Cristiano, M.L.S. Molecular structure of nitrogen-linked methyltetrazole-saccharinates. *J. Mol. Struct.* **2012**, *1023*, 128–142. [CrossRef]

59. Cabral, L.; Brás, E.; Henriques, M.; Marques, C.; Frija, L.M.T.; Barreira, L.; Paixão, J.A.; Fausto, R.; Cristiano, M.L.S. Synthesis, Structure, and Cytotoxicity of a New Sulphanyl-Bridged Thiadiazolyl-Saccharinate Conjugate: The Relevance of S···N Interaction. *Chem. Eur. J.* **2018**, *24*, 3251–3262. [CrossRef] [PubMed]

60. Rijo, P.; Duarte, A.; Francisco, A.P.; Semedo-Lemsaddek, T.; Simões, M.F. In vitro antimicrobial activity of royleanone derivatives against Gram-positive bacterial pathogens. *Phytother. Res.* **2014**, *8*, 76–81. [CrossRef] [PubMed]

61. Malik, E.; Dennison, S.R.; Harris, F.; Phoenix, D.A. pH Dependent Antimicrobial Peptides and Proteins, Their Mechanisms of Action and Potential as Therapeutic Agents. *Pharmaceuticals* **2016**, *9*, 67. [CrossRef] [PubMed]

62. Rijo, P.; Falé, P.L.; Serralheiro, M.L.; Simões, M.F.; Gomes, A.; Reis, C. Optimization of medicinal plant extraction methods and their encapsulation through extrusion technology. *Measurement* **2014**, *58*, 249–255. [CrossRef]

63. Alanís-Garza, B.A.; González-González, G.M.; Salazar-Aranda, R.; Waksman de Torres, N.; Rivas-Galindo, V.M. Screening of antifungal activity of plants from the northeast of Mexico. *J. Ethnopharmacol.* **2007**, *114*, 468–471. [CrossRef] [PubMed]

7

Atopic Dermatitis as a Multifactorial Skin Disorder. Can the Analysis of Pathophysiological Targets Represent the Winning Therapeutic Strategy?

Irene Magnifico [1], Giulio Petronio Petronio [1,*] , Noemi Venditti [1], Marco Alfio Cutuli [1], Laura Pietrangelo [1], Franca Vergalito [2], Katia Mangano [3] , Davide Zella [4] and Roberto Di Marco [1]

[1] Department of Health and Medical Sciences "V. Tiberio" Università degli Studi del Molise, 8600 Campobasso, Italy; i.magnifico@studenti.unimol.it (I.M.); n.venditti@studenti.unimol.it (N.V.); m.cutuli@studenti.unimol.it (M.A.C.); laura.pietrangelo@unimol.it (L.P.); roberto.dimarco@unimol.it (R.D.M.)

[2] Department of Agricultural, Environmental and Food Sciences (DiAAA), Università degli Studi del Molise, 86100 Campobasso, Italy; franca.vergalito@unimol.it

[3] Department of Biomedical and Biotechnological Sciences, Universitá degli Studi di Catania, 95123 Catania, Italy; kmangano@unict.it

[4] Department of Biochemistry and Molecular Biology, School of Medicine, Institute of Human Virology, University of Maryland, Baltimore, MD 21201, USA; DZella@ihv.umaryland.edu

* Correspondence: giulio.petroniopetronio@unimol.it

Abstract: Atopic dermatitis (AD) is a pathological skin condition with complex aetiological mechanisms that are difficult to fully understand. Scientific evidence suggests that of all the causes, the impairment of the skin barrier and cutaneous dysbiosis together with immunological dysfunction can be considered as the two main factors involved in this pathological skin condition. The loss of the skin barrier function is often linked to dysbiosis and immunological dysfunction, with an imbalance in the ratio between the pathogen *Staphylococcus aureus* and/or other microorganisms residing in the skin. The bibliographic research was conducted on PubMed, using the following keywords: 'atopic dermatitis', 'bacterial therapy', 'drug delivery system' and 'alternative therapy'. The main studies concerning microbial therapy, such as the use of bacteria and/or part thereof with microbiota transplantation, and drug delivery systems to recover skin barrier function have been summarized. The studies examined show great potential in the development of effective therapeutic strategies for AD and AD-like symptoms. Despite this promise, however, future investigative efforts should focus both on the replication of some of these studies on a larger scale, with clinical and demographic characteristics that reflect the general AD population, and on the process of standardisation, in order to produce reliable data.

Keywords: atopic dermatitis; skin barrier; cutaneous dysbiosis; *Staphylococcus aureus*; microbial therapy; drug delivery systems

1. Introduction

Atopic dermatitis (AD) is a chronic relapsing inflammatory skin disorder, affecting 7–10% of the adult population and 15–30% of children, and is associated with significant morbidity and decreased quality of life [1]. Although AD can occur at any age, the incidence peaks in infancy with approximately 45% of all cases beginning within the first six months of life, 60% during the first year, and 80–90% by an individual's fifth birthday [2]. The general term 'eczema' was initially used to describe the condition.

Subsequently, the correlation between eczema and other atopic disorders led to the coining of the term 'atopic dermatitis' in 1933 by Wise and Sulzberger [3]. The AD clinical pattern includes both pruritic and eczematous lesions and the pathophysiology is complex and multifactorial [3–6]. Current knowledge indicates that the main pathogenetic factors of AD are skin barrier dysfunction and dysbiosis of resident microbiota [7]. To these main factors, immunological dysregulation must be added. Skin barrier dysfunction induces immune dysregulation and immune dysregulation alters skin barrier function. Skin microbial dysbiosis also alters immune responses in AD ([8–10]). Therefore, the interaction between barrier dysfunction, microbial dysbiosis and immune dysregulation is at the basis of the worsening of the disease [8]. The skin barrier is localised to the uppermost area of the epidermis, which is the cornified layer (stratum corneum) forming by the migration of keratinocytes from the basal to the upper layers. Keratinocytes produce lipids, cyclic adenosine monophosphate (cyclic AMP), cathelicidin and beta-defensins, which form extracellular lipid-enriched layers, kill pathogens and play essential roles in maintaining skin homeostasis [11]. Epidermal barrier proteins, including filaggrin (FLG), keratins, loricrin, involucrin and intercellular proteins, are cross-linked to form an impermeable skin barrier [12]. The alteration in the protein and lipid content of the skin contributes to skin barrier dysfunction. The loss of the function of FLG and other proteins is strongly associated with the development of AD [13]. The overexpression of Th2 and Th22 cytokines altering the protein and lipid content of the skin contributes to skin barrier dysfunction [14]. When developing drug delivery systems (DDSs) for dermatological disorders such as AD, different features of the compromised skin should be considered. In infected, broken or damaged skin where the integrity of the stratum corneum is compromised, DDSs improve the efficiency of the formulation [15]. Numerous studies have shown how these systems can aid the delivery of payloads to target sites in dermatological disorder treatment. In particular, the potential for nanocarriers to serve as DDSs for effective AD management has been investigated [15,16].

In addition, an imbalance between Staphylococcus aureus (S. aureus) and the resident skin microbiota can generate a dysbiosis state that induces an alteration in the immune response and compromises the skin barrier [17]. The skin microbiota plays a role in protecting against infection and inflammation because they guarantee the normal function of the skin barrier. Indeed, viruses, fungi, and bacteria residing on the skin metabolise host proteins and lipids and produce bioactive molecules. These include free fatty acids, cAMP, phenol-soluble modulins (PSMs), microbial cell wall components and antibiotics like bacteriocins that can act on other microbes to inhibit pathogen invasion. All these substances target the host epithelium and stimulate keratinocyte-derived immune mediators such as complement and IL-1, or immune cells in the epidermis and dermis [18–20]. For instance, Staphylococcus epidermidis (S. epidermidis) suppresses inflammation by inducing the secretion of interleukin-10, an anti-inflammatory cytokine, from antigen-presenting cells [21,22]. In addition, is able to secrete a unique lipoteic acid that suppress both keratinocytes' inflammatory cytokines and inflammation through a TLR2-dependent mechanism [22,23].

The skin dysbiosis that occurs through an increase in the pathogen S. aureus and a variation in the composition and number of skin commensal bacteria also contributes to skin barrier defects and can be a trigger for AD [24]. Indeed, a recent analysis highlighted a prevalence of S. aureus on the skin of subjects with AD, with an abundance rate of 70% compared to 39% in the control group [25]. We now have a better understanding of the pathogenetic mechanism of S. aureus. This pathogen has numerous virulence factors that contribute to its pathogenesis.

Among these, those most commonly involved in the etiopathogenesis of AD are δ-toxin, phenol-soluble modulins, superantigens, protein A, pro-inflammatory lipoproteins and proteases [26].

In addition to S. aureus, skin dysbiosis may occur through an increase in the relative abundance of other species of the genus Staphylococcus, such as S. haemolyticus. Furthermore, reductions in microorganisms belonging to the genera Streptococcus spp., Propionibacterium spp., Acinetobacter spp., Corynebacterium spp. and Prevotella spp. have also been observed, which cannot be attributed to an increase in S. aureus [27]; on the other hand, Propionibacterium acnes was found less frequently on the skin of AD and it was inversely correlated to disease severity [28,29]. After a flare, the species that saw a reduction in their levels then saw an increase in relative abundance [27,29]. An important role is also played by fungal microbiota, which lead to a reduction in the relative abundance of *Malassezia* spp. and an increase in the enrichment of the *M. dermatis* and fungi not belonging to the genus *Malassezia*, *Aspergillus*, *Candida* and *Cryptococcus* [29–31]. The reconstitution of healthy microbial diversity, presumably by removing *S. aureus* and allowing the skin to repopulate with physiological microbiota, can restore the protective function of the skin and promote the healing process [7,32]. Within the scientific literature, clinical severity has been evaluated using the objective SCORAD index (scoring AD), which was developed by the European Task Force on Atopic Dermatitis (ETFAD) to create a consensus on assessment methods for AD. This system considers both objective signs (severity and extension) and subjective signs (pruritus and loss of sleep). The SCORAD (AD SCORing) allows a unique classification of the disease: mild, moderate or severe. In addition, a complete diagnosis also includes the evaluation of the intensity of the itching [33]. The European guidelines for the management of AD in adults and children are different for the each level of severity: baseline—emollients and bath oils; mild topical glucocorticosteroids; moderate topical tacrolimus or glucocorticosteroids; and severe systemic immunosuppression [34].

In this case, the new treatment options with antibodies (Ab), especially with the Ab Dupilumab, against interleukin-4 receptor revealed great potential without serious side effects [35–38]

Currently, available drugs are influenced by bioavailability and may give rise to severe adverse events. For example, the use of topical corticosteroids can improve the condition of AD patients, but over-use of corticosteroids during a long bout of sickness can cause some side effects such as hypertension, atrophy and tachyphylaxis result in cumulative toxicity [39]. Although the use of corticosteroids, supported by the use of emollient creams, are widely used in combination to improve symptoms, they do not ensure the complete elimination of AD [40]. The lack of a curative treatment has led to the search for alternative and/or complementary therapies. Microbial therapy and DDSs can help to restore healthy skin microbiota, which have been altered due to skin dysbiosis, and efficiently deliver drugs to skin compromised by AD in order to re-establish the normal function of the skin barrier [41].

This review aims to provide, for the first time, a broad view of AD in light of the newest scientific evidence correlating the two most relevant aspects of this pathology: restoration of healthy skin microbiota and DDSs.

2. Results

2.1. Microbial Therapy: Restoration of Healthy Skin Microbiota

The use of live/heat-killed or inactivated microorganism, the substances with microorganism-derivatives, and the rebalancing of the physiological skin microbiota through skin bacterial transplant may be considered the therapeutic landscape for AD, since they promote the correct functioning of the skin barrier [7,32,42]. Current scientific evidence shows the role of probiotics in improving the clinical course of AD by restoring skin microbiota homeostasis, maintaining lipid barrier functions and modulating the immune system [43]. In addition, some bacterial compounds such as cell wall fragments and their metabolites demonstrate greater stability than viable cells when kept at room temperature, making them more suitable for the formulation of topical preparations. For example, microbe free cultures are still able to exert antimicrobial and immunomodulatory activity in the same way as vital forms [44]. Lastly, studies on the effects of bacterial skin transplant (SBT), an intriguing treatment for the restoration of a healthy skin microbiome in AD patients, have yielded promising results in human and animal models [45]. Together, these approaches have low costs, few side effects, a more relaxed therapy (no daily application necessary) and a more lasting effect.

2.1.1. Live Microorganisms

The use of living microorganisms as food supplements or in medical practices for the treatment of bacterial vaginosis, vaginitis, childhood colic, obesity, type 2 diabetes and pharingotonsillitis is already well known [46,47]. Clinical and experimental research extensively documents the capacity for probiotics to go beyond positively influencing the intestinal functions, and to exert their benefits at the skin level thanks to their peculiar properties [43]. The topical administration of probiotics can increase skin ceramides, improve erythema, scaling and pruritus, and decrease the concentration of the pathogenic *S. aureus* [48].

There have been several studies into the use of live microorganisms for the treatment of AD, using both human and animal models. Seven of these studies are reviewed: three employed animal models; four involved clinical trials, of which three involved children and one adults (see Table S1A in the Supplementary Electronic Material for details).

Firstly, an in vivo study using Sprague-Dawley rats and ddY mice, and the oral administration of *Lactobacillus plantarum*. It has been proven that food supplementation of β-1,3/1,6-glucan and/or *L. plantarum* LM1004 can reduce vasodilation, itching, oedema and regulates the immune response [49].

In a double-blind clinical trial on 50 children with moderate AD, the oral administration of a mixture of the probiotics *Bifidobacterium lactis*, *Bifidobacterium longum* and *Lactobacillus casei* was effective in reducing SCORAD index scores and reducing the use of topical steroids to treat flares when compared to the control arm. These findings suggest that such a mixture of probiotics can be used for the treatment of AD [50].

An in vivo study on SKH-1 hairless mice aimed to test a probiotic mixture of five bacterial strains, *Bifidobacterium longum*, *Lactobacillus helveticus*, *Lactococcus lactis*, *Streptococcus thermophilus* and *Lactobacillus rhamnosus*, in preserving skin integrity and homeostasis. It has been observed that daily oral treatment with the probiotic mixture, through modulation of the immune response, has significantly limited chronic skin inflammation, demonstrating its use in pathological dermatological conditions such as AD and psoriasis [51].

The oral administration of *Weissella cibaria* WIKIM28 in a mouse model of AD induced in BALB/c mice has shown that this bacterial strain can be a good candidate as a probiotic for AD prevention and improvement. Thus, the intake of this live microorganism improved AD-like skin lesions and exhibited excellent immunomodulatory activity [52].

A randomised, double-blind study carried out on 220 children affected by moderate/severe AD, showed that the oral administration of *Lactobacillus paracasei* and *Lactobacillus fermentum*, for 3 weeks led to decreased IgE, TNF-α, urine eosinophilic protein X and SCORAD scores. Thus indicating that supplementation of a probiotic mixture of *L. plantarum* and *L. fermentum* is associated with clinical improvement of AD [53].

Another trial on 43 children tested *Lactobacillus salivarius*, which, when orally administered, showed a significant improvement in clinical parameters, SCORAD scores and itch values [54].

In a prospective controlled pilot trial on 25 adults, the oral administration of the probiotic strain *L. salivarius* LS01 in association with *Streptococcus thermophilus*, significantly improved both SCORAD scores and the *S. aureus* count. Moreover, the combination of *S. thermophilus* ST10 with *L. salivarius* LS01 improved the overall effectiveness of the formulation by reducing the recovery time [55].

2.1.2. Heat-Killed or Inactivated Microorganisms.

The growing interest in the biological effects of heat-killed or inactivated microorganisms is already well documented. In particular, the use of heat-treated probiotic bacteria (lactic and bifidobacteria), together with their cell-free supernatants or selected purified cellular components in immunomodulation and maintaining the integrity of the intestinal barrier against enteropathogens is well known to the scientific community. Only recently, numerous scientific studies have investigated the role of these non-viable microorganisms in the management of dermatological diseases [56]. There are several studies that have investigated the potential of heat-killed or inactivated microorganisms for the treatment of AD, which have used both human and animal models. The findings of seven of these studies are reported herein. One employed animal models, five involved clinical trials, of which two were in children, and finally one was conducted within an in vitro reconstructed human epidermis (RHE) (see Table S1B in the Supplementary Electronic Material for details).

Topical application of a formulation containing heat-treated *Lactobacillus johnsonii* NCC 533 (HT La1) was able to modulate endogenous antimicrobial peptides (AMP) expression and to inhibit the binding of *S. aureus* in an in vitro reconstructed human epidermis model (RHE). These results highlight the role of innate skin immunity in reducing *S. aureus* colonization in atopic skin [57].

An open-label clinical study in AD patients showed that the application of a lotion containing a heat-treated *Lactobacillus johnsonii* NCC 533 (HT La1) led to a decrease in the SCORAD score. This clinical improvement was associated with a reduction in the *S. aureus* viable count. In addition, the authors were able to establish a directly proportional correlation between the *S. aureus* skin concentrations and the lotion response [58].

In a double-blind clinical trial conducted on 60 patients suffering from moderate AD, topical application of an emollient containing biomass from the non-pathogenic bacteria *Vitreoscilla filiformis* lysate one month after the end of the treatment ameliorated the evolution of the average SCORAD score, which was significantly lower than that of the control patients treated with a generic emollient.

During one month of treatment, the level of *Staphylococcus* spp. decreased in treated subjects with the formulation enriched by *V. filiformis* biomass, demonstrating the normalization of the skin microbiota and the significant reduction in the number and severity of flare-ups compared to another formulation without bacterial biomass [59].

In a clinical trial on 179 children, oral administration of the bacterial lysate OM-85 of 21 strains from eight common respiratory pathogenic microorganisms (i.e., *Haemophilus influenzae*, *Streptococcus pneumoniae*, *Klebsiella ozaenae and pneumoniae*, *S. aureus*, *Streptococcus viridans* and *pyogenes* and *Neisseria catarrhalis*) showed an adjuvant therapeutic effect which led to significantly fewer new flares and delayed their onset. Indeed, these results showed an adjuvant therapeutic effect of a well-standardised bacterial lysate OM-85 on established AD [60].

An in vivo study on NC/Nga mice demonstrated that the oral administration of *Lactobacillus plantarum* lysates was able to restore the skin homeostasis of the treated animals. Indeed, after two months of treatment, there was a reduction in the formation of the horny layer and a decrease in skin thickening compared to untreated mice [61].

Kim et al. stressed the importance of clinical research in the study of AD. In their study, the authors tested *L. plantarum* K8 lysates formulation, both with in vitro/in vivo experiments, and in a clinical trial with the healthy volunteer. Preliminary data obtained in vitro with HaCaT cells and after 2 months of in vivo treatment with on DNCB-treated SKH-1 hairless mice demonstrated an attenuation of the stratum corneum formation and epidermal thickening of AD mice skin. These data were supported by the clinical study, where an improvement in the barrier function of the epidermis was observed in subjects who ate candies containing L. plantarum K8 lysate [62].

In a clinical trial, 606 infants at risk of atopy were treated with an oral application of bacterial lysate containing heat-killed *Escherichia coli* and *Enterococcus faecalis*. The results showed a reduced possibility of developing AD, suggesting that bacterial lysates prevent the development of this skin condition in children [63].

2.1.3. Microorganism-Derived Substances

The capacity of microorganism-derived compounds to inhibit allergic inflammation make them candidates for novel therapies for allergic diseases [64]. Among these compounds are bacteriocins, proteins and enzymes [65]. Several studies have highlighted the beneficial role of skin commensals due to the production of bacteriocins. Indeed, many members of the cutaneous microbiome can metabolise glycerol into antimicrobial compounds, such as bacteriocin, that inhibit *S. aureus* growth. Skin commensal coagulase-negative staphylococci (CoNS) are the primary producers, but there are also other microorganisms able to produce these compounds [66,67]. There are several studies, both in human and animal models. In this section, seven studies concerning the use of microorganism-derived substances for AD treatment are presented. Of these, four employed animal models, two were conducted in vitro, and one were conducted both in vitro and in vivo (see Table S1C in the Supplementary Electronic Material for details).

An in vitro study showed that cytoplasmic bacteriocins isolated from *S. epidermidis* selectively exhibited antimicrobial activity against *S. aureus* and methicillin-resistant *S. aureus* (MRSA). These findings suggest that these cytoplasmic bacteriocin compounds could potentially inhibit the growth of *S. aureus* and be used as a topical AD treatment [68].

In an in vivo model of AD on BALB/cAJcl mice, the oral administration of an exopolysaccharide (EPS) produced by *Lactobacillus paracasei* reduced ear swelling, produced a repression of ear interleukin-4 (T helper (Th) 2 cytokine) mRNA and decreased serum immunoglobulin E levels. These results suggest that *Lactobacillus paracasei*-derived EPS inhibits the catalytic activity of hyaluronidase promoting inflammatory reactions and is useful for improving type I and type IV allergies, including AD [69].

The commensal yeast *Malassezia globosa*, secretes a protease called '*Malassezia globosa* secreted Aspartyl Protease 1 (MgSAP1)', which, in vitro, can disrupt *S. aureus* biofilms by hydrolysing protein A. This study defined a role for the skin fungus Malassezia in inter-kingdom interactions and suggested that this fungus enzyme may be beneficial for skin health [70].

In a mouse model the topical application of p40, a particulate fraction from *Corynebacterium granulosum*, used in a formula with hyaluronic acid produced a significant reduction in ear thickness, weight, oedema, and leukocyte recruitment. These results suggest that p40-conjugated with hyaluronic acid may constitute an outstanding innovative dermatitis treatment [71].

In addition, other bacteria not belonging to the skin microbiota are able to produce antibiotics with properties useful for treating AD. An example would be the topical application of josamycin, a macrolide antibiotic derived from *Streptomyces narbonensis* subsp. *josamyceticus* which was applied to NC/Nga mice. In this case, the topical application of this antibiotic reduced the expression of proinflammatory cytokines demonstrating antimicrobial activity against *S. aureus* present on the skin of AD mice [72].

Another molecule with antibacterial activity, produced by *S. lugdunensis*, lugdunine, was tested in an in vivo experiment with shaved black-6 (C57BL/6) mice and it was able to reduce or completely eradicate *S. aureus* viable count both on the surface and in the deeper layers of the skin. The isolation and study of other lugdunin- or lugdunin-like molecules isolated from s commensal bacteria could represent a new therapeutic approach in the prevention and management of staphylococcal infections [73].

Similarly, an AD-like in vivo NC/Nga mice model demonstrated that the protein P14, isolated from *Lactobacillus casei*, can be used as an active immunomodulatory agent for treating patients with AD [74].

2.1.4. Skin Bacterial Transplantation

Although there are still few studies on the transplantation of skin bacteria (SBT), this particular type of bacteriotherapy that involves transplanting several skin microbiota from one individual to another has already provided promising results in both human clinical trials and in animal models [45]. Indeed this intriguing therapeutic potential has earned it the definition of the "future of eczema therapy" [75]. Herein, three human studies are reported focusing on skin microbiota transplantation for the treatment AD. Of these studies, one involved a clinical trial conducted on healthy volunteers to develop the technique for transferring the entire skin microbiota, another was carried out on adults, and the last one involved both adults and paediatric patients (see Table S1D in the Supplementary Electronic Material for details).

In a recent prospective pilot study, researchers attempted to perform a complete skin microbiota transplant that shifted the entire bacterial skin community of healthy volunteers from the forearm to the back in a unidirectional manner. Evidence of the transfer of a partial DNA signature was seen by comparing the bacterial species present in the arm with the mixed communities ('transplantation') that were absent in the back. This technique aimed to move viable skin organisms from one site to another and is worthy of further investigation [76].

The successful transplantation of *Roseomonas mucosa* was conducted in an open-label phase I/II safety and activity trial with adults and pediatric patients. The results demonstrated a significant decrease in disease severity, a reduction in steroid administration, and a viable *S. aureus* count [77]. All these finds were supported by a previous study in mice conducted by the same authors [20].

Najatsuji et al. conducted a clinical study by autologous CoNS transplantation isolated from AD patients *S. aureus* culture positive. After isolation, CoNS strains (*S. epidermidis* and *S. hominis*) were formulated in a cream base vehicle and applied to the forearm of the same subjects for 24 h. The results showed a significant decrease in *S. aureus* colonization at the microbial transplant site compared to the contralateral forearm treated with the bacteria-free vehicle alone. These observations were also confirmed by in vivo experiments on the back of C57BL6 mice. These findings show, once again, the role of commensal skin bacteria in protecting against colonisation by pathogens and how dysbiosis of the skin microbiome can contribute to the onset of the disease [19].

2.2. Drug Delivery Systems

It is often preferable to use non-invasive delivery to provide relief for AD [78]. Topical treatment is preferential to parenteral or oral administration because of better compliance and the reduction in drug concentrations and side effects [79]. Topically, DDSs deliver therapeutic agents or natural active compounds directly to the target site to maximise the benefits and minimise the risks associated with drugs. In this regard, in the last two decades, an interest in nano-based DDSs has developed. The latter have already been applied in the treatment of various diseases ranging from cancer to Alzheimer's [80].

The most common nano-based DDS carriers addressed in this manuscript, include polymeric nanoparticles (NPs), solid lipid nanoparticles (SLNs), lLiposomes, ethosomes, and elastic vesicles due to their small size (range from 1 to 1000 nm). They can penetrate through the *stratum corneum* and accumulate in the target site, improving the delivery of transported bioactive compounds and favouring higher drug retention, demonstrated by drug diffusion and permeation study profiles [79–82]. Although the dimensions are variable, desired therapeutic benefits, avoidance of off-target effects, and optimal localised delivery of drugs are achieved using nanocarriers <200 nm in size. Nanocarrier-mediated interventions have been well-reported for topical and transdermal applications [83]. Together, these approaches offer novel solutions, allowing: (i) the management of severe forms of AD, especially those not responsive to steroid therapy; (ii) improved performance of pharmacokinetic parameters such as permeation and controlled release; (iii) significant improvements in the patient's state of health; iv) a reduction in the dosage of the active ingredient with a consequent reduction in toxicity and an improved safety profile [84,85].

2.2.1. Nanoparticles

Nanoparticles (NP) are a broad class of DSS in the order of 100 nanometres with optimal rheological properties, antimicrobial effects and the ability to restore skin conditions [16,86]. For instance, NPs loaded with a lipid drug and/or made by lipophilic compounds (i.e., lipid NPs) ensure skin hydration and the occlusion effect in a size-dependent manner and can form a thin film on the skin surface, which allows for rehydration [87]. The complete biodegradation of lipid NPs and their biocompatible chemical features have secured them the title of nano-safe carriers [84]. Twelve studies concerning the use of NPs in AD treatment were identified for review. Only in vivo studies using animals were selected. Of the seventeen studies, one employed only in vivo animal models, four were conducted in vitro and ex vivo, six were conducted in vitro and in vivo, and one was conducted in vitro, ex vivo and in vivo. In vitro tests provided a characterisation and evaluation of the formulation (see Table S2A in the Supplementary Electronic Material for details).

An in vitro and ex vivo drug test performed using a jacketed Franz diffusion cell showed that nanoencapsulation of betamethasone valerate (BMV) into the chitosan nanoparticles (CS-NPs) displayed a Fickian diffusion type mechanism of release in the simulated skin surface. Drug permeation efficiency and the amount of BMV retained in the epidermis and the dermis was higher when compared to BMV solution alone. These results suggest that this formulation of betamethasone improved the therapeutic efficacy of the treatment of AD [88].

Tacrolimus-loaded thermosensitive solid lipid nanoparticles (TCR-SLN) in the dorsal skin of Sprague Dawley rats penetrated to a deeper layer than the control formula. The penetration test in vivo of the skin of white rabbits demonstrated that TCR-SLNs delivered more drug into deeper skin layers than the control, suggesting that thermosensitive SLNs could be employed for the delivery of difficult-to-permeate, poorly water-soluble drugs into deep skin layers [89].

In an in vitro test with a Franz static diffusion cell system and ex vivo on skin from Wistar albino rats, the application of 'hyaluronic acid-modified betamethasone encapsulated polymeric nanoparticles' (HA-BMV-CS-NPs) revealed that drug permeation efficiency of betamethasone was higher in the case of BMV-CS-NPs and that there was a greater amount of drug retained in the epidermis and the dermis. This complex could be a promising nano delivery system for efficient dermal targeting of BMV and improved anti-AD efficacy [90].

In a clinical trial that enrolled healthy volunteers treated with hydrocortisone hydroxytyrosol anti-oxidant-loaded chitosan nanoparticles (HA-HT-CSNPs) to evaluate systemic toxicity, the results of blood haematology, blood biochemistry, and adrenal cortico-thyroid hormone levels were not significant. This indicated non-systemic toxicity and supports the view that this formula could be used for AD treatment [91].

In vitro and in vivo permeation studies on Sprague Dawley rats with tacrolimus nanoparticles based on chitosan and combined with nicotinamide (FK506-NIC-CS-NPs), demonstrated that these nanoparticles significantly enhance tacrolimus permeation through and into the skin, and deposited more tacrolimus into the skin. Moreover, this system enhances the permeability of tacrolimus and plays an adjuvant role in anti-AD, reducing the dose of tacrolimus in treating AD, and is, therefore, a promising nanoscale system of tacrolimus for the effective treatment of AD [92].

Betamethasone Valerate incorporates in a lipidic carrier revealed an enhancement of the Betamethasone Valerate ratio in comparison with the control group and had an anti-inflammatory effect. The outcome of complete characterisation suggests that the developed formulation is efficient in a single daily dosage in the therapy of AD [93].

An in vitro/ex vivo test on NC/Nga mice skin demonstrated the anti-AD efficacy of tacrolimus-hyaluronic acid-charged nanoparticles. According to the author's findings, this formulation can be used as a promising therapeutic approach for patients who cannot be treated with steroid therapy, such as children and adults with steroid intolerance [94].

In an in vivo test with SKH-1 mice, the topical application of dendritic nano-multi-shell dendritic nanocarriers was evaluated as a deposit formulation for anti-inflammatory drugs in the skin. Both in vitro release and toxicological studies have confirmed the biocompatibility of the formulation, providing evidence of prolonged release of the active substance especially for anti-inflammatory drugs like those used in AD. Furthermore, no evidence of local or systemic toxic/adverse effects was observed [95].

An in vivo test on Wistar albino rats evaluated the penetration into the deep skin layers of cationic polymeric chitosan nanoparticles loaded with anti-inflammatory (hydrocortisone) and antimicrobial (hydroxytyrosol,) anti-inflammatory agents compared to a similar commercial formulation. The results proved a better performance in the local release of the active ingredients without involving the underlying tissues. In addition, no toxicity was found compared to the commercial formulation, providing substantial safety benefits [96].

In an in vivo test with NC/Nga mice, transcutaneous co-delivery based on nanocarrier hydrocortisone and hydroxytyrosol was studied as a possible therapy for the management of the immunological and histological issues of AD. The results of immunological and histological experiments conducted on the sera and biopsies of the tested mice confirmed this hypothesis [97].

Furthermore, a Silver-nano lipid complex incorporated into an o/w cream and a lotion showed a high adhesivity to the skin and bacterial surfaces, leading to a locally high concentration of silver ion killing bacteria, restoring the distorted skin barrier, and being much more useful than silver alone. Data were generated either by in vitro tests determining the colony-forming unit (CFU) count over time of *S. aureus* ATCC25923, or in vivo on BALB/c mice. This formula makes the drug more effective in terms of enhanced penetration and exploits the skin normalisation ability of the skincare sNLC formulation [16].

Another in vivo study in NC/Nga mice aimed to assess whether the transcutaneous administration of hydrocortisone nanoparticle could be considered a valid therapeutic approach in the management of dermatitis suggested a substantial reduction in inflammatory cascade mediators, accompanied by positive histological results on fibroblast infiltration and elastic fiber fragmentation, demonstrating how these formulations can promote and maintain the integrity of connective tissues especially in an injured skin like AD [98].

2.2.2. Liposomes, Ethosomes, and Elastic Vesicles

Liposomes and ethosomes can be defined as vesicular DDSs. Liposomes are spherical vesicles with particle sizes ranging from 30 nm to several micrometres consisting of single or multiple concentric lipid bilayers encapsulating an aqueous compartment. These formulations have been successfully applied for the management of AD due to their moisturising effect on the *stratum corneum* and their ability to act as bioactive compound carriers [85]. Rigid liposomes remain confined to the *stratum corneum*, resulting in the formation of a drug reservoir in the upper skin layers, and do not allow percutaneous absorption. More recently, efforts have been made to investigate vesicular lipid systems capable of facilitating drug penetration to the underlying skin layers, allowing transdermal absorption [99].

In contrast, ethosomes are made mainly of phospholipids with a high concentration of ethanol (20–50%) and water. Due to this composition, they have demonstrated remarkably high deformability features [100]. Moreover, ethosomes guarantee a more efficient transfer of the active principle through the skin (epidermis and dermis) than liposomes [15].

Finally, a further advance in the field of DDS is represented by the elastic vesicles used as a new topical and transdermal delivery system. Although the manufacturing method of these vehicles is very similar to that of liposomes, the presence of an 'activating' agent in the phospholipid bilayer gives it a high degree of elasticity. It has been demonstrated that the topical administration of elastic vesicles does not occlude the skin and easily permeates through the *stratum corneum* lipid lamellar regions due to skin hydration or by osmotic force. Furthermore, this DDS can be loaded with a wide range of small molecules, peptides and proteins [101].

Six applications of liposomes, ethosomes, and elastic vesicles in AD treatment are herein reported Of them, one was conducted using only in vitro methods, one enrolled patients with AD, one were conducted by in vitro and ex vivo studies, one by in vitro and in vivo and in the last two an in vitro, ex vivo and in vivo methodology was adopted. In vitro tests have provided a characterisation and evaluation of the formulation (see Table S2B in the Supplementary Electronic Material for details).

In an in vitro test with a static Franz diffusion cell setup on the heat-separated human epidermis, the use of ultra-flexible lipid vesicles effectively delivered cyclosporin A into the skin. This study introduces a promising approach to the topical treatment of skin pathologies with an immune component [102].

In an in vitro test with a dialysis membrane and ex vivo with Wistar rat skin, the application of cyclo-ethosomes with fluocinolone acetonide (FA) showed maximum permeability as compared with an optimised reference ethosomal gel and control gel. These results suggest that β-cyclo-ethosomes could be a promising carrier for improvised penetration of fluocinolone acetonide via topical gel [103].

In an open-label pilot study of 20 patients with AD, the application of liposomal polyvinylpyrrolidone-iodine hydrogel showed that this strategy was well tolerated and led to an improvement in pain, quality of life, eczema area and severity. This formula has potential utility as an effective treatment for inflammatory skin conditions associated with bacterial colonisation [104].

An in vitro test with a dialysis membrane and ex vivo with Wistar rat skin revealed that nano ethosomal glycolic vesicles of triamcinolone acetonide have excellent permeation. Besides the histological analysis, the study confirmed the non-irritant potential. These results suggest that nano-ethosomal glycolic vesicles can be active non-irritant carriers for the improvised penetration of triamcinolone acetonide for potential topical therapeutics [105].

The pharmaco-dynamic evaluation of the ethosome-based topical delivery system of the antihistaminic drug cetirizine (measured by in vivo and ex vivo tests on BALB/c mice) showed a reduction in the scratching score, the erythema score, skin hyperplasia and the dermal eosinophil count. The data suggest that this formula could be an effective carrier for the dermal delivery of the antihistaminic drug, cetirizine, for the treatment of AD [106].

An in vivo and ex vivo tests on BALB/c mice, a topical formulation of levocetirizine based on flexible vesicles (FVs) showed a reduction in the scratching score and the erythema score in addition to the dermal eosinophil count [107].

3. Discussion

AD is a pathological skin condition that is becoming increasingly common in clinical dermatological practice. The pathogenesis is exacerbated by its complex aetiological mechanisms that are not yet fully understood, providing many opportunities for misinterpretation [108]. Among the different hypotheses, numerous studies have demonstrated that dysbiosis and skin barrier dysfunction contribute to the pathobiology of AD [109]. Immune dysregulation is another factor involved in the pathogenesis of AD and is closely related to the previous ones. Indeed skin colonisation of Staphylococcus aureus damages the skin barrier and induces inflammatory responses, on the other hand, local Th2 immune responses diminish barrier function, promoting bacterial dysbiosis [9].

Although it is common to associate skin dysbiosis with an increase in *S. aureus* abundance, more recent studies are converging on the opinion that AD skin microbiota is characterised by low bacterial diversity. The relative abundance of both *S. aureus* and *S. epidermidis* are elevated and the presence of *Propionibacterium* spp. is reduced, along with other genera (*Streptococcus, Acinetobacter, Corynebacterium* and *Prevotella*). Moreover, the absence of early colonisation with commensal staphylococci might precede AD presentation [31]. Skin dysbiosis contributes to skin barrier defects [12]. The latter promote easy penetration of numerous insults relevant to the development of the disease i.e., pathogens, toxins, allergens, irritants and pollutants. Accordingly, all the treatments (pharmacological and adjuvants) aim to minimise the number of exacerbations, the so-called 'flares', and reduce their duration and intensity [110]. To date, there is not a resolutive therapy that can take into account the complex pathogenic interplay between a patient's susceptible genes, their skin barrier abnormalities and their immune dysregulation [15].

The majority of AD patients are paediatric and when moderate-to-severe symptoms occur, current therapies have proven to be of limited efficacy and have several side effects [111–113]. For all these reasons, there has been a surge of interest from clinicians and the lay public in exploring targeted bacteriotherapy to treat this pathological skin condition [76]. Microbic therapies with microorganisms that are commensal of the healthy skin microbiota, or probiotics in conjunction with transplantation, could represent a new diagnostic and therapeutic target for AD [114–116]. Several studies have demonstrated that probiotic use has led to increased skin ceramides and has improved erythema, scaling and pruritus, suggesting that probiotics may be useful for the treatment of AD, especially for moderate to severe AD in children and adults [48,51,53,116]. Furthermore, specific probiotic strains have shown active immunomodulatory properties [59,117].

Restoring the skin microbiota homeostasis could also represent a new era in AD treatment [118]. The reconstitution of healthy microbial diversity can boost the right immune response and normal barrier function [7,32,119,120]. Similarly, other studies have demonstrated that commensal microorganisms can reduce *S. aureus* by bacteriocin production or competition mechanisms, improving AD symptoms. In this context, the development of antibiotic resistance by the *S. aureus* methicillin-resistant (MRSA) strain has considerable importance, not only from the point of view of infectious disease but also as it can influence the course of the disease. Bacteriocins from CoNS also exhibit antimicrobial activity against MRSA [72,121]. The clinical promise of transplanting commensal skin organisms from healthy individuals onto diseased skin, together with faecal microbiota transplantation to selectively target pathogenic *S. aureus*, thus modifying the diseased skin microbiome to attenuate the course of the disease, have been investigated, with promising results [16,76].

Furthermore, the therapeutic potential of DDSs based on nano-products has provided a new avenue for the prevention and treatment of inflammation and sequelae of skin diseases. Several studies have shown the effectiveness of nanoparticles, liposomes, ethosomes and vesicles in AD. This was particularly valid in recalcitrant form treatments, due to their unique characteristics, such as the improvement in pharmacokinetic parameters (targeted transdermal release of the active ingredient, permeation, retention, and diffusion) and physicochemical properties. These advances in pharmaceutical technology have led to improvements in both clinical symptoms and immune responses, along with better inhibition of inflammatory cascades mediators that positively impact patients' quality of life, with fewer adverse events reported and increased patient compliance [85,110,122,123].

4. Materials and Methods

The interest of the scientific community in research into novel targets for the development of effective therapeutic strategies in AD management has dramatically increased. For this reason, the bibliographic research for scientific papers specialised in the field of interest was conducted from 2014 to March 2020 on PubMed (the MEDLINE database), using the following keywords: 'atopic dermatitis', 'bacterial therapy', 'drug delivery system' and 'alternative therapy' alone and/or in combination. As a preliminary result, more than 300 documents were found. Of these, 24 papers on microbial therapy and 15 on nano-based DDSs were selected for review due to their relevance.

5. Conclusions

All the studies reviewed show enormous potential for AD treatment, so we can state that research into novel targets is key to the development of effective therapeutic strategies. Nevertheless, some limitations still need to be overcome. An aspect of primary importance in the advancement of scientific and technological innovation is the possibility of marketing the new formulations. To this end, there are different international regulations regarding bacterial formulations for medical use. The European Medical Device Directive (MD) (DDM 93/42) and subsequent amendments include MDs containing live microorganisms (especially those containing probiotics) for the management of AD [124]. On the other hand, the US Food and Drug Administration (FDA) has not approved any oral or topical microbial-based formulations for the treatment of dermatological condition [125].

Although the potential of bacteriotherapy for the treatment of AD seems to be clear, further studies will need to be conducted with the goals of recruiting more patients with different clinical characteristics and standardising the process to produce reliable data. Put differently, even if the topically used DDSs offer promising opportunities in dermal delivery, many questions arise, which remain to be explored and addressed, concerning, for example, their toxicological characteristics and the long-term safety of these technologies.

In vivo and in vitro assays are useful to identify the toxicity of dds because they help to establish the dose–response relationship [126]

However despite in vitro tests are useful for bypassing cell interactions that exist in vivo, in vivo toxicity testing is needed due to the difference between in vitro dosimetry and real topical exposure and additional innovative research is needed to address the cost-effectiveness and long-term safety of these nanoparticles [127].

Author Contributions: Conceptualization: I.M., G.P.P., R.D.M.; Methodology: I.M. and G.P.P.; Investigation: I.M., G.P.P., M.A.C., N.V., L.P.; Resources: I.M., G.P.P., F.V., K.M.; Writing—original draft preparation: I.M. and G.P.P.; Writing—review and editing, I.M., G.P.P., K.M., D.Z., R.D.M.; Supervision: D.Z. and R.D.M.; Project administration: R.D.M. All authors have read and agreed to the published version of the manuscript.

Acknowledgments: The authors thank Aileens Pharma s.r.l for founding the journal APC and Professor Amy Muschamp for the language revision.

References

1. Weidinger, S.; Beck, L.; Bieber, T.; Kabashima, K.; Irvine, A. Atopic dermatitis. *Nat. Rev. Dis. Primers* **2018**, *4*, 1. [CrossRef]

2. Abuabara, K.; Yu, A.; Okhovat, J.P.; Allen, I.; Langan, S.M. The prevalence of atopic dermatitis beyond childhood: A systematic review and meta-analysis of longitudinal studies. *Allergy* **2018**, *73*, 696–704. [CrossRef]

3. Patel, N.; Feldman, S.R. Adherence in atopic dermatitis. In *Management of Atopic Dermatitis*; Springer: Berlin, Germany, 2017; pp. 139–159.

4. Wollenberg, A.; Schnopp, C. Evolution of conventional therapy in atopic dermatitis. *Immunol. Allergy Clin.* **2010**, *30*, 351–368. [CrossRef]

5. Guttman-Yassky, E.; Waldman, A.; Ahluwalia, J.; Ong, P.Y.; Eichenfield, L.F. Atopic dermatitis: Pathogenesis. *Semin. Cutan. Med. Surg.* **2017**, *36*, 100–103. [CrossRef] [PubMed]

6. Spergel, J.M. From atopic dermatitis to asthma: The atopic march. *Ann. Allergy Asthma Immunol.* **2010**, *105*, 99–106. [CrossRef] [PubMed]

7. Seite, S.; Bieber, T. Barrier function and microbiotic dysbiosis in atopic dermatitis. *Clin. Cosmet. Investig. Dermatol.* **2015**, *8*, 479. [CrossRef] [PubMed]

8. Patrick, G.J.; Archer, N.K.; Miller, L.S. Which Way Do We Go? Complex Interactions in Atopic Dermatitis Pathogenesis. *J. Investig. Dermatol.* **2020**, *396*, P345–P360.

9. Langan, S.M.; Irvine, A.D.; Weidinger, S. Atopic dermatitis. *Lancet* **2020**, *396*, 345–360. [CrossRef]

10. Nakahara, T.; Kido-Nakahara, M.; Tsuji, G.; Furue, M. Basics and recent advances in the pathophysiology of atopic dermatitis. *J. Dermatol.* **2020**. [CrossRef]

11. Proksch, E.; Brandner, J.M.; Jensen, J.M. The skin: An indispensable barrier. *Exp. Dermatol.* **2008**, *17*, 1063–1072. [CrossRef]

12. Kim, B.E.; Leung, D.Y. Significance of skin barrier dysfunction in atopic dermatitis. *Allergy Asthma Immunol. Res.* **2018**, *10*, 207–215. [CrossRef] [PubMed]

13. Drislane, C.; Irvine, A.D. The role of filaggrin in atopic dermatitis and allergic disease. *Ann. Allergy Asthma Immunol.* **2020**, *124*, 36–43. [CrossRef] [PubMed]

14. Hamid, Q.; Boguniewicz, M.; Leung, D. Differential in situ cytokine gene expression in acute versus chronic atopic dermatitis. *J. Clin. Investig.* **1994**, *94*, 870–876. [CrossRef] [PubMed]

15. Shao, M.; Hussain, Z.; Thu, H.E.; Khan, S.; Katas, H.; Ahmed, T.A.; Tripathy, M.; Leng, J.; Qin, H.-L.; Bukhari, S.N.A. Drug nanocarrier, the future of atopic diseases: Advanced drug delivery systems and smart management of disease. *Colloids Surf. B Biointerfaces* **2016**, *147*, 475–491. [CrossRef] [PubMed]

16. Keck, C.; Anantaworasakul, P.; Patel, M.; Okonogi, S.; Singh, K.; Roessner, D.; Scherrers, R.; Schwabe, K.; Rimpler, C.; Müller, R. A new concept for the treatment of atopic dermatitis: Silver–nanolipid complex (sNLC). *Int. J. Pharm.* **2014**, *462*, 44–51. [CrossRef]

17. Tham, E.H.; Koh, E.; Common, J.E.; Hwang, I.Y. Biotherapeutic Approaches in Atopic Dermatitis. *Biotechnol. J.* **2020**, e1900322. [CrossRef]

18. Chen, Y.E.; Fischbach, M.A.; Belkaid, Y. Skin microbiota–host interactions. *Nature* **2018**, *553*, 427–436. [CrossRef]

19. Nakatsuji, T.; Chen, T.H.; Narala, S.; Chun, K.A.; Two, A.M.; Yun, T.; Shafiq, F.; Kotol, P.F.; Bouslimani, A.; Melnik, A.V. Antimicrobials from human skin commensal bacteria protect against Staphylococcus aureus and are deficient in atopic dermatitis. *Sci. Transl. Med.* **2017**, *9*, 4680. [CrossRef]

20. Myles, I.A.; Williams, K.W.; Reckhow, J.D.; Jammeh, M.L.; Pincus, N.B.; Sastalla, I.; Saleem, D.; Stone, K.D.; Datta, S.K. Transplantation of human skin microbiota in models of atopic dermatitis. *JCI Insight* **2016**, *1*, e86955. [CrossRef]

21. Chau, T.A.; McCully, M.L.; Brintnell, W.; An, G.; Kasper, K.J.; Vinés, E.D.; Kubes, P.; Haeryfar, S.M.; McCormick, J.K.; Cairns, E. Toll-like receptor 2 ligands on the staphylococcal cell wall downregulate superantigen-induced T cell activation and prevent toxic shock syndrome. *Nat. Med.* **2009**, *15*, 641. [CrossRef]

22. Lai, Y.; Di Nardo, A.; Nakatsuji, T.; Leichtle, A.; Yang, Y.; Cogen, A.L.; Wu, Z.-R.; Hooper, L.V.; Schmidt, R.R.; Von Aulock, S. Commensal bacteria regulate Toll-like receptor 3–dependent inflammation after skin injury. *Nat. Med.* **2009**, *15*, 1377. [CrossRef] [PubMed]

23. Gallo, R.L.; Nakatsuji, T. Microbial symbiosis with the innate immune defense system of the skin. *J. Investig. Dermatol.* **2011**, *131*, 1974–1980. [CrossRef] [PubMed]

24. Williams, M.R.; Gallo, R.L. Evidence that human skin microbiome dysbiosis promotes atopic dermatitis. *J. Investig. Dermatol.* **2017**, *137*, 2460–2461. [CrossRef] [PubMed]

25. Totté, J.; Van Der Feltz, W.; Hennekam, M.; van Belkum, A.; Van Zuuren, E.; Pasmans, S. Prevalence and odds of Staphylococcus aureus carriage in atopic dermatitis: A systematic review and meta-analysis. *Br. J. Dermatol.* **2016**, *175*, 687–695. [CrossRef] [PubMed]

26. Geoghegan, J.A.; Irvine, A.D.; Foster, T.J. Staphylococcus aureus and atopic dermatitis: A complex and evolving relationship. *Trends Microbiol.* **2018**, *26*, 484–497. [CrossRef]

27. Kong, H.H.; Oh, J.; Deming, C.; Conlan, S.; Grice, E.A.; Beatson, M.A.; Nomicos, E.; Polley, E.C.; Komarow, H.D.; Murray, P.R. Temporal shifts in the skin microbiome associated with disease flares and treatment in children with atopic dermatitis. *Genome Res.* **2012**, *22*, 850–859. [CrossRef]

28. Dekio, I.; Sakamoto, M.; Hayashi, H.; Amagai, M.; Suematsu, M.; Benno, Y. Characterization of skin microbiota in patients with atopic dermatitis and in normal subjects using 16S rRNA gene-based comprehensive analysis. *J. Med. Microbiol.* **2007**, *56*, 1675–1683. [CrossRef]

29. Oh, J.; Freeman, A.F.; Park, M.; Sokolic, R.; Candotti, F.; Holland, S.M.; Segre, J.A.; Kong, H.H. The altered landscape of the human skin microbiome in patients with primary immunodeficiencies. *Genome Res.* **2013**, *23*, 2103–2114. [CrossRef]

30. Chng, K.R.; Tay, A.S.L.; Li, C.; Ng, A.H.Q.; Wang, J.; Suri, B.K.; Matta, S.A.; McGovern, N.; Janela, B.; Wong, X.F.C.C. Whole metagenome profiling reveals skin microbiome-dependent susceptibility to atopic dermatitis flare. *Nat. Microbiol.* **2016**, *1*, 16106. [CrossRef]

31. Bjerre, R.; Bandier, J.; Skov, L.; Engstrand, L.; Johansen, J. The role of the skin microbiome in atopic dermatitis: A systematic review. *Br. J. Dermatol.* **2017**, *177*, 1272–1278. [CrossRef]

32. Wollina, U. Microbiome in atopic dermatitis. *Clin. Cosmet. Investig. Dermatol.* **2017**, *10*, 51. [CrossRef] [PubMed]

33. Gelmetti, C.; Colonna, C. The value of SCORAD and beyond. Towards a standardized evaluation of severity? *Allergy* **2004**, *59* (Suppl. 78), 61–65. [CrossRef]

34. Wollenberg, A.; Barbarot, S.; Bieber, T.; Christen-Zaech, S.; Deleuran, M.; Fink-Wagner, A.; Gieler, U.; Girolomoni, G.; Lau, S.; Muraro, A. Consensus-based European guidelines for treatment of atopic eczema (atopic dermatitis) in adults and children: Part II. *J. Eur. Acad. Dermatol. Venereol.* **2018**, *32*, 850–878. [CrossRef] [PubMed]

35. Chun, P.I.F.; Lehman, H. Current and Future Monoclonal Antibodies in the Treatment of Atopic Dermatitis. *Clin. Rev. Allergy Immunol.* **2020**, *59*, 208–219. [CrossRef] [PubMed]

36. Boguniewicz, M. Biologics for Atopic Dermatitis. *Immunol. Allergy Clin.* **2020**, *40*, 593–607. [CrossRef] [PubMed]

37. Katoh, N.; Kataoka, Y.; Saeki, H.; Hide, M.; Kabashima, K.; Etoh, T.; Igarashi, A.; Imafuku, S.; Kawashima, M.; Ohtsuki, M. Efficacy and safety of dupilumab in Japanese adults with moderate-to-severe atopic dermatitis: A subanalysis of three clinical trials. *Br. J. Dermatol.* **2020**, *183*, 39–51. [CrossRef] [PubMed]

38. Newsom, M.; Bashyam, A.M.; Balogh, E.A.; Feldman, S.R.; Strowd, L.C. New and Emerging Systemic Treatments for Atopic Dermatitis. *Drugs* **2020**, *1*, 1–12.

39. Chatterjee, S.; Hui, P.C.-L.; Wat, E.; Kan, C.-W.; Leung, P.-C.; Wang, W. Drug delivery system of dual-responsive PF127 hydrogel with polysaccharide-based nano-conjugate for textile-based transdermal therapy. *Carbohydr. Polym.* **2020**, *236*, 116074. [CrossRef]

40. Eichenfield, L.F.; Tom, W.L.; Berger, T.G.; Krol, A.; Paller, A.S.; Schwarzenberger, K.; Bergman, J.N.; Chamlin, S.L.; Cohen, D.E.; Cooper, K.D. Guidelines of care for the management of atopic dermatitis: Section 2. Management and treatment of atopic dermatitis with topical therapies. *J. Am. Acad. Dermatol.* **2014**, *71*, 116–132. [CrossRef]

41. Shi, K.; Lio, P.A. Alternative treatments for atopic dermatitis: An update. *Am. J. Clin. Dermatol.* **2019**, *20*, 251–266. [CrossRef]

42. Olle, B. Medicines from microbiota. *Nat. Biotechnol.* **2013**, *31*, 309–315. [CrossRef] [PubMed]

43. Cinque, B.; La Torre, C.; Melchiorre, E.; Marchesani, G.; Zoccali, G.; Palumbo, P.; Di Marzio, L.; Masci, A.; Mosca, L.; Mastromarino, P. Use of probiotics for dermal applications. In *Probiotics*; Springer: Berlin, Germany, 2011; pp. 221–241.

44. Lew, L.; Liong, M. Bioactives from probiotics for dermal health: Functions and benefits. *J. Appl. Microbiol.* **2013**, *114*, 1241–1253. [CrossRef] [PubMed]

45. Hendricks, A.J.; Mills, B.W.; Shi, V.Y. Skin bacterial transplant in atopic dermatitis: Knowns, unknowns and emerging trends. *J. Dermatol. Sci.* **2019**, *95*, 56–61. [CrossRef] [PubMed]

46. Verrucci, M.; Iacobino, A.; Fattorini, L.; Marcoaldi, R.; Maggio, A.; Piccaro, G. Use of probiotics in medical devices applied to some common pathologies. *Ann. dell'Ist. Super. Sanità* **2019**, *55*, 380–385.

47. Blandino, G.; Fazio, D.; Di Marco, R. Probiotics: Overview of microbiological and immunological characteristics. *Expert Rev. Anti-Infect. Ther.* **2008**, *6*, 497–508. [CrossRef] [PubMed]

48. Knackstedt, R.; Knackstedt, T.; Gatherwright, J. The role of topical probiotics on skin conditions: A systematic review of animal and human studies and implications for future therapies. *Exp. Dermatol.* **2019**, *29*, 15–21. [CrossRef]

49. Kim, I.S.; Lee, S.H.; Kwon, Y.M.; Adhikari, B.; Kim, J.A.; Yu, D.Y.; Kim, G.I.; Lim, J.M.; Kim, S.H.; Lee, S.S. Oral Administration of β-Glucan and Lactobacillus plantarum Alleviates Atopic Dermatitis-Like Symptoms. *J. Microbiol. Biotechnol.* **2019**, *29*, 1693–1706. [CrossRef]

50. Navarro-López, V.; Ramírez-Boscá, A.; Ramón-Vidal, D.; Ruzafa-Costas, B.; Genovés-Martínez, S.; Chenoll-Cuadros, E.; Carrión-Gutiérrez, M.; de la Parte, J.H.; Prieto-Merino, D.; Codoñer-Cortés, F.M. Effect of oral administration of a mixture of probiotic strains on SCORAD index and use of topical steroids in young patients with moderate atopic dermatitis: A randomized clinical trial. *JAMA Dermatol.* **2018**, *154*, 37–43. [CrossRef]

51. Holowacz, S.; Guinobert, I.; Guilbot, A.; Hidalgo, S.; Bisson, J. A Mixture of Five Bacterial Strains Attenuates Skin Inflammation in Mice. *Anti-Inflamm. Anti-Allergy Agents Med. Chem.* **2018**, *17*, 125–137. [CrossRef]

52. Lim, S.K.; Kwon, M.-S.; Lee, J.; Oh, Y.J.; Jang, J.-Y.; Lee, J.-H.; Park, H.W.; Nam, Y.-D.; Seo, M.-J.; Roh, S.W. Weissella cibaria WIKIM28 ameliorates atopic dermatitis-like skin lesions by inducing tolerogenic dendritic cells and regulatory T cells in BALB/c mice. *Sci. Rep.* **2017**, *7*, 1–9. [CrossRef]

53. Wang, I.J.; Wang, J.Y. Children with atopic dermatitis show clinical improvement after Lactobacillus exposure. *Clin. Exp. Allergy* **2015**, *45*, 779–787. [CrossRef] [PubMed]

54. Niccoli, A.A.; Artesi, A.L.; Candio, F.; Ceccarelli, S.; Cozzali, R.; Ferraro, L.; Fiumana, D.; Mencacci, M.; Morlupo, M.; Pazzelli, P. Preliminary results on clinical effects of probiotic Lactobacillus salivarius LS01 in children affected by atopic dermatitis. *J. Clin. Gastroenterol.* **2014**, *48*, S34–S36. [CrossRef] [PubMed]

55. Drago, L.; De Vecchi, E.; Toscano, M.; Vassena, C.; Altomare, G.; Pigatto, P. Treatment of atopic dermatitis eczema with a high concentration of Lactobacillus salivarius LS01 associated with an innovative gelling complex: A pilot study on adults. *J. Clin. Gastroenterol.* **2014**, *48*, S47–S51. [CrossRef] [PubMed]

56. Piqué, N.; Berlanga, M.; Miñana-Galbis, D. Health benefits of heat-killed (Tyndallized) probiotics: An overview. *Int. J. Mol. Sci.* **2019**, *20*, 2534. [CrossRef] [PubMed]

57. Rosignoli, C.; Thibaut de Ménonville, S.; Orfila, D.; Béal, M.; Bertino, B.; Aubert, J.; Mercenier, A.; Piwnica, D. A topical treatment containing heat-treated Lactobacillus johnsonii NCC 533 reduces Staphylococcus aureus adhesion and induces antimicrobial peptide expression in an in vitro reconstructed human epidermis model. *Exp. Dermatol.* **2018**, *27*, 358–365. [CrossRef] [PubMed]

58. Blanchet-Réthoré, S.; Bourdès, V.; Mercenier, A.; Haddar, C.H.; Verhoeven, P.O.; Andres, P. Effect of a lotion containing the heat-treated probiotic strain Lactobacillus johnsonii NCC 533 on Staphylococcus aureus colonization in atopic dermatitis. *Clin. Cosmet. Investig. Dermatol.* **2017**, *10*, 249. [CrossRef] [PubMed]

59. Seité, S.; Zelenkova, H.; Martin, R. Clinical efficacy of emollients in atopic dermatitis patients–relationship with the skin microbiota modification. *Clin. Cosmet. Investig. Dermatol.* **2017**, *10*, 25. [CrossRef]

60. Bodemer, C.; Guillet, G.; Cambazard, F.; Boralevi, F.; Ballarini, S.; Milliet, C.; Bertuccio, P.; La Vecchia, C.; Bach, J.-F.; de Prost, Y. Adjuvant treatment with the bacterial lysate (OM-85) improves management of atopic dermatitis: A randomized study. *PLoS ONE* **2017**, *12*, e0161555. [CrossRef]

61. Kim, H.; Kim, H.R.; Kim, N.-R.; Jeong, B.J.; Lee, J.S.; Jang, S.; Chung, D.K. Oral administration of Lactobacillus plantarum lysates attenuates the development of atopic dermatitis lesions in mouse models. *J. Microbiol.* **2015**, *53*, 47–52. [CrossRef]

62. Kim, H.; Kim, H.R.; Jeong, B.J.; Lee, S.S.; Kim, T.-R.; Jeong, J.H.; Lee, M.; Lee, S.; Lee, J.S.; Chung, D.K. Effects of oral intake of kimchi-derived Lactobacillus plantarum K8 lysates on skin moisturizing. *J. Microbiol. Biotechnol.* **2015**, *25*, 74–80. [CrossRef]

63. Lau, S. Oral application of bacterial lysate in infancy diminishes the prevalence of atopic dermatitis in children at risk for atopy. *Benef. Microbes* **2014**, *5*, 147–149. [CrossRef] [PubMed]

64. Dunstan, J.; Brothers, S.; Bauer, J.; Hodder, M.; Jaksic, M.; Asher, M.; Prescott, S. The effects of Mycobacteria vaccae derivative on allergen-specific responses in children with atopic dermatitis. *Clin. Exp. Immunol.* **2011**, *164*, 321–329. [CrossRef] [PubMed]

65. Gupta, C.; Prakash, D.; Gupta, S. Natural useful therapeutic products from microbes. *Microbiol. Exp.* **2014**, *1*, 00006. [CrossRef]

66. Woo, T.E.; Sibley, C.D. The emerging utility of the cutaneous microbiome in the treatment of acne and atopic dermatitis. *J. Am. Acad. Dermatol.* **2019**. [CrossRef] [PubMed]

67. O'Sullivan, J.N.; Rea, M.C.; O'Connor, P.M.; Hill, C.; Ross, R.P. Human skin microbiota is a rich source of bacteriocin-producing staphylococci that kill human pathogens. *FEMS Microbiol. Ecol.* **2019**, *95*, fiy241. [CrossRef] [PubMed]

68. Jang, I.-T.; Yang, M.; Kim, H.-J.; Park, J.-K. Novel Cytoplasmic Bacteriocin Compounds Derived from Staphylococcus epidermidis Selectively Kill Staphylococcus aureus, Including Methicillin-Resistant Staphylococcus aureus (MRSA). *Pathogens* **2020**, *9*, 87. [CrossRef]

69. Noda, M.; Sultana, N.; Hayashi, I.; Fukamachi, M.; Sugiyama, M. Exopolysaccharide Produced by Lactobacillus paracasei IJH-SONE68 Prevents and Improves the Picryl Chloride-Induced Contact Dermatitis. *Molecules* **2019**, *24*, 2970. [CrossRef]

70. Li, H.; Goh, B.N.; Teh, W.K.; Jiang, Z.; Goh, J.P.Z.; Goh, A.; Wu, G.; Hoon, S.S.; Raida, M.; Camattari, A. Skin commensal Malassezia globosa secreted protease attenuates Staphylococcus aureus biofilm formation. *J. Investig. Dermatol.* **2018**, *138*, 1137–1145. [CrossRef]

71. Mangano, K.; Vergalito, F.; Mammana, S.; Mariano, A.; De Pasquale, R.; Meloscia, A.; Bartollino, S.; Guerra, G.; Nicoletti, F.; Di Marco, R. Evaluation of hyaluronic acid-P40 conjugated cream in a mouse model of dermatitis induced by oxazolone. *Exp. Ther. Med.* **2017**, *14*, 2439–2444. [CrossRef]

72. Matsui, K.; Tachioka, K.; Onodera, K.; Ikeda, R. Topical application of josamycin inhibits development of atopic dermatitis-like skin lesions in NC/Nga mice. *J. Pharm. Pharm. Sci.* **2017**, *20*, 38–47. [CrossRef]

73. Zipperer, A.; Konnerth, M.C.; Laux, C.; Berscheid, A.; Janek, D.; Weidenmaier, C.; Burian, M.; Schilling, N.A.; Slavetinsky, C.; Marschal, M. Human commensals producing a novel antibiotic impair pathogen colonization. *Nature* **2016**, *535*, 511–516. [CrossRef] [PubMed]

74. Kim, M.-S.; Kim, J.-E.; Yoon, Y.-S.; Kim, T.H.; Seo, J.-G.; Chung, M.-J.; Yum, D.-Y. Improvement of atopic dermatitis-like skin lesions by IL-4 inhibition of P14 protein isolated from Lactobacillus casei in NC/Nga mice. *Appl. Microbiol. Biotechnol.* **2015**, *99*, 7089–7099. [CrossRef] [PubMed]

75. Abbasi, J. Are bacteria transplants the future of eczema therapy? *JAMA* **2018**, *320*, 1094–1095. [CrossRef] [PubMed]

76. Perin, B.; Addetia, A.; Qin, X. Transfer of skin microbiota between two dissimilar autologous microenvironments: A pilot study. *PLoS ONE* **2019**, *14*, e0226857. [CrossRef] [PubMed]

77. Myles, I.A.; Earland, N.J.; Anderson, E.D.; Moore, I.N.; Kieh, M.D.; Williams, K.W.; Saleem, A.; Fontecilla, N.M.; Welch, P.A.; Darnell, D.A. First-in-human topical microbiome transplantation with Roseomonas mucosa for atopic dermatitis. *JCI Insight* **2018**, *3*, e120608. [CrossRef]

78. Wang, J.; Hui, P.; Kan, C.-W. Functionalized Textile Based Therapy for the Treatment of Atopic Dermatitis. *Coatings* **2017**, *7*, 82. [CrossRef]

79. Kakkar, V.; Saini, K. Scope of nano delivery for atopic dermatitis. *Ann. Pharmacol. Pharm.* **2017**, *2*, 1038.

80. Patra, J.K.; Das, G.; Fraceto, L.F.; Campos, E.V.R.; del Pilar Rodriguez-Torres, M.; Acosta-Torres, L.S.; Diaz-Torres, L.A.; Grillo, R.; Swamy, M.K.; Sharma, S.J. Nano based drug delivery systems: Recent developments and future prospects. *J. Nanobiotechnol.* **2018**, *16*, 71. [CrossRef]

81. Souto, E.B.; Dias-Ferreira, J.; Oliveira, J.; Sanchez-Lopez, E.; Lopez-Machado, A.; Espina, M.; Garcia, M.L.; Souto, S.B.; Martins-Gomes, C.; Silva, A.M. Trends in Atopic Dermatitis—From Standard Pharmacotherapy to Novel Drug Delivery Systems. *Int. J. Mol. Sci.* **2019**, *20*, 5659. [CrossRef]

82. Gupta, M.; Agrawal, U.; Vyas, S.P. Nanocarrier-based topical drug delivery for the treatment of skin diseases. *Expert Opin. Drug Deliv.* **2012**, *9*, 783–804. [CrossRef]

83. Dubey, V.; Mishra, D.; Dutta, T.; Nahar, M.; Saraf, D.; Jain, N. Dermal and transdermal delivery of an anti-psoriatic agent via ethanolic liposomes. *J. Control. Release* **2007**, *123*, 148–154. [CrossRef] [PubMed]

84. Puglia, C.; Bonina, F. Lipid nanoparticles as novel delivery systems for cosmetics and dermal pharmaceuticals. *Expert Opin. Drug Deliv.* **2012**, *9*, 429–441. [CrossRef] [PubMed]

85. Damiani, G.; Eggenhöffner, R.; Pigatto, P.D.M.; Bragazzi, N.L. Nanotechnology meets atopic dermatitis: Current solutions, challenges and future prospects. Insights and implications from a systematic review of the literature. *Bioact. Mater.* **2019**, *4*, 380–386. [CrossRef] [PubMed]

86. Khan, I.; Saeed, K.; Khan, I. Nanoparticles: Properties, applications and toxicities. *Arab. J. Chem.* **2019**, *12*, 908–931. [CrossRef]

87. Schäfer-Korting, M.; Mehnert, W.; Korting, H.-C. Lipid nanoparticles for improved topical application of drugs for skin diseases. *Adv. Drug Deliv. Rev.* **2007**, *59*, 427–443. [CrossRef]

88. Md, S.; Kuldeep Singh, J.K.A.P.; Waqas, M.; Pandey, M.; Choudhury, H.; Habib, H.; Hussain, F.; Hussain, Z. Nanoencapsulation of betamethasone valerate using high pressure homogenization–solvent evaporation technique: Optimization of formulation and process parameters for efficient dermal targeting. *Drug Dev. Ind. Pharm.* **2019**, *45*, 323–332. [CrossRef]

89. Kang, J.-H.; Chon, J.; Kim, Y.-I.; Lee, H.-J.; Oh, D.-W.; Lee, H.-G.; Han, C.-S.; Kim, D.-W.; Park, C.-W. Preparation and evaluation of tacrolimus-loaded thermosensitive solid lipid nanoparticles for improved dermal distribution. *Int. J. Nanomed.* **2019**, *14*, 5381. [CrossRef]

90. Pandey, M.; Choudhury, H.; Gunasegaran, T.A.; Nathan, S.S.; Md, S.; Gorain, B.; Tripathy, M.; Hussain, Z. Hyaluronic acid-modified betamethasone encapsulated polymeric nanoparticles: Fabrication, characterisation, in vitro release kinetics, and dermal targeting. *Drug Deliv. Transl. Res.* **2019**, *9*, 520–533. [CrossRef]

91. Siddique, M.I.; Katas, H.; Jamil, A.; Amin, M.C.I.M.; Ng, S.-F.; Zulfakar, M.H.; Nadeem, S.M. Potential treatment of atopic dermatitis: Tolerability and safety of cream containing nanoparticles loaded with hydrocortisone and hydroxytyrosol in human subjects. *Drug Deliv. Transl. Res.* **2019**, *9*, 469–481. [CrossRef]

92. Yu, K.; Wang, Y.; Wan, T.; Zhai, Y.; Cao, S.; Ruan, W.; Wu, C.; Xu, Y. Tacrolimus nanoparticles based on chitosan combined with nicotinamide: Enhancing percutaneous delivery and treatment efficacy for atopic dermatitis and reducing dose. *Int. J. Nanomed.* **2018**, *13*, 129. [CrossRef]

93. Nagaich, U.; Gulati, N. Preclinical assessment of steroidal nanostructured lipid carriers based gels for atopic dermatitis: Optimization and product development. *Curr. Drug Deliv.* **2018**, *15*, 641–651. [CrossRef] [PubMed]

94. Zhuo, F.; Abourehab, M.A.; Hussain, Z.J.C.P. Hyaluronic acid decorated tacrolimus-loaded nanoparticles: Efficient approach to maximize dermal targeting and anti-dermatitis efficacy. *Carbohydr. Polym.* **2018**, *197*, 478–489. [CrossRef] [PubMed]

95. Radbruch, M.; Pischon, H.; Ostrowski, A.; Volz, P.; Brodwolf, R.; Neumann, F.; Unbehauen, M.; Kleuser, B.; Haag, R.; Ma, N. Dendritic core-multishell nanocarriers in murine models of healthy and atopic skin. *Nanoscale Res. Lett.* **2017**, *12*, 1–12. [CrossRef] [PubMed]

96. Siddique, M.I.; Katas, H.; Amin, M.C.I.M.; Ng, S.-F.; Zulfakar, M.H.; Jamil, A. In-vivo dermal pharmacokinetics, efficacy, and safety of skin targeting nanoparticles for corticosteroid treatment of atopic dermatitis. *Int. J. Pharm.* **2016**, *507*, 72–82. [CrossRef]

97. Hussain, Z.; Katas, H.; Amin, M.C.I.M.; Kumolosasi, E. Efficient immuno-modulation of TH1/TH2 biomarkers in 2, 4-dinitrofluorobenzene-induced atopic dermatitis: Nanocarrier-mediated transcutaneous co-delivery of anti-inflammatory and antioxidant drugs. *PLoS ONE* **2014**, *9*, e113143. [CrossRef]

98. Hussain, Z.; Katas, H.; Amin, M.C.I.M.; Kumolosasi, E.; Sahudin, S. Downregulation of immunological mediators in 2, 4-dinitrofluorobenzene-induced atopic dermatitis-like skin lesions by hydrocortisone-loaded chitosan nanoparticles. *Int. J. Nanomed.* **2014**, *9*, 5143.

99. Peralta, M.F.; Guzmán, M.L.; Pérez, A.; Apezteguia, G.A.; Fórmica, M.L.; Romero, E.L.; Olivera, M.E.; Carrer, D.C. Liposomes can both enhance or reduce drugs penetration through the skin. *Sci. Rep.* **2018**, *8*, 1–11. [CrossRef]

100. Godin, B.; Touitou, E. Ethosomes: New prospects in transdermal delivery. *Crit. Rev. Ther. Drug Carr. Syst.* **2003**, *20*, 63–102. [CrossRef]

101. Benson, H.A. Vesicles for transdermal delivery of peptides and proteins. In *Percutaneous Penetration Enhancers Chemical Methods in Penetration Enhancement*; Springer: Berlin, Germany, 2016; pp. 297–307.

102. Carreras, J.J.; Tapia-Ramirez, W.E.; Sala, A.; Guillot, A.J.; Garrigues, T.M.; Melero, A. Ultraflexible lipid vesicles allow topical absorption of cyclosporin A. *Drug Deliv. Transl. Res.* **2019**, *24*, 1–12. [CrossRef]

103. Akhtar, N.; Verma, A.; Pathak, K. Investigating the penetrating potential of nanocomposite β-cycloethosomes: Development using central composite design, in vitro and ex vivo characterization. *J. Liposome Res.* **2018**, *28*, 35–48. [CrossRef]

104. Augustin, M.; Goepel, L.; Jacobi, A.; Bosse, B.; Mueller, S.; Hopp, M. Efficacy and tolerability of liposomal polyvinylpyrrolidone-iodine hydrogel for the localized treatment of chronic infective, inflammatory, dermatoses: An uncontrolled pilot study. *Clin. Cosmet. Investig. Dermatol.* **2017**, *10*, 373. [CrossRef] [PubMed]

105. Akhtar, N.; Verma, A.; Pathak, K. Feasibility of binary composition in development of nanoethosomal glycolic vesicles of triamcinolone acetonide using Box-behnken design: In vitro and ex vivo characterization. *Artif. Cells Nanomed. Biotechnol.* **2017**, *45*, 1123–1131. [CrossRef] [PubMed]

106. Goindi, S.; Dhatt, B.; Kaur, A. Ethosomes-based topical delivery system of antihistaminic drug for treatment of skin allergies. *J. Microencapsul.* **2014**, *31*, 716–724. [CrossRef] [PubMed]

107. Goindi, S.; Kumar, G.; Kaur, A. Novel flexible vesicles based topical formulation of levocetirizine: In vivo evaluation using oxazolone-induced atopic dermatitis in murine model. *J. Liposome Res.* **2014**, *24*, 249–257. [CrossRef] [PubMed]

108. Goddard, A.L.; Lio, P.A. Alternative, complementary, and forgotten remedies for atopic dermatitis. *Evid. Based Complement. Altern. Med.* **2015**, *2015*, 676897. [CrossRef] [PubMed]

109. Kim, J.; Kim, B.E.; Leung, D.Y. Pathophysiology of atopic dermatitis: Clinical implications. *Proc. Allergy Asthma Proc.* **2019**, *40*, 84–92. [CrossRef]

110. Kakkar, V.; Kumar, M.; Saini, K. An Overview of Atopic Dermatitis with a Focus on Nano-Interventions. *Innovations* **2019**, *1*, 2019.

111. Schneider, L.; Tilles, S.; Lio, P.; Boguniewicz, M.; Beck, L.; LeBovidge, J.; Novak, N.; Bernstein, D.; Blessing-Moore, J.; Khan, D. Atopic dermatitis: A practice parameter update 2012. *J. Allergy Clin. Immunol.* **2013**, *131*, 295–299.e227. [CrossRef]

112. Ring, J.; Alomar, A.; Bieber, T.; Deleuran, M.; Fink-Wagner, A.; Gelmetti, C.; Gieler, U.; Lipozencic, J.; Luger, T.; Oranje, A. Guidelines for treatment of atopic eczema (atopic dermatitis) part I. *J. Eur. Acad. Dermatol. Venereol.* **2012**, *26*, 1045–1060. [CrossRef]

113. Silverberg, J.I. Public health burden and epidemiology of atopic dermatitis. *Dermatol. Clin.* **2017**, *35*, 283–289. [CrossRef]

114. Balato, A.; Cacciapuoti, S.; Caprio, R.; Marasca, C.; Masarà, A.; Raimondo, A.; Fabbrocini, G. Human Microbiome: Composition and Role in Inflammatory Skin Diseases. *Arch. Immunol. Ther. Exp.* **2018**. [CrossRef] [PubMed]

115. Lacour, J.-P. Skin microbiota and atopic dermatitis: Toward new therapeutic options? In Proceedings of Annales de dermatologie et de venereologie. *Ann. Dermatol. Venereol.* **2015**, *142*, S18–S22. [CrossRef]

116. Kim, S.-O.; Ah, Y.-M.; Yu, Y.M.; Choi, K.H.; Shin, W.-G.; Lee, J.-Y. Effects of probiotics for the treatment of atopic dermatitis: A meta-analysis of randomized controlled trials. *Ann. Allergy Asthma Immunol.* **2014**, *113*, 217–226. [CrossRef] [PubMed]

117. Kano, H.; Kita, J.; Makino, S.; Ikegami, S.; Itoh, H. Oral administration of Lactobacillus delbrueckii subspecies bulgaricus OLL1073R-1 suppresses inflammation by decreasing interleukin-6 responses in a murine model of atopic dermatitis. *J. Dairy Sci.* **2013**, *96*, 3525–3534. [CrossRef]

118. Brandwein, M.; Fuks, G.; Israel, A.; Sabbah, F.; Hodak, E.; Szitenberg, A.; Harari, M.; Steinberg, D.; Bentwich, Z.; Shental, N. Skin Microbiome Compositional Changes in Atopic Dermatitis Accompany Dead Sea Climatotherapy. *Photochem. Photobiol.* **2019**, *95*, 1446–1453. [CrossRef]

119. Baviera, G.; Leoni, M.C.; Capra, L.; Cipriani, F.; Longo, G.; Maiello, N.; Ricci, G.; Galli, E. Microbiota in healthy skin and in atopic eczema. *BioMed Res. Int.* **2014**, *2014*, 436921. [CrossRef]

120. Paller, A.S.; Kong, H.H.; Seed, P.; Naik, S.; Scharschmidt, T.C.; Gallo, R.L.; Luger, T.; Irvine, A.D. The microbiome in patients with atopic dermatitis. *J. Allergy Clin. Immunol.* **2019**, *143*, 26–35. [CrossRef]

121. Okuda, K.-I.; Zendo, T.; Sugimoto, S.; Iwase, T.; Tajima, A.; Yamada, S.; Sonomoto, K.; Mizunoe, Y. Effects of bacteriocins on methicillin-resistant Staphylococcus aureus biofilm. *Antimicrob. Agents Chemother.* **2013**, *57*, 5572–5579. [CrossRef]

122. Sun, L.; Liu, Z.; Cun, D.; HY Tong, H.; Zheng, Y. Application of nano-and micro-particles on the topical therapy of skin-related immune disorders. *Curr. Pharm. Des.* **2015**, *21*, 2643–2667. [CrossRef]

123. Okada, H. Drug discovery by formulation design and innovative drug delivery systems (DDS). *Yakugaku Zasshi J. Pharm. Soc. JPN* **2011**, *131*, 1271–1287. [CrossRef]

124. Directive, C. 93/42/EEC of 14 June 1993 Concerning Medical Devices. *Official Journal of the European Communities*, 12 July 1993; OJ L 169.

125. Gottlieb, S. Statement from FDA Commissioner Scott Gottlieb, MD, on the Agency's Scientific Evidence on the Presence of Opioid Compounds in Kratom, Underscoring Its Potential for Abuse. Silver Spring MD Food Drug Adm. 2018. Available online: https://www.fda.gov/news-events/press-announcements/statement-fda-commissioner-scott-gottlieb-md-agencys-scientific-evidence-presence-opioid-compounds (accessed on 22 November 2020).

126. Dickinson, A.M.; Godden, J.M.; Lanovyk, K.; Ahmed, S.S. Assessing the safety of nanomedicines: A mini review. *Appl. In Vitro Toxicol.* **2019**, *5*, 114–122. [CrossRef]

127. Palmer, B.C.; DeLouise, L.A. Nanoparticle-enabled transdermal drug delivery systems for enhanced dose control and tissue targeting. *Molecules* **2016**, *21*, 1719. [CrossRef] [PubMed]

8

3-Amino-5-(indol-3-yl)methylene-4-oxo-2-thioxothiazolidine Derivatives as Antimicrobial Agents: Synthesis, Computational and Biological Evaluation

Volodymyr Horishny [1], Victor Kartsev [2], Vasyl Matiychuk [3], Athina Geronikaki [4,*][ID], Petrou Anthi [4][ID], Pavel Pogodin [5], Vladimir Poroikov [5][ID], Marija Ivanov [6][ID], Marina Kostic [6], Marina D. Soković [6][ID] and Phaedra Eleftheriou [7]

[1] Department of Chemistry, Danylo Halytsky Lviv National Medical University, Pekarska 69, 79010 Lviv, Ukraine; vgor58@ukr.net

[2] InterBioScreen, 142432 Chernogolovka, Moscow Region, Russia; vkartsev@ibscreen.chg.ru

[3] Department of Chemistry, Ivan Franko National University of Lviv, Kyryla i Mefodia 6, 79005 Lviv, Ukraine; v_matiychuk@ukr.net

[4] School of Pharmacy, Aristotle University of Thessaloniki, 54124 Thessaloniki, Greece; anthi.petrou.thessaloniki1@gmail.com

[5] Institute of Biomedical Chemistry, Pogodinskaya Street 10 Bldg.8, 119121 Moscow, Russia; pogodinpv@gmail.com (P.P.); vladimir.poroikov@ibmc.msk.ru (V.P.)

[6] Mycological Laboratory, Department of Plant Physiology, Institute for Biological Research, Siniša, Stanković-National Institute of Republic of Serbia, University of Belgrade, Bulevar Despota Stefana 142, 11000 Belgrade, Serbia; marija.smiljkovic@ibiss.bg.ac.rs (M.I.); marina.kostic@ibiss.bg.ac.rs (M.K.); mris@ibiss.bg.ac.rs (M.D.S.)

[7] Department of Biomedical Sciences, School of Health Sciences, International Hellenic University, Sindos, 57400 Thessaloniki, Greece; eleftheriouphaedra@gmail.com

* Correspondence: geronik@pharm.auth.gr

Abstract: Herein we report the design, synthesis, computational, and experimental evaluation of the antimicrobial activity of fourteen new 3-amino-5-(indol-3-yl) methylene-4-oxo-2-thioxothiazolidine derivatives. The structures were designed, and their antimicrobial activity and toxicity were predicted in silico. All synthesized compounds exhibited antibacterial activity against eight Gram-positive and Gram-negative bacteria. Their activity exceeded those of ampicillin and (for the majority of compounds) streptomycin. The most sensitive bacterium was *S. aureus* (American Type Culture Collection ATCC 6538), while *L. monocytogenes* (NCTC 7973) was the most resistant. The best antibacterial activity was observed for compound **5d** (Z)-N-(5-((1H-indol-3-yl)methylene)-4-oxo-2-thioxothiazolidin-3-yl)-4-hydroxybenzamide (Minimal inhibitory concentration, MIC at 37.9–113.8 µM, and Minimal bactericidal concentration MBC at 57.8–118.3 µM). Three most active compounds **5d, 5g,** and **5k** being evaluated against three resistant strains, Methicillin resistant *Staphilococcus aureus* (MRSA), *P. aeruginosa*, and *E. coli*, were more potent against MRSA than ampicillin (MIC at 248–372 µM, MBC at 372–1240 µM). At the same time, streptomycin (MIC at 43–172 µM, MBC at 86–344 µM) did not show bactericidal activity at all. The compound **5d** was also more active than ampicillin towards resistant *P. aeruginosa* strain. Antifungal activity of all compounds exceeded those of the reference antifungal agents bifonazole (MIC at 480–640 µM, and MFC at 640–800 µM) and ketoconazole (MIC 285–475 µM and MFC 380–950 µM). The best activity was exhibited by compound **5g**. The most sensitive fungal was *T. viride* (IAM 5061), while *A. fumigatus* (human isolate) was the most resistant. Low cytotoxicity against HEK-293 human embryonic kidney cell line and reasonable selectivity indices were shown for the most active compounds **5d, 5g, 5k, 7c** using thiazolyl blue tetrazolium bromide MTT assay.

The docking studies indicated a probable involvement of *E. coli* Mur B inhibition in the antibacterial action, while CYP51 inhibition is likely responsible for the antifungal activity of the tested compounds.

Keywords: indole; thioxothiazolidine; antibacterial activity; antifungal activity; computer-aided prediction; docking; Mur B; CYP 51

1. Introduction

Infectious diseases affect large populations and cause significant morbidity and mortality [1]. They represent a global indirect load on public health security and an impact on socio-economic stability worldwide. Bacterial, fungal, and viral infections have monopolized the dominant factors of death and disability of millions of humans for centuries. They are presently plaguing and even ravaging populations worldwide each year with performances far surpassing wars [2].

It should be mentioned that several dozen new infections have grown and affected the health of billions of people over the world, mainly in developing countries [3]. Unfortunately, there are no successful pharmaceuticals or vaccines for many of these new infections [3].

The treatment of infectious disease is still an imperative and demanding problem due to the growing number of multi-drug resistant pathogens, especially Gram-positive bacteria. Due to this, the lack of effective antimicrobial drugs, morbidity, and mortality notably increased [4].

Drug resistance causes vast human suffering, and now it is one of the most significant challenges of the twenty-first century. Species such as the methicillin-resistant *S. aureus* and vancomycin-resistant enterococci have emerged due to the irrational or overuse of antimicrobial agents [5].

The pathogens, including *Enterococcus faecium*, *Staphylococcus aureus*, *Klebsiella pneumoniae*, *Acinetobacter baumannii*, *Pseudomonas aeruginosa*, and *Enterobacter spp.* which also called ESCAPE pathogens, are of particular importance since they play a significant role affecting several human organs including the lung and urinary system. Besides, they exhibited increased resistance to clinically used antibiotics [6].

Numerous of these pathogens are Gram-negative bacteria, which are of specific concern due to their resistance of up to 50% against carbapenems that have been reported in some developing countries [6]. Despite the availability of some new antibiotics against Gram-positive pathogens, no treatment of these pathogens with a new class of compounds has been introduced in the last 40 years. Therefore, to overcome the resistance, the discovery of safer and more effective antimicrobial agents with a different mechanism of action is still an urgent need [7].

The interest in thiazolidine-based compounds attracted the attention of medicinal chemists, and a plethora of them have been studied to evaluate pharmacological properties [8–10]. Despite the appearance of some controversial opinions regarding the analysis of the molecular mechanism of their action, prominent representatives among the developed drug-like molecules are thiazolidinone derivatives [11,12] since they are a valuable source of building blocks for the development of novel molecules [13–15].

N-(4-oxo-2-thioxothiazolidin-3-yl)carboxamides exhibit antimicrobial [16–20] and antitumor [21–23] actions, are dual COX-1/2 and 5-LOX inhibitors [24,25], non-nucleoside inhibitors of Hepatitis C NS5b RNA polymerase [26,27] and HIV-1 reverse transcriptase inhibitors [28].

The combination of the thiazolidinone ring with other pharmacologically promising heterocycles has been a warranted approach for developing new "drug-like" molecules with the desired activity profile [29–31]. Our previous studies showed that thiazolidinone core with indole fragment in one molecule gave the compounds with high antimicrobial activity [19].

On the other hand, indole derivatives represent another scaffold widely spread in nature with a broad spectrum of biological activities. The indole ring was found not only in natural compounds but also in diverse semisynthetic and synthetic drug-like molecules [32,33].

They exhibit antimicrobial [34–39], anti-inflammatory [40,41], COX inhibitory [42,43] anticancer [44–46], antiviral [47,48], anti-HIV [49,50], and antidiabetic [51] activities. Among the natural compounds containing the indolene fragment, several imidazoline and imidazolidine alkaloids are known, which have a wide spectrum of biological activity, including antibacterial. Thus, indole-containing azahydantoins 1-6 from sponges and streptomycetes have a potent antibacterial and antiseptic action (Figure 1) [52–54]:

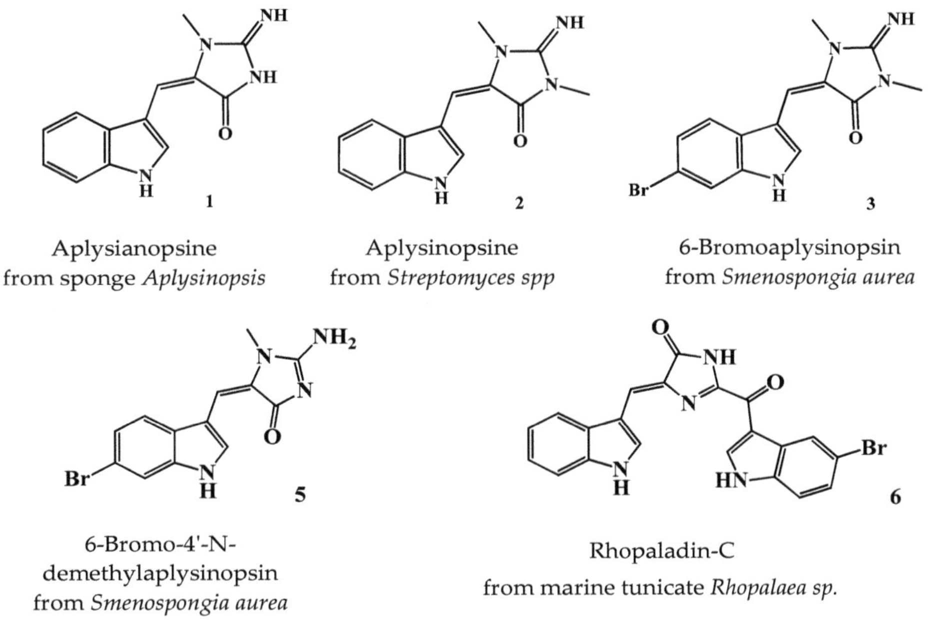

Figure 1. Structure of indole-containing azahydantoins 1-5 from sponges and streptomycetes.

It is also known that synthetic thiohydantoin (rhodanine) analogs 7, 8 (Figure 2), exhibit pronounced antibacterial properties [55].

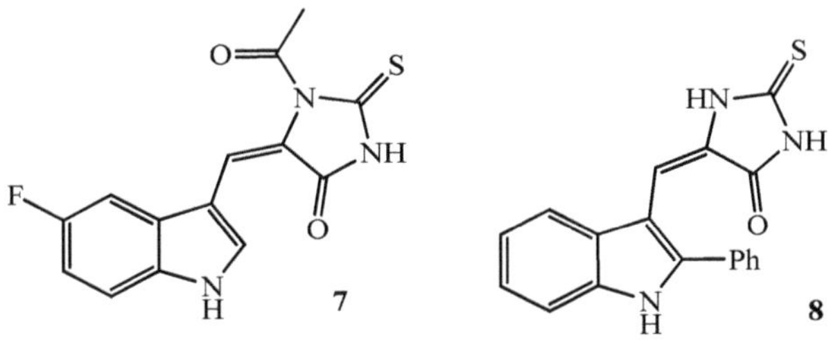

Figure 2. Synthetic thiohydantoin analogues.

Therefore, the design and development of hybrid molecules combining thiazolidinone and indole cores in the same structure is a promising approach. Taking into account all issues mentioned above and encouraging results obtained in our earlier studies [19], in this paper, we present the synthesis and biological evaluation of new (1H-indole-3-yl-methylene)-4-oxo-2-thioxothiazolidin derivatives with potent antimicrobial activity.

2. Results and Discussion

2.1. In Silico Antimicrobial Activity Estimation

2.1.1. Antibacterial Activity

Using AntiBac-Pred [56] one of the predictive web services of Way2Drug platform [57], activity against at least one strain of bacteria was predicted for each of the fourteen designed compounds with Pa-Pi values in the range from 0.001 to 0.309. According to the prediction results, the highest probability of antibacterial activity against the *Bacillus subtilis subsp. subtilis* str. 168 was estimated for derivatives **7a** and **5b** (Pa-Pi values are 0.309 and 0.305, respectively).

Similarly, we estimated in silico the probability of antibacterial activity for the reference drugs streptomycin and ampicillin. For both reference drugs, wide antibacterial action was predicted. For the top-10 predictions of streptomycin Pa-Pi values vary from 0.905 to 0.947; for ampicillin—from 0.712 to 0.989. Contrary, for relatively new antibacterial agent trifolirhizin, which structure was disclosed only on July 7, 2020 (Clarivate Analytics Integrity [58]), the top-10 predictions Pa-Pi values vary from 0.369 to 0.552.

2.1.2. Antifungal Activity

Using web service AntiFun-Pred [59], activity against at least one of the fungal species was predicted for six of the fourteen studied compounds with Pa-Pi values ranging from 0.001 to 0.112. The results show that among the studied compounds, derivatives 5a (Pa-Pi against *Trichophyton mentagrophytes* equals 0.112) and 7a (Pa-Pi against *Candida equals* 0.101) have better chances to be found active in biological evaluation of the antifungal activity.

The results of in silico antimicrobial activity assessment are given in the supplementary file PASSweb_results_13mols.xlsx. Small Pa-Pi values reflect the novelty of the analyzed compounds compared to those included in the PASS training set.

Similarly, for the reference drug ketoconazole wide antifungal action was predicted with Pa-Pi values in the range 0.622–0.812 (top-10 predictions), while for the new antifungal agent drimenin disclosed on 12 June 2020 (Clarivate Analytics Integrity [58]), only two antifungal activity were predicted with Pa-Pi values 0.007 and 0.030.

2.1.3. Acute Rat Toxicity

Using web service based on GUSAR software [60,61], acute rat toxicity with regards to different administration routes was estimated for the studied compounds. LD50 values and toxicity classes are given in Table 1. Most of the predictions indicate that the studied compounds belong to the fifth or fourth rodent toxicity classes.

Table 1. In silico assessments of acute rat toxicity.

Compound ID	LD_{50}, mg/kg				Toxicity Class			
	IP	IV	Oral	SC	IP	IV	Oral	SC
5a	809.8	402.5	1218	780.4 *	5	5	4	4 *
5b	680.4	309	1266	1434	5	5	4	5
5c	980.3	311.5	1325	619.9 *	5	5	4	4 *
5d								
5e	1263	466	843.9	440 *	NT	5	4	4 *
5f	1266	502.2	469.2	477.7 *	NT	5	4	4 *
5g	1010 *	371.9	192.4 *	397.6 *	5 *	5	3 *	4 *
5h	1282	448.5	1001	1588	NT	5	4	5
5i	1299	476.5	732.3	545.4 *	NT	5	4	4 *
5j	1258	381.6	196.2 *	422 *	NT	5	3 *	4 *
5k	1031 *	398.3	202.8 *	442 *	5 *	5	3 *	4 *
7a	1033	236.6	593.7	1644 *	5	4	4	5 *
7b	1061	287.2	720 *	862.1 *	5	4	4 *	4 *
7c	1180 *	210.7	765.1 *	682 *	5 *	4	4 *	4 *

Notes: *: Calculated for compounds that do not correspond to the model's applicability domain; thus, they are less reliable than unmarked ones. NT: Non-Toxic.

2.2. Chemistry

The starting N-(4-oxo-2-thioxothiazolidin-3-yl) -carbamides **3a-d** was prepared by reacting the acid hydrazides **1a-d** with trithiocarbonyl diglycolic acid (Scheme 1). The reaction was carried out in a medium of boiling aqueous alcohol. The yield of the products was 83–97%.

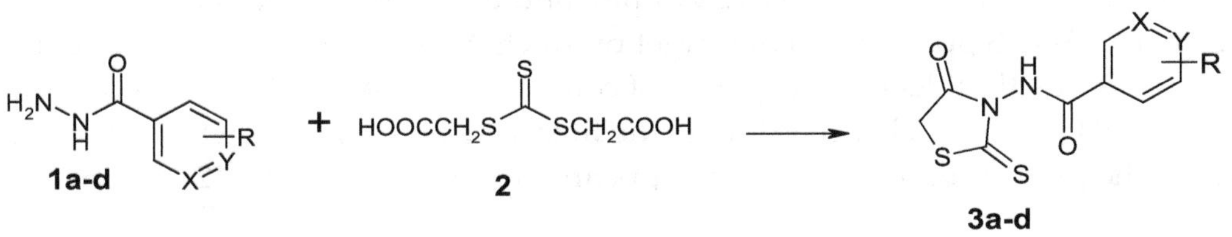

1a, 3a R = 2-OH, X = Y = CH; **1b, 3b** R = 4-OH, X = Y = CH; **1c, 3c** X = N, R = H, Y = CH;
1d, 3d Y = N, R = H, X = CH

Scheme 1. Synthesis of initial compounds.

The titled compounds were synthesized according to the process shown in Scheme 2.

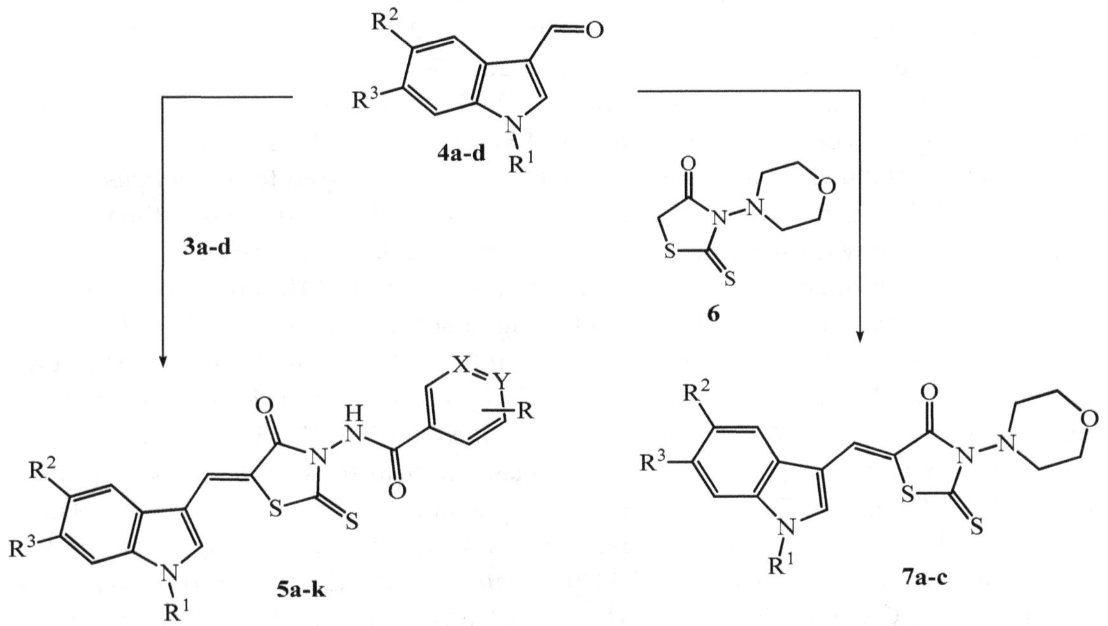

4a R^1 = R^2 = R^3 = H; **4b** R^1 = CH$_3$, R^2= R^3 = H; **4c** R^2 = OCH$_3$ R^1 = R^3 = H; **4d** R^3 = OCH$_3$ R^1 = R^2 = H.
5a R = 2-OH, R^1 = CH$_3$, R^2 = R^3 = H, X = Y = CH; **5b** R = 2-OH, R^2 = OCH$_3$, R^1 = R^3 = H, X = Y = CH;
5c R = 2-OH,R^3 = OCH$_3$, R^1 = R^2 = H, X = Y = CH; **5d** R = 4-OH, R^1 = R^2 = R^3 = H, X = Y = CH;
5e X = N, R = R^1 = R^2 = R^3 = H, Y = CH; **5f** X = N, R^1 = CH$_3$, R = R^2 = R^3 = H, Y = CH;
5g X = N, R^2 = OCH$_3$, R = R^1 = R^3 = H, Y = CH; **5h** Y = N, R = R^1 = R^2 = R^3 = H, X = CH;
5i Y = N, R^1 = CH$_3$, R = R^2 = R^3 = H, X = CH; **5j** Y = N, R^2 = OCH$_3$, R = R^1 = R^3 = H, X = CH;
5k Y = N, R^3 = OCH$_3$, R = R^1= R^2 = H, X = CH.
7a R^1 = R^2 = R^3 = H, **7b** R^1 = CH$_3$, R^2 = R^3= H; **7c** R^2 = OCH$_3$, R^1 = R^3 = H.

Scheme 2. Synthesis of final compounds.

The reaction of N-(4-oxo-2-thioxothiazolidin-3-yl)carbamides **3a–d** with indole-3-carbaldehydes **4a-d** in acetic acid in the presence of an ammonium acetate catalyst afforded with high yield 5-[(R-1*H*-indol-3-yl)methylene]-4-oxo-2-thioxothiazolidin-3-ylcarbamides **5a–k**, while upon reaction of indole-3-carbaldehydes **4a–d** with 3-morpholino-2-thioxothiazolidin-4-one **6** in the same conditions 5-[(R-1*H*-indol-3-yl) methylene] -3-morpholin-4-yl-2-thioxothiazolidin-4-ones **7a–c** were obtained.

All compounds were characterized by IR, ^{1}H and ^{13}C NMR spectroscopy. In the IR spectra of compounds **3a–d, 5a–k,** and **7a, 7c**, the carbonyl group of the 4-thiazolidone ring absorbs at 1753.21–1690.53 cm^{-1}, and the thiocarbonyl group—at 1608.56–1556.48 cm^{-1}. The absorption band of the carbonyl group of the amide fragment of **3a–d** and **5a–k** is located at 1689.56–1654.84 cm^{-1}.

In the starting 3-substituted 2-thione-4-thiazolidones, the amide proton NH-CO of the compounds **3a–d** appears as a singlet in the range 11.95-10.91 ppm, and the cyclic methylene group resonates as a singlet or quartet at 4.55–4.48 ppm. etc. In the target products **5a–k**, the amide proton is in the range of 11.85–11.12 ppm. The 5-methylidene proton CH = of compounds **5a–k** and **7a, 7c** resonates in the form of a singlet at 8.20–7.94 ppm, which, according to the literature [9,62], is characteristic of the Z isomer. The singlet NH of the protons of the indole ring appeared in the range 12.31–12.06 ppm.

2.3. Biological Evaluation

2.3.1. Antibacterial Activity

Compounds **5a–k** and **7a–c** were evaluated for antibacterial activity, by microdilution method to determine the minimal bacteriostatic and bactericidal concentrations. As reference compounds, we used ampicillin and streptomycin, which are both broad-spectrum antibiotics commonly applied to treat different conditions. Antibacterial activity of tested compounds is shown in Table 2 with MIC values in the range of 36.5–211.5 µM and MBC at 73.3–282.0 µM. According to the order of activity which can be presented as: **5d > 5g > 5k > 5j > 5c > 5h > 5e > 5f > 5a > 7c > 7b > 5b > 7a > 5i** the best activity is achieved for compound **5d** with MIC at 37.9–113.8 µM and MBC at 75.9–151.7 µM. The lowest antibacterial activity was observed for compound **5i** with MIC values in the range of 76.1–152.1 µM and MBC at 152.1–304.2 µM. The most sensitive bacterium appeared to be *S.aureus* (ATCC 6538), *En. cloacae* (ATCC 35,030) was the second most sensitive, while *S.Typhimirium* was the most resistant one. Another resistant strain was Gram-negative bacterium *S. Typhimurium* (ATCC 13,311).

Compound **7b** exhibited good activity against *B. cereus* with MIC and MBC at 41.7 and 83.4 µM respectively. Compound **5d** appeared to be potent against *S. aureus* (ATCC 6538), *P. aeruginosa* (ATCC 27,853), and *En. cloacaei* (ATCC 35,030) with MIC at 37.9 µM and MBC at 75.9 µM. It also showed good activity against *B. cereus* with MIC and MBC at 55.6 and 75.9 µM respectively. Compound **5h** appeared to be potent against *En. cloacae* and *P. aeruginosa* (ATCC 27,853) with MIC and MBC at 39.4 and 78.9 µM. Good activity against these two species and *S. aureus* (ATCC 6538) was also shown by compound 5j (MIC/MBC 58.6/73.1 µM). Good activity against *S. aureus* (ATCC 6538), also exhibited by compound **7b** with MIC at 41.7 µM and MBC at 83.4 µM. On the other hand, compound **5g** exhibited good activity against *En. cloacae* (ATCC 35030), *S. aureus* (ATCC 6538), and *S. typhimurium* (ATCC 13311) with MIC/MBC values 36.5/73.1 and 53.6/73.1 µM, respectively. It is worth to notice that all compounds appeared to be more potent than ampicillin against all bacteria used and more active than streptomycin against all bacteria except *B. cereus* and *S. typhimurium* (ATCC 13,311).

The structure-activity studies revealed that the most beneficial for antibacterial activity is the presence of hydroxybenzamide (**5d**) on the N-atom of (Z)-5-((5-methoxy-1H-indol-3-yl)methylene)-3-morpholino-2-thioxothiazolidin-4-one. Introduction of the 5-methoxy group to indole ring and replacement of hydroxybenzamide by nicotinamide (**5g**) decreased a little activity while shifting of methoxy group from position 5 to position 6 of indole ring and replacement of nicotinamide by isonicotinamide led to less active compound **5k** compared to compound **5g**.

On the other hand, the isonicotinamide derivative of (Z)-5-((1-methyl-indol-3-yl)methylene)-2-thioxothiazolidin-4-one (**5i**) appeared to be the less active compound. It was observed that for (Z)-5- [(1H-indol-3-yl)methylene]-2-thioxothiazolidin-4-one (**5h**) as well as for (Z)-N-5-[(1-methyl-1H-indol-3-yl)methylene]-4-oxo-2-thioxothiazolidin-4-one (**5g**) derivatives isonicotinamide substituent is endowed with better activity. The opposite was observed for 6-methoxy indole derivatives where more preferable is nicotinamide as a substituent (**5k**). Between methylindole derivatives (**5a, 5f, 5i**), more favorable for activity was nicotinamide substituent (**5f**), followed by benzamide, (**5a**) while isonicotinamide (**5i**) had a negative effect on antibacterial activity. For -2-hydroxybenzamides derivatives more preferable for antibacterial activity appeared to be 6-methoxy substitution of indole ring (**5c**) followed by methylidole (**5a**) while 5-methoxy substitution on indole ring was negative leading to one of the less active compounds (**5b**). In the case of 3-morpholino-2-thioxothiazolidin-4- one derivatives (**7a–c**), which were among the less active compound, it seems that 5-methoxy substitution on indole ring is preferable than methylindole or indole ring.

Thus, it can be concluded that the most favorable effect on the antibacterial activity of the target compounds is provided by the introduction into the molecule of an unsubstituted indolidene and 6-methoxyindolidene fragment. In addition, the nature of the substituent at position 3 of the thiazolidine ring has a direct influence on the enhancement of the antibacterial action. An increase in the antibacterial effect is observed from the use of 4-hydroxybenzamide and isonicotinamide substitutes.

From all mentioned above, it is evident that the antibacterial activity of these compounds depends not only on substituent and its position in the indole ring but also on substituent on the N-atom of 2-thioxothiazolidin-4-one ring.

Table 2. Antibacterial activity of compounds **5a–k** and **7a–c** (MIC/MBC in μM).

Com/d ID		B.c	M.f	S.a	L.m	En.cl	P.a	S.T	E.coli
5a	MIC	73.3 ± 0.4	109.9 ± 0.1	73.3 ± 0.3	146.5 ± 1.0	73.3 ± 0.8	73.3 ± 0.08	73.3 ± 0.08	109.9 ± 0.1
	MBC	146.5 ± 1.0	146.5 ± 2.0	146.5 ± 2.0	293.0 ± 4.0	146.5 ± 1.0	146.5 ± 1.0	146.5 ± 1.0	146.5 ± 2.0
5b	MIC	70.5 ± 0.4	105.8 ± 0.8	70.5 ± 0.8	105.8 ± 1.5	70.5 ± 0.8	70.5 ± 0.8	141.0 ± 1.2	211.5 ± 2.0
	MBC	141.0 ± 1.0	141.0 ± 2.0	141.0 ± 1.0	141.0 ± 2.0	141.0 ± 1.0	141.0 ± 0.1	282.0 ± 3.0	282.0 ± 2.0
5c	MIC	68.2 ± 0.8	102.6 ± 1.0	68.4 ± 0.5	68.4 ± 0.4	68.4 ± 0.4	68.4 ± 0.4	102.6 ± 1.0	102.6 ± 1.5
	MBC	136.8 ± 1.0	136.8 ± 1.5	136.8 ± .1.0	136.8 ± 1.0	136.8 ± 1.0	136.8 ± 1.0	136.8 ± 1.5	136.8 ± 2.0
5d	MIC	55.6 ± 0.2	113.8 ± 0.8	37.9 ± 0.2	113.8 ± 0.8	37.9 ± 0.4	37.9 ± 0.2	113.8 ± 1.0	75.6 ± 0.4
	MBC	75.9 ± 0.4	151.7 ± 2.0	75.9 ± 0.5	151.7 ± 2.0	75.9 ± 0.8	75.9 ± 0.6	151.7 ± 1.0	151.7 ± 1.0
5e	MIC	78.9 ± 0.2	118.3 ± 1.0	57.8 ± 0.4	78.9 ± 0.5	78.9 ± 0.1	78.9 ± 0.6	78.9 ± 0.8	118.3 ± 1.0
	MBC	157.7 ± 0.8	157.7 ± 2.0	78.9 ± 0.8	157.7 ± 1.5	157.7 ± 2.0	157.7 ± 1.5	157.7 ± 1.0	157.7 ± 2.0
5f	MIC	114.1 ± 1.0	114.1 ± 8.0	114.1 ± 1.0	76.1 ± 0.4	76.1 ± 0.8	76.1 ± 0.3	114.1 ± 1.5	114.1 ± 1.0
	MBC	152.1 ± 2.0	152.1 ± 1.0	152.1 ± 1.5	152.1 ± 1.0	152.1 ± 1.0	152.1 ± 1.0	152.1 ± 2.0	152.1 ± 1.0
5g	MIC	73.1 ± 1.0	73.1 ± 1.0	53.6 ± 0.4	73.1 ± 0.8	36.5 ± 0.5	109.6 ± 1.0	53.6 ± 0.6	109.6 ± 1.0
	MBC	146.2 ± 1.0	146.2 ± 1.0	73.1 ± 0.8	146.2 ± 1.6	73.1 ± 1.0	146.2 ± 1.2	73.1 ± 1.0	146.2 ± 2.0
5h	MIC	78.9 ± 0.5	118.3 ± 1.5	118.3 ± 1.0	78.9 ± 0.8	39.4 ± 0.5	39.4 ± 0.6	78.9 ± 0.6	118.3 ± 1.5
	MBC	157.7 ± 1.0	157.7 ± 2.0	157.7 ± 2.0	157.7 ± 1.0	78.9 ± 0.8	78.9 ± 0.8	157.7 ± 1.2	157.7 ± 1.0
5i	MIC	114.1 ± 1.0	114.1 ± 1.5	76.1 ± 0.8	152.1 ± 1.0	76.1 ± 0.8	76.1 ± 0.8	152.1 ± 1.0	114.1 ± 1.0
	MBC	152.1 ± 1.0	152.1 ± 2.0	152.1 ± 2.0	304.2 ± 4.0	152.1 ± 1.2	152.1 ± 1.2	304.2 ± 2.0	152.1 ± 1.0
5j	MIC	73.1 ± 0.5	109.6 ± 1.0	58.6 ± 0.4	146.2 ± 0.8	58.6 ± 0.6	58.6 ± 0.8	109.6 ± 1.0	109.6 ± 1.0
	MBC	146.2 ± 1.0	146.2 ± 2.0	73.1 ± 0.8	292.3 ± 0.2	73.1 ± 0.6	73.1 ± 0.06	146.2 ± 1.0	146.2 ± 2.0
5k	MIC	73.1 ± 0.5	109.6 ± 1.0	58.6 ± 0.4	109.6 ± 1.5	58.6 ± 0.6	58.6 ± 0.6	109.6 ± 1.5	109.6 ± 2.0
	MBC	146.2 ± 1.0	146.2 ± 2.0	73.1 ± 0.8	146.2 ± 1.0	73.1 ± 0.8	73.1 ± 0.8	146.2 ± 2.0	146.2 ± 2.0
7a	MIC	130.3 ± 1.0	130.3 ± 1.5	63.7 ± 0.4	86.9 ± 0.4	86.9 ± 1.0	86.9 ± 1.0	173.7 ± 2.0	130.3 ± 2.0
	MBC	173.7 ± 2.0	173.7 ± 2.0	86.9 ± 0.8	173.7 ± 1.5	173.7 ± 1.5	173.7 ± 1.5	347.4 ± 4.0	173.7 ± 1.5
7b	MIC	41.7 ± 0.2	125.2 ± 1.0	41.7 ± 0.2	166.9 ± 1.0	83.4 ± 0.9	61.2 ± 0.5	166.9 ± 2.0	125.2 ± .1.0
	MBC	83.4 ± 0.4	166.9 ± 2.0	83.4 ± 0.8	333.9 ± .2.0	166.9 ± 1.0	83.4 ± 1.0	333.9 ± 4.0	166.9 ± 2.0
7c	MIC	79.9 ± 0.4	119.8 ± 1.5	79.9 ± 1.0	159.8 ± 1.0	58.6 ± 0.4	58.6 ± 0.4	119.8 ± 1.0	119.8 ± 1.5
	MBC	159.8 ± 1.0	159.8 ± 2.0	159.8 ± 1.4	319.6 ± 2.0	79.9 ± 1.0	79.9 ± 1.0	159.8 ± 2.0	159.8 ± .2.0
Am.	MIC	248.0 ± 3.0	248.0 ± 2.0	248.0 ± 2.0	372.0 ± 4.0	248.0 ± 3.0	744.0 ± 9.0	248.0 ± 3.0	372.0 ± 4.0
	MBC	372.0 ± 4.0	372.0 ± 4.0	372.0 ± 2.0	744.0 ± 8.0	372.0 ± 3.0	1240 ± 2	492.0 ± 6.0	492.0 ± 8.0
Str.	MIC	43.0 ± 0.8	86.0 ± 1.0	172.0 ± 2.0	258.0 ± 4.0	43.0 ± 0.3	172.0 ± 3.0	172.0 ± 3.0	172.0 ± 2.0
	MBC	86.0 ± 1.0	172.0 ± 2.0	344.0 ± 4.0	516.0 ± 4.0	86.0 ± 0.6	344.0 ± 3.0	344.0 ± 3.0	344.0 ± 2.0

MIC–minimal inhibitory concentration, MBC–minimal bactericidal concentration, *B.c.-B.cereus* (clinical isolate), *M.f.-M.flavus* (ATCC 10,240), *S.a.-S.aurues* (ATCC 6538), *l.m.-L.monocytogenes* (NCTC 7973), *E.c.-E.coli* (ATTC 35210, *En.c.-En.cloaca* (ATCC 3503), *P.a.-P.aeruginosa* (ATCC 27,853), *S.T.-S.Typhimurium* (ATCC 13,311).

Three most active compounds were also evaluated against the resistant strains, including MRSA, *P. aeruginosa*, and *E. coli*, (Table 3). From the obtained results, it is evident that all three compounds were more active against MRSA than ampicillin, while streptomycin did not show any bactericidal activity. The compound **5d** was also more active than ampicillin towards resistant *P. aeruginosa* strain.

Table 3. Antibacterial activity against resistant strains (MIC/MBC in μM).

Compound ID		Resistant Strains		
		MRSA	P.aeruginosa	E.coli
5d	MIC	1260 ± 0.8	315 ± 9.0	1260 ± 21
	MBC	2520 ± 0.1	630 ± 8.0	2502 ± 22
5g	MIC	1220 ± 18	610 ± 5.0	1220 ± 19
	MBC	2440 ± 0.2	1202 ± 21	2440 ± 16
5k	MIC	1220 ± 0.6	610 ± 10	1220 ± 0.6
	MBC	2440 ± 22	1220 ± 21	2440 ± 22
Streptomycin	MIC	172.0 ± 21	86 ± 12	172 ± 21
	MBC	-	172 ± 14	344 ± 42
Ampicilline	MIC	-	572 ± 64	572 ± 78
	MBC	/	/	/

2.3.2. Antifungal Activity

All compounds also showed antifungal activity with MIC values ranging from 9.7 to 347.4 μM and MFC at 19.5–694.8 μM. The antifungal activity of compounds is shown in Table 4 and follows the order: **5g > 7c > 7b > 5d > 5b > 5e > 5k > 5f > 5j > 5c > 5i > 5a > 7a > 5h**. Compound **5g** displayed the best activity with MIC values in the range of 9.7–73.1 μM and MFC at 36.5–146.2 μM, while compound **5h** exhibited the lowest potential with MIC and MFC at 28.9–315.5 μM and 39.4–630.9 μM respectively. It was observed that similar to bacteria, fungi showed different sensitivity towards compounds tested. Thus, the most sensitive fungal strain appeared to be *T. viride* (IAM 5061), while the most resistant filamentous A. fumigatus. The behavior of compounds towards fungi species was different, too.

Several compounds showed very good activity against some species. For example, compound **5d** exhibited good activity against the most resistant *A. fumigatus* (MIC/MFC at .20.2/37.9 μM, while compound **7b** against *T. viride* (IAM 5061), *P. cyclpoium var verucosum* (food isolate) and all Aspergillus species except *A. fumigatus* (human isolate) with MIC at 22.3 μM and MFC at 41.4 μM. Compound **5g** exhibited excellent activity against *T. viride* (IAM 5061) (MIC/MFC at 0.97/1.95 μmol/mL × 10^{-2}). Additionally, good activity was achieved for compound **5g** against *A. versicolor* (ATCC 11730), *A. ochraceus* (ATCC 12066), *P. funiculosum* (ATCC 36839) with MIC and MFC at 19.5 μM and 36.5 μM respectively. Compound **5c** appeared to be potent against *A. ochraceus* (ATCC 12066) and *T. viride* (IAM 5061) (MIC/MFC at 18.8/35.3 μM whereas compound **7c** exhibited very good activity against *T. viride* (IAM 5061) with MIC at 10.7 μM and MFC at 21.3 μM and also good activity against *A. ochraceus* (ATCC 12066) and *P. funiculosum* (ATCC 36839 (MC/MFC at 23.1/39.9 μM. The potential of ketoconazole was at MIC 285-475 μM and MFC at 380–950 μM. Bifonazole displayed MIC at 480-640 μM and MFC at 640–800 μM. It should be mentioned that all compounds appeared to be more potent than ketoconazole and bifonazole. Only compound **7a** against *A. fumigatus (human isolate)* was less active than bifonazole.

According to the analysis of the structure-activity relationships, the most beneficial for antifungal activity is the presence of the 5-methoxy group in indole ring as well as nicotinamide as a substituent of the side chain (**5g**). In contrast, the presence of isonicotinamide in methylindole (**5i**) derivative appeared to be detrimental. Shifting of 5-OMe of compound **5g** to position 6 of indole and replacement of nicotinamide by 2-hydroxybenzamide resulted in compound **5c** with decreased activity. Removal of methoxy group and introduction of morpholino moiety to the N atom of thioxothiazolidinone **(7a)** decreased more activity.

In indole derivatives (**5d, 5e, 5h**), the presence of 4-hydroxybenzamide was favorable for antifungal activity, while isonicotinamide substituent had a negative effect. On the contrary, for methylindole derivatives (**5a, 5f, 5i**), the negative impact was observed with the presence of 2-hydroxybenzamide, while in the case of the 5-methoxy indole derivatives (**5b, 5j**) it was the opposite. Finally, for the derivatives with morpholino moiety, the best activity was observed with the presence of the 5-methoxy group in the indole ring. The indole derivative was one of the less potent.

Thus, as in the case of antibacterial activity, antifungal activity depends not only on substitution in the indole ring but also on substituent on the N-atom of the 2-thioxothiazolidinone ring. In the series of (Z)-5-((5-methoxy-1H-indol-3-yl)methylene)-3-morpholino-2-thioxothiazolidin-4-one derivatives the most important structural features which enhanced the antifungal activity are again 4-hydroxybenzamide and 1H-indole moiety as well as nicotinamide and 5- and 6-methoxyindole moieties. On the other hand, in the series of indole 3-methylene morpholino-2-thioxothiazolidin-4-one derivatives, the presence of the 5-OCH3 group in the indole ring enhance the antifungal activity.

Table 4. Antifungal activity of compounds **5a–k** and **7a–c** (MIC/MFC in μM).

Com. ID		A.f	A.v	A.o	A.n	T.v	P.o	P.f	Pvc
5a	MIC	293.0 ± 2.2	36.6 ± 0.4	26.9 ± 0.1	53.7 ± 0.6	26.9 ± 0.1	36.6 ± 0.2	36.6 ± 0.2	109.9 ± 0.1
	MFC	586.1 ± 7.0	73.3 ± 0.8	36.6 ± 0.2	73.3 ± 0.8	36.6 ± 0.3	73.3 ± 0.5	73.3 ± 0.8	146.5 ± 0.2
5b	MIC	35.2 ± 0.6	35.2 ± 0.2	25.9 ± 0.2	35.2 ± 0.2	25.9 ± 0.2	35.2 ± 0.5	51.7 ± 0.5	35.2 ± 0.2
	MFC	70.5 ± 0.6	70.5 ± 0.4	35.2 ± 0.4	70.5 ± 0.8	35.2 ± 0.2	70.5 ± 0.5	70.5 ± 0.5	70.5 ± 0.5
5c	MIC	282.0 ± .2.0	35.3 ± 0.2	18.8 ± 0.2	25.9 ± 0.1	18.8 ± 0.2	35.3 ± 0.2	35.3 ± 0.2	35.3 ± 0.2
	MFC	564.1 ± 4.0	68.2 ± 0.4	35.3 ± 0.2	35.3 ± 0.2	35.3 ± 0.5	68.2 ± 0.5	68.2 ± 0.5	68.2 ± 0.5
5d	MIC	202 ± 0.1	37.9 ± 0.2	27.8 ± 0.1	37.9 ± 0.0	27.8 ± 0.2	37.9 ± 0.5	37.9 ± 0.2	37.9 ± 0.2
	MFC	37.9 ± 0.2	75.6 ± 0.4	37.9 ± 0.5	75.6 ± 0.5	37.9 ± 0.5	75.6 ± 0.5	75.6 ± 0.5	75.6 ± 0.5
5e	MIC	39.4 ± 0.2	39.4 ± 0.2	21.0 ± 0.1	39.4 ± 0.5	21.0 ± 0.1	39.4 ± 0.5	39.4 ± 0.5	39.4 ± 0.5
	MFC	78.9 ± 0.4	78.9 ± 0.4	39.4 ± 0.2	78.9 ± 1.0	39.4 ± 0.5	78.9 ± 0.5	78.9 ± 0.5	78.9 ± 0.5
5f	MIC	76.1 ± 0.4	38.0 ± 0.2	27.9 ± 0.1	38.0 ± 0.5	27.9 ± 0.2	55.8 ± 0.5	55.8 ± 0.5	55.8 ± 0.5
	MFC	152.1 ± 0.1	76.1 ± 0.4	38.0 ± 0.5	76.1 ± 0.8	38.0 ± 0.5	76.1 ± 1.0	76.1 ± 0.8	76.1 ± 1.0
5g	MIC	73.1 ± 0.4	19.5 ± 0.2	19.5 ± 0.1	14.6 ± 0.1	9.7 ± 0.01	36.5 ± 0.5	19.5 ± 0.1	26.8 ± 0.1
	MFC	146.2 ± 0.1	36.5 ± 0.4	36.5 ± 0.5	19.5 ± 0.1	19.5 ± 0.08	73.1 ± 0.8	36.5 ± 0.5	36.5 ± 0.2
5h	MIC	315.5 ± 2.5	78.9 ± 1.0	39.4 ± 0.2	78.9 ± 0.5	28.9 ± 0.1	39.4 ± 0.5	78.9 ± 0.5	118.3 ± 1.0
	MFC	630.9 ± 8.0	157.7 ± 1.0	78.9 ± 0.8	157.7 ± 1.0	39.4 ± 0.2	78.9 ± 0.5	157.7 ± 1.0	157.7 ± 2.0
5i	MIC	152.1 ± 1.0	38.0 ± 0.4	38.0 ± 0.0	38.0 ± 0.0	27.9 ± 0.2	76.1 ± 0.5	55.8 ± 0.5	76.1 ± 0.5
	MFC	304.2 ± .2.0	76.1 ± 0.0	76.1 ± 1.0	76.1 ± 0.8	38.0 ± 0.5	152.1 ± 1.0	76.1 ± 0.8	152.1 ± 1.0
5j	MIC	146.2 ± 1.0	35.5 ± 0.2	53.6 ± 0.4	26.8 ± 0.2	35.5 ± 0.5	35.5 ± 0.4	35.5 ± 0.4	35.5 ± 0.6
	MFC	292.3 ± .2.0	73.1 ± 0.8	73.1 ± 0.8	35.5 ± 0.5	73.1 ± 1.0	73.1 ± 0.4	73.1 ± 1.0	73.1 ± 1.0
5k	MIC	35.5 ± 0.4	35.5 ± 0.2	35.5 ± 0.2	35.5 ± 0.5	35.5 ± 0.2	35.5 ± 0.5	35.5 ± 0.4	35.5 ± 0.2
	MFC	73.1 ± 0.8	73.1 ± 0.8	73.1 ± 1.0	73.1 ± 0.5	73.1 ± 0.8	73.1 ± 0.8	73.1 ± 0.8	73.1 ± 0.8
7a	MIC	347.4 ± 2.0	43.4 ± 0.2	43.4 ± 0.2	43.4 ± 0.2	31.8 ± 0.2	43.4 ± 0.2	43.4 ± 0.4	86.9 ± 1.0
	MFC	694.8 ± 4.0	86.9 ± 1.0	86.9 ± 0.5	86.9 ± 1.0	43.4 ± 0.5	86.9 ± 1.0	86.9 ± 1.0	173.7 ± 2.0
7b	MIC	22.3 ± 0.1	22.3 ± 0.1	22.3 ± 0.1	41.7 ± 0.5	22.3 ± 0.2	41.7 ± 0.5	41.7 ± 1.0	22.3 ± 0.1
	MFC	41.7 ± 0.2	41.7 ± 0.2	41.7 ± 0.5	83.4 ± .1.0	41.7 ± 0.8	83.4 ± 1.0	83.4 ± 1.0	41.7 ± 0.4
7c	MIC	79.9 ± 0.4	21.3 ± 0.1	16.0 ± 0.1	21.3 ± 0.2	10.7 ± 0.2	21.3 ± 0.1	21.3 ± 1.0	58.6 ± 0.4
	MFC	159.8 ± 1.0	39.9 ± 0.5	21.3 ± 0.1	39.9 ± 0.2	21.3 ± 0.5	39.9 ± 0.2	39.9 ± 1.0	79.9 ± 1.0
Ket.	MIC	380 ± 12	2850 ± 68	380 ± 12	380 ± 8.0	475 ± 58	3800 ± 58	380 ± 16	380 ± 12
	MFC	950 ± 23	3800 ± 84	950 ± 12	950 ± 6.0	570 ± 86	3800 ± 48	950 ± 26	950 ± 23
Bif.	MIC	480 ± 22	480 ± .2	480 ± 28	480 ± 12	640 ± 28	480 ± 20	640 ± 12	480 ± 22
	MFC	640 ± 3.4	640 ± 0.8	800 ± 1.8	640 ± 2.3	800 ± 3.8	640 ± 1.6	800 ± 2.1	640 ± 3.4

MIC–minimal inhibitory concentration, MFC–minimal fungicidal concentration. *A.fum.-A.fumigatus* (human isolate), *A.v.-A.versicolor* (ATCC 11730), *A.o.-A.ochraceus* (ATCC 12066), *A.n.-A.niger* (ATCC 6275), *T.v.-T.viride* (IAM 5061), *P.f.-P.funiculosum* (ATCC 36839), *P.o.-P.ochrochloron* (ATCC 9112), *P.v.c.-P.cyclpoium var. verucosum* (food isolate).

2.3.3. Cytotoxicity Assessment

Low toxicity and selectivity of action of antimicrobial compounds is a crucial pre-requisite for further development. Thus, we studied the cytotoxicity of the most active compounds. MTT analysis was performed on the HEK-293 human embryonic kidney cell line. The cells were cultured in DMEM medium supplemented with 10% fetal bovine serum. The cells were inoculated into a 96-well plate at a concentration of $5 \cdot 10^4$/mL ($5 \cdot 10^3$ per well, 100 μL each). After one day of culture, compound preparations were added, and the results were obtained after a 72 h culture period. The compounds were added at four concentrations (25, 50, 100, and 250 μM). Since compound solutions contained DMSO, control cultures containing only DMSO at the final concentration obtained when the appropriate volume of compound solution was added were performed.

Although the compounds do not exhibit statistically significant concentration-dependent toxicity up to 100 μM (Figure 3), they show some toxicity at higher concentrations. The average CC_{50} values obtained from three different experiments are given in Tables 5 and 6. The SI index is also shown in Tables 5 and 6.

Compound **5g** and **7c** exhibited the best SI index for anti-fungal activity while compound **5d** exhibited the best SI index for anti-bacterial activity.

We compared the CC_{50} values of compounds **5d**, **5k**, **5g**, **7c** with cytotoxicity of the reference drugs obtained in the HEK-293 human embryonic kidney cell line. For antibacterials streptomycin, ampicillin and antifungal bifonazole CC_{50} exceeded 100 μM [63,64]; for antifungal ketoconazole CC_{50} = 60 μM [65]. Thus, cytotoxicity of the most active compounds in our study is comparable or lower than cytotoxicity of the reference antimicrobial drugs.

Table 5. Antibacterial activity (MIC), cytotoxicity (CC_{50}), and selectivity indices (SI) of compounds **5d, 5g, 5k, 7c.**

ID	CC_{50}		B.c	M.f	S.a	L.m	En.cl	P.a	S.T	E.coli
5d		MIC	55.6 ± 0.2	113.8 ± 0.8	37.9 ± 0.2	113.8 ± 0.8	37.9 ± 0.4	37.9 ± 0.2	113.8 ± 1.0	75.6 ± 0.4
	252 ± 1.5	SI	4.5	2.2	6.7	2.2	6.7	6.7	2.2	3.3
5g		MIC	73.1 ± 0.1	73.1 ± 1.0	53.6 ± 0.4	73.1 ± 0.8	36.5 ± 0.5	109.6 ± 1.0	53.6 ± 0.6	109.6 ± 1.0
	256 ± 6.21	SI	3.5	3.5	4.8	3.5	7.0	2.3	4.8	2.3
5k		MIC	73.1 ± 0.5	109.6 ± 1.0	58.6 ± 0.4	109.6 ± 1.5	58.6 ± 0.6	58.6 ± 0.6	109.6 ± 1.5	109.6 ± 2.0
	252 ± 1.89	SI	3.5	2.3	4.3	2.3	4.3	4.3	2.3	2.3
7c		MIC	79.9 ± 0.4	119.8 ± 1.5	79.9 ± 1.0	159.8 ± 1.0	58.6 ± 0.4	58.6 ± 0.4	119.8 ± 1.0	119.8 ± 1.5
	225± 1.87	SI	2.8	1.9	2.8	1.4	3.8	3.8	1.9	1.9

Table 6. Antifungal activity (MIC), cytotoxicity (CC_{50}), and selectivity indices (SI) of compounds **5d, 5g, 5k, 7c.**

Com.	CC_{50} (μM)		A.f	A.v	A.o	A.n	T.v	P.o	P.f	Pvc
5d		MIC	202 ± 0.1	37.9 ± 0.2	27.8 ± 0.1	37.9 ± 0.2	27.8 ± 0.2	37.9 ± 0.5	37.9 ± 0.2	37.9 ± 0.2
	252 ± 1.5	SI	1.3	6.7	9.1	6.7	9.1	6.7	6.7	6.7
5g		MIC	73.1 ± 0.2	19.5 ± 0.2	19.5 ± 0.2	14.6 ± 0.1	9.7 ± 0.1	36.5 ± 0.5	19.5 ± 0.1	26.8 ± 0.1
	256 ± 6.21	SI	3.5	13.1	13.1	17.5	26.4	7.0	13.1	9.6
5k		MIC	35.5 ± 0.4	35.5 ± 0.2	35.5 ± 0.2	35.5 ± 0.5	35.5 ± 0.2	35.5 ± 0.5	35.5 ± 0.4	35.5 ± 0.2
	252 ± 1.89	SI	7.1	7.1	7.1	7.1	7.1	7.1	7.1	7.1
7c		MIC	79.9 ± 0.4	21.3 ± 0.1	16.0 ± 0.1	21.3 ± 0.2	10.7 ± 0.2	21.3 ± 0.1	21.3 ± 1.0	58.6 ± 0.4
	225 ± 1.87	SI	2.8	10.6	14.1	10.6	21.0	10.6	10.6	3.8
Ket.		MIC	380 ± 12	285 ± 68	380 ± 12	380 ± 8.0	475 ± 58	380 ± 58	380 ± 16	380 ± 12
	60 *	SI	0.158	0.210	0.158	0.158	0.126	0.158	0.158	0.158

* 24 h.

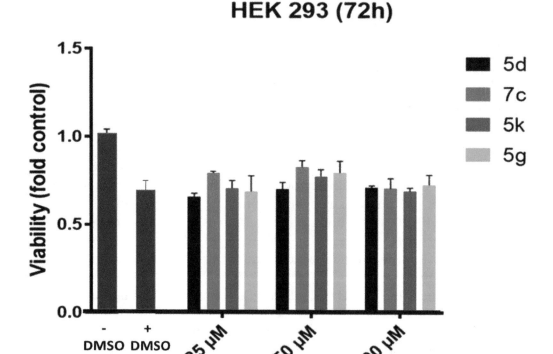

Figure 3. MTT assay results for compounds **5d, 5k, 5g, 7c.** According to the results, all compounds did not show statistically significant, concentration-dependent cytotoxicity at concentrations up to 100 μM. The stable decrease in viability observed can be attributed to dimethyl soulfoxide (DMSO,) present at stable concentration at all compound samples.

2.4. Docking Studies

Since the mechanism of antimicrobial action of our compounds is not known, to choose the proteins as potential targets, we based on the literature. It was found that benzothiazole derivatives are mentioned as Gyrase inhibitors [66–68]. On the other hand, according to the literature, thiazolidinones act as MurB inhibitors [69–72]. Furthermore, prediction of the mechanism of action by computer program PASS indicated Thymidylate kinase as the probable antibacterial target. On the other hand, several publications mentioned thiazolidinone and indole derivatives as 14$^\alpha$-lanosterol demethylase inhibitors [73–75]. Thus, taking all these into account, we proposed E. coli DNA Gyrase, Thymidylate kinase, and E. coli MurB enzymes as antibacterial targets, with CYP51 as the antifungal target.

2.4.1. Docking to Antibacterial Targets

The docking studies revealed that estimated binding energy to E. coli DNA Gyrase (−2.59 to −6.54 kcal/mol) as well as to thymidylate kinase (−1.55 to −4.12 kcal/mol), were higher than that to E. coli MurB (−7.07 to −10.93 kcal/mol). Therefore, it may be resolved that E. coli MurB is the most suitable enzyme where binding scores were consistent with biological activity (Table 7).

Table 7. Molecular docking binding energies.

Comp.	Est. Binding Energy (kcal/mol)			I-H E. coli MurB	Residues E. coli MurB
	E.coli DNA Gyrase 1KZN	Thymidylate Kinase 4QGG	E. coli MurB 2Q85		
5a	−4.63	-	−8.22	2	Gly122, Ser228
5b	−3.12	-	−7.70	2	Arg213, Asn232
5c	−5.39	−2.13	-9.16	2	Gly122, Ser228
5d	−6.21	−4.12	−10.93	2	Ser228, Arg326
5e	−6.28	−2.39	−8.97	2	Arg213, Ser228
5f	−5.46	−1.55	−8.74	2	Gly122, Ser228
5g	−6.54	−3.26	−10.88	3	Gly122, Ser228, Asn232
5h	−6.11	−1.24	−9.12	2	Gly122, Ser228
5i	−3.69	−1.15	−7.07	2	Arg213, Arg326
5j	−5.52	−3.25	−9.21	2	Gly122, Ser228
5k	−5.63	−2.96	−9.83	2	Arg213, Ser228
7a	−2.59	-	−7.28	2	Gly122, Arg213
7b	−3.67	-	−7.75	2	Ser228, Asn232
7c	−4.28	-	−7.88	2	Gly122, Ser228

The docking pose of the most active compound **5d** in E. coli MurB enzyme showed two favorable hydrogen bond interactions. The first one is between the oxygen atom of the C–O group of the compound and the hydrogen of the side chain of Ser228. The second one between the oxygen atom of -OH group of the compound and the side chain of Arg326 (distances 2.17 Å and 1.99 Å, respectively). The fused rings interact hydrophobically with the residues Tyr189, Asn232, Leu289, Ala123, Leu217, and Arg213, while the benzene ring interacts hydrophobically with the residues Asn50, Ser115, Ile118, Ile121, Gln119 and Glu324 (Figure 4). These interactions stabilize the complex compound-enzyme and play a crucial role in the increased inhibitory activity of compound **5d** Moreover, the hydrogen bond formation with the residue Ser228 is essential for the inhibitory action of the compounds; thus, this residue takes part in the proton transfer at the second stage of peptidoglycan synthesis [76].

The second most active compound, **5g,** also forms the hydrogen bond interaction with the residue Ser228 that explains its high inhibitory action (Figure 2). Detailed analysis of the docking pose of the two most active compounds showed that they similarly bind MurB, and they insert deeper to the binding center of the enzyme than FAD, forming a hydrogen bond with the residue Ser228 (Figure 5).

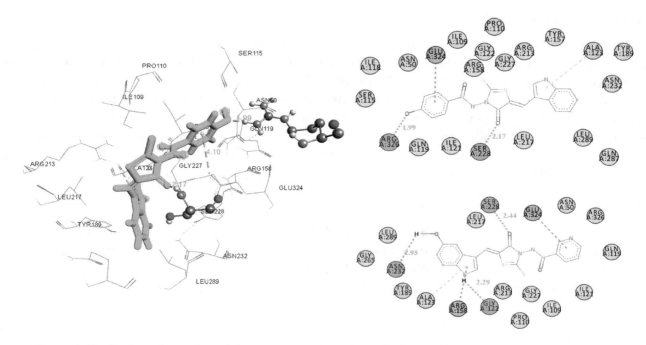

Figure 4. Docked conformation of the most active compound **5d** in *E.coli* MurB **(Left)**. 2D diagrams of the most active compounds **5d** (up) and **5g** (down) in *E.coli* MurB **(Right)**.

The same behavior was observed in the case of docking of the most active compound among 5-(1*H*-indol-3-ylmethylene)-4-oxo-2-thioxothiazolidin-3-yl)alkane carboxylic acids [19] and 5-adamantane thiadiazole-based thiazolidinones [70]. Again, the formation of the hydrogen bond between the C=O group and Ser228 was observed. Thus, the obtained results support previous data [69–72] that MurB maybe is the most appropriate target for the antibacterial activity for this chemical series.

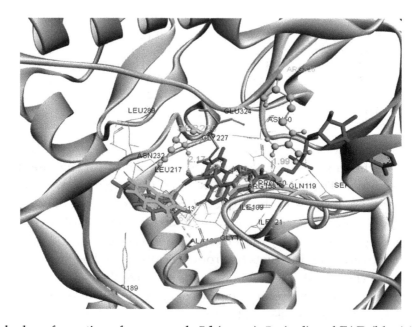

Figure 5. Docked conformation of compounds **5d** (green), **5g** (red) and FAD (blue) in *E.Coli* MurB.

2.4.2. Docking to Lanosterol 14α-demethylase of *C. albicans*

All the synthesized compounds and the reference drug ketoconazole were docked to lanosterol 14α-demethylase of *C. albicans* (Table 8).

Table 8. Molecular docking binding energies.

N/N	Est. Binding Energy (kcal/mol) CYP51 of *C. albicans* PDB ID: 5V5Z	I-H	Residues CYP51 of *C. albicans* PDB ID: 5V5Z	Interactions with HEM601
5a	−7.65	1	Tyr132	Hydrophobic
5b	−9.74	1	Tyr132	Ionizable, Hydrophobic
5c	−8.13	2	Tyr64, Tyr132	Hydrophobic
5d	−10.22	2	Tyr118, Tyr132	Ionizable, Hydrophobic
5e	−9.15	1	Tyr132	Ionizable, Hydrophobic
5f	−8.79	2	Tyr118, Tyr132	Hydrophobic
5g	−11.55	1	Tyr132	Fe binding, Ionizable, Hydrophobic
5h	−7.11	-	-	Ionizable, Hydrophobic
5i	−7.84	1	Tyr132	Ionizable, Hydrophobic
5j	−8.72	2	Tyr118, Met508	Hydrophobic
5k	−9.24	2	Tyr64, Tyr118	Hydrophobic
7a	−7.08	1	Tyr132	Hydrophobic
7b	−10.36	1	Tyr132	Ionizable, Hydrophobic
7c	−10.84	2	Tyr118, Tyr132	Ionizable, Hydrophobic
ketoconazole	−8.23	1	Tyr64	Ionizable, Hydrophobic

Docking results showed that all the synthesized compounds might bind to CYP51$_{Ca}$ close to those of the reference drug ketoconazole. Compound **5g** is located inside the enzyme alongside to heme group, interacting with the Fe of the heme group of CYP51$_{Ca}$ throughout its atom N of the pyridine ring. Moreover, compound **5g** forms a hydrogen bond between the oxygen of –OCH$_3$ substituent and the hydrogen of the side chain of Tyr132. Hydrophobic interactions were detected between residues Thr122, Phe126, Tyr132, and Ile131 and the fused rings of the compound **5g**, also between Leu376, Thr311 and the benzene ring of the compound. Furthermore, compound **5g** interacts hydrophobically throughout its benzene ring with the heme group of the enzyme, and also it forms a positive ionizable bond with it (Figure 6). Interaction with the heme group was also observed with the benzene ring of ketoconazole, which forms positive ionizable interactions (Figures 6 and 7). However, compound **5g** forms a more stable complex of the ligand with enzyme indicating its interaction with the Fe, which is probably why compound **5g** showed high antifungal activity.

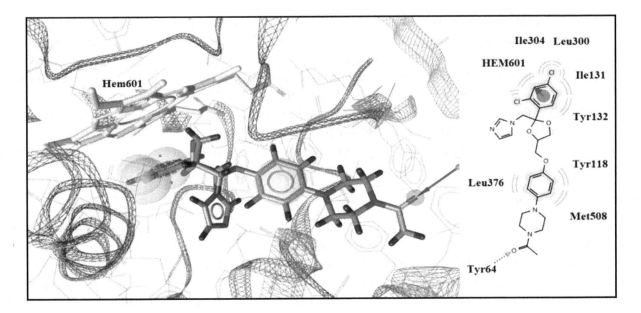

Figure 6. Docked conformation of ketoconazole in lanosterol 14alpha-demethylase of *C. albicans* (CYP51$_{ca}$).

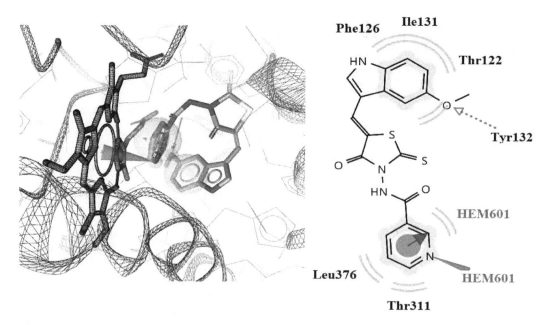

Figure 7. Docked conformation of compound **5g** in lanosterol 14alpha-demethylase of *C. albicans* (CYP51$_{ca}$).

It should be mentioned that the tested compounds interact more strongly with the heme group of the enzyme CYP51$_{Ca}$ because the heme's Fe is involved in this interaction. In the case of our previous work [19], the most active compound interacts with the heme but throughout its benzene ring and the –NO_2 group, forming pi and negative ionizable interactions with the heme group, respectively. In the case of 5-adamantane thiadiazole-based thiazolidinones [72], again, the most active compound form positive interactions between the heme group and heterocyclic rings of the compound. Thus, it can be concluded that thiazolidinone derivatives, in general, can interact with the heme of CYP51$_{Ca}$ in the same way as ketoconazole interacts.

3. Materials and Methods

All starting materials were purchased from Merck and used without purification. NMR spectra were determined with Varian Mercury VX-400" (Varian Co., Palo Alto, CA, USA) and AM-300 Bruker 300 MHz. spectrometers in DMSO-d$_6$. MS (ESI) spectra were recorded on an LC-MS system-HPLC Agilent 1100 (Agilent Technologies Inc., Santa, Clara, CA USA) equipped with a diode array detector Agilent LC\MSD SL. Parameters of analysis: Zorbax SB-C18 column (1.8 µM, 4.6–15 mm, PN 821975-932), solvent water–acetonitrile mixture (95:5), 0.1% of aqueous trifluoroacetic acid; eluent flow 3 mL min^{-1}; injection volume 1 µL; IR spectra were recorded on a Vertex 70 Bruker" (Bruker, Karlsruhe, Germany) spectrometer in KBr pellets. Melting points were determined in open capillary tubes and are uncorrected.

3.1. In Silico Biological Activity Evaluation

Antimicrobial activity and toxicity of the designed compounds have been estimated in silico using web services available on the Way2Drug portal [56]. These services are based on the PASS (Prediction of Activity Spectra for Substances) and GUSAR (General Unrestricted Structure-Activity Relationships) software, which is described in detail elsewhere [60,61]. It is essential to mention that PASS-based services provide the assessments of the compound's activity as the difference between the probabilities for the chemical compound with a particular structure to display activity (Pa) and do not display this activity (Pi). By default, in PASS, all activities with Pa > Pi are considered as probable. High Pa-Pi values reflect the high structural similarity of the analyzed compound to the structures included in the training set with those activities. Since our goal was not finding close analogs of the earlier discovered antimicrobial agents, we considered compounds with small Pa-Pi values as the promising hits for experimental testing. If the experiment will confirm their activity, there is a chance to find a New Chemical Entity. GUSAR-based service [60,61] provides the quantitative assessment of acute rat toxicity expressed as LD_{50} values for four routes of administration: intraperitoneal (IP), intravenous (IV), oral, and subcutaneous (SC).

3.2. Chemistry

3.2.1. General Procedure for the Preparation of N-(4-oxo-2-thioxothiazolidin-3-yl) carbamides 3a–d

In a round-bottom flask equipped with a reflux condenser, 0.05 mol of trithiocarbonyl diglycolic acid, 0.05 mol of the corresponding hydrazide and alcohol-water mixture (1:1) were placed and boiled for 3 h. The reaction mixture is cooled, the precipitate is filtered off and recrystallized.

2-Hydroxy-N-(4-oxo-2-thioxothiazolidin-3-yl)benzamide 3a. Yield 97%; m.p. 104–106 °C (CH_3COOH-H_2O 2:1). IR (cm^{-1}): 3342.48 (OH), 1751.28 (C=O), 1657.74 (C=O), 1608.56 (C=S).). ^1H NMR (400 MHz, DMSO-d_6, ppm) δ 11.62–10.91 (br.s, 2H, NH, OH), 7.88 (dd, J = 8.0, 1.6 Hz, 1H, H_6 benzene), 7.52–7.46 (m, 1H, H_3 benzene), 7.05–6.95 (m, 1H, 2H, H_4 +H_5, aromatic), 4.48 (q, J = 18.7 Hz, 2H, CH_2). ^{13}C NMR (101 MHz, DMSO, ppm) δ 199.90, 170.25, 164.91, 157.93, 134.62, 129.83, 119.44, 117.19, 115.07, 33.38. Anal. Calcd. for $C_{10}H_8N_2O_3S_2$ (%): C, 44.77; H, 3.01; N, 10.44; S, 23.90 Found (%):C, 44.88; H, 3.09; N, 10.37; S, 23.95.

4-Hydroxy-N-(4-oxo-2-thioxothiazolidin-3-yl)benzamide 3b. Yield 87%; m.p. 207–209 °C (CH_3COOH).). IR (cm^{-1}): 3259.54 (OH), 3166(NH), 1739.71 (C=O), 1667.38(C=O), 1583.48 (C=S). ^1H NMR (400 MHz, DMSO-d_6, ppm) δ 11.25 (s, 1H, NH), 10.29 (s, 1H, OH), 7.81 (dd, J = 9.1, 2.3 Hz, 2H, H_2 +H_6, benzene), 6.88 (dd, J = 9.1, 2.3 Hz, 2H, H_3 +H_5, benzene), 4.51 (s, 2H, CH_2). ^{13}C NMR (101 MHz, DMSO, ppm) δ 200.33, 170.54, 163.93, 161.44, 129.96, 121.44, 115.24, 33.32. Anal. Calcd. for $C_{10}H_8N_2O_3S_2$ (%): C, 44.77; H, 3.01; N, 10.44; S, 23.90 Found (%):C, 44.69; H, 2.95; N, 10.36; S, 23.81.

N-(4-Oxo-2-thioxothiazolidin-3-yl)nicotinamide 3c. Yield 83%; m.p. 190 °C decomp.(C_2H_5OH). IR (cm^{-1}): 1753.21 (C=O), 1687.63 (C=O), 1556.48 (C=S). ^1H NMR (400 MHz, DMSO-d_6, ppm) δ 11.95 (s, 1H, NH), 8.97–8.73 (m, 2H, H_2 +H_4, pyridine), 7.99–7.70 (m, 2H, H_5 +H_6, pyridine), 4.55 (s, 2H, CH_2).). ^{13}C NMR (101 MHz, DMSO, ppm) δ 199.81, 170.20, 163.25, 150.76, 137.93, 121.31, 119.56, 33.55. Anal. Calcd. for $C_9H_7N_3O_2S_2$ (%): C, 42.68; H, 2.79; N, 16.59; S, 25.32 Found (%):C, 42.79; H, 2.70; N, 16.48; S, 25.45.

N-(4-Oxo-2-thioxothiazolidin-3-yl)isonicotinamide 3d. Yield 85%; m.p. 193 °C decomp. (C_2H_5OH). IR (cm^{-1}): 1753.21(C=O), 1678.95 (C=O), 1556.48 (C=S). ^1H NMR (400 MHz, DMSO-d_6, ppm) δ 11.95 (s, 1H, NH), 8.87–8.79 (m, 2H, H_3 +H_5, pyridine), 7.85–7.80 (m, 2H, H_2 +H_6, pyridine), 4.55 (s, 2H, CH_2). ^{13}C NMR (101 MHz, DMSO, ppm) δ 199.81, 170.19, 163.25, 150.76, 137.93, 121.39, 119.56, 33.58. Anal. Calcd. for $C_9H_7N_3O_2S_2$ (%): C, 42.68; H, 2.79; N, 16.59; S, 25.32 Found (%):C, 42.77; H, 2.85; N, 16.76; S, 25.26.

3.2.2. General Procedure 5-[(R-1H-indol-3-ylmethylene)-4-oxo-2-thioxothiazolidin-3-yl] carbamides 5a–k and 5-(R-1H-indol-3-ylmethylene)-3-morpholin-4-yl-2-thioxothiazolidin-4-ones 7a–c

In a round-bottom flask equipped with a reflux condenser, 2.5 mmol of 3-substituted 2-thioxo-4-oxothiazolidine 3a-d or 6, 3.3 mmol of the corresponding aldehyde 1a-d, 2.5 mmol of ammonium acetate and 5 mL of acetic acid are placed. The reaction mixture is boiled for 2 h, cooled, the precipitate is filtered off, washed with acetic acid and water, dried and recrystallized.

2-Hydroxy-N-{(5Z)-5-[(1-methyl-1H-indol-3-yl)methylene]-4-oxo-2-thioxothiazolidin-3-yl}benzamide 5a. Yield 98%; m.p. 265–267 °C (DMFA-CH_3COOH). IR (cm^{-1}): 3272.08 (OH), 1700.17 (C=O), 1656.77 (C=O), 1588.3 (C=C), 1573.84 (C=S). ^1H-NMR (300 MHz, DMSO-d_6, ppm) δ 11.40 (s, 1H, NH-CO), 11.31 (s, 1H, OH), 8.12 (s, 1H, CH=), 8.01 (d, J = 7.9 Hz, 1H, H_6 benzene), 7.91 (d, J = 4.2 Hz, 2H, H_4 +H_7, indole), 7.54–7.41 (m, 2H, H_3 benzene + H_2 indole), 7.37–7.22 (m, 2H, H_5 +H_6, indole), 6.97 (dd, J = 17.3, 8.1 Hz, 2H, H_4 +H_5, benzene), 4.00 (s, 3H, CH_3N). ^{13}C NMR

(101 MHz, DMSO, ppm) δ 189.71, 164.99, 163.08, 158.00, 136.96, 134.65, 134.45, 129.90, 127.29, 127.01, 123.54, 122.01, 119.46, 118.78, 117.22, 115.13, 111.01, 109.93, 33.50. ESI-MS [m/z]: [M + H]$^+$ = 411.0; [M − H]$^-$ = 408.2. Anal. Calcd. for $C_{20}H_{15}N_3O_3S_2$ (%): C, 58.66; H, 3.69; N, 10.26; S, 15.66 Found (%): 58.75 H, 3.62; N, 10.21; S, 15.52.

2-Hydroxy-N-{(5Z)-5-[(5-methoxy-1H-indol-3-yl)methylene]-4-oxo-2-thioxothiazolidin-3-yl}benzamide 5b. Yield 77%; m.p. 239–241 °C (DMFA-CH$_3$COOH).). IR (cm^{-1}): 3234.47 (OH), 1699.21 (C=O), 1654.84 (C=O), 1585.41 (C=C, C=S). ^{1}H-NMR (300 MHz, DMSO-d$_6$, ppm) δ 12.15 (s, 1H, NH), 11.45 (s, 1H, NH-CO), 11.35 (s, 1H, OH), 8.18 (s, 1H, CH=), 8.00 (d, J = 7.8 Hz, 1H, H$_6$ benzene), 7.74 (d, J = 2.2 Hz, 1H, H$_4$ indole), 7.50–7.33 (m, 3H, H$_3$ benzene + H$_2$ +H$_7$, indole), 7.04–6.90 (m, 2H, H$_4$ +H$_5$, benzene), 6.83 (d, J = 8.4 Hz, 1H, H$_6$ indole), 3.87 (s, 3H, CH$_3$O ^{13}C NMR (101 MHz, DMSO, ppm) δ 189.72, 165.10, 163.07, 158.10, 155.45, 134.64, 131.12, 131.09, 129.80, 128.22, 127.84, 119.43, 117.25, 115.07, 113.67, 113.38, 111.09, 110.44, 100.58, 55.85. ESI-MS [m/z]: [M + H]$^+$ = 426.0; [M − H]$^-$ = 424.0. Anal. Calcd. for $C_{20}H_{15}N_3O_4S_2$ (%): C, 56.46; H, 3.55; N, 9.88; S, 15.07 Found (%):C, 56.57; H, 3.49; N, 9.96; S, 15.15.

2-Hydroxy-N-{(5Z)-5-[(6-methoxy-1H-indol-3-yl)methylene]-4-oxo-2-thioxothiazolidin-3-yl}benzamide 5c. Yield 80%; m.p. 268–270 °C (DMFA-CH$_3$COOH). IR (cm^{-1}): 3227.72 (OH), 1705.96 (C=O), 1670.27 (C=O), 1591.2 (C=C), 1576.73 (C=S). ^{1}H-NMR (300 MHz, DMSO-d$_6$, ppm) δ 12.06 (s, 1H, NH), 11.45 (s, 1H, NH-CO),), 11.34 (s, 1H, OH), 8.10 (s, 1H, CH=), 7.99 (d, J = 7.9 Hz, 1H, H$_6$ benzene), 7.75 (d, J = 8.7 Hz, 1H, H$_4$ indole), 7.69 (d, J = 1.9 Hz, 1H, H$_3$ benzene), 7.48-7,42 (m, 1H, H$_2$ indole), 7.05–6.91 (m, 3H, H$_7$ indole +H$_4$ + H$_5$, benzene), 6. 83 (d, J = 8.5 Hz, 1H, H$_5$ indole), 3.84 (s, 3H, CH$_3$O^{13}C NMR (101 MHz, DMSO, ppm) δ 189.71, 165.00, 163.10, 158.01, 156.93, 137.32, 134.64, 130.31, 129.87, 127.93, 120.68, 119.49, 119.44, 117.22, 115.11, 111.63, 111.13, 111.06, 95.41, 55.28. ESI-MS [m/z]: [M + H]$^+$ = 426.0; [M − H]$^-$ = 424.0.. Anal. Calcd. for $C_{20}H_{15}N_3O_4S_2$ (%): C, 56.46; H, 3.55; N, 9.88; S, 15.07 Found (%):C, 56.39; H, 3.51; N, 9.80; S, 15.01.

4-Hydroxy-N-[(5Z)-5-(1H-indol-3-ylmethylene)-4-oxo-2-thioxothiazolidin-3-yl]benzamide 5d. Yield 90%; m.p. > 275 °C (DMFA-CH$_3$COOH). IR (cm^{-1}): 3369.48 (OH), 3225.79 (NH), 1694.38 (C=O), 1668.35 (C=O), 1591.2 (C=C), 1573.84 (C=S). ^{1}H-NMR (300 MHz, DMSO-d$_6$, ppm) δ 12.23 (s, 1H, NH), 11.12 (s, 1H, NH-CO), 9.89 (s, 1H, OH), 8.13 (s, 1H, CH=), 7.92–7.81 (m, 3H, H$_2$ + H$_6$, benzene + H$_4$ indole), 7.79 (d, J = 3.0 Hz, 1H, H$_7$ indole), 7.53–7.45 (m, 1H, H$_2$ indole), 7.28–7.15 (m, 2H, H$_5$ + H$_6$, indole), 6.85 (d, J = 8.7 Hz, 2H, H$_3$ +H$_5$, benzene). ^{13}C NMR (101 MHz, DMSO, ppm) δ 190.12, 164.06, 163.36, 161.49, 136.48, 131.20, 129.97, 127.80, 126.77, 123.49, 121.69, 121.50, 118.64, 115.30, 112.61, 111.16, 110.97. ESI-MS [m/z]: [M + H]$^+$ = 396.0; [M − H]$^-$ = 394.0. Anal. Calcd. for $C_{19}H_{13}N_3O_3S_2$ (%): C, 57.71; H, 3.31; N, 10.63; S, 16.22 Found (%):C, 57.62; H, 3.37; N, 10.55; S, 16.16.

N-[(5Z)-5-(1H-Indol-3-ylmethylene)-4-oxo-2-thioxothiazolidin-3-yl]nicotinamide 5e. Yield 90%; m.p. > 275 °C (DMFA-CH$_3$COOH). IR (cm^{-1}): 3485.2 (NH), 1696.31 (C=O), 1674.13 (C=O), 1596.98 (C=C), 1577.7 (C=S). ^{1}H-NMR (500 MHz, DMSO-d$_6$, ppm) δ 12.31 (s, 1H, NH), 11.75 (s, 1H, NH-CO), 9.15 (d, J = 1.7 Hz, 1H, H$_4$ pyridine), 8.77 (dd, J = 4.8, 1.4 Hz, 1H, H$_2$ pyridine), 8.33 (d, J = 8.0 Hz, 1H, H$_6$ pyridine), 8.17 (s, 1H, CH=), 7.90 (d, J = 7.6 Hz, 1H, H$_5$ pyridine), 7.84 (d, J = 3.0 Hz, 1H, H$_4$ indole), 7.57–7.48 (m, 2H, H$_2$ +H$_7$, indole), 7.27–7.18 (m, 2H, H$_5$ +H$_6$, indole). ^{13}C NMR (101 MHz, DMSO, ppm) δ 189.54, 163.32, 162.94, 150.78, 137.89, 136.41, 131.49, 128.38, 126.78, 123.56, 121.78, 121.38, 118.68, 112.65, 110.98, 110.72. ESI-MS [m/z]: [M + H]$^+$ = 381.0; Anal. Calcd. for $C_{18}H_{12}N_4O_2S_2$ (%): C, 56.83; H, 3.18; N, 14.73; S, 16.86 Found (%):C, 56.71; H, 3.24; N, 14.80; S, 16.79.

N-{(5Z)-5-[(1-Methyl-1H-indol-3-yl)methylene]-4-oxo-2-thioxothiazolidin-3-yl}nicotinamide 5f. Yield 94%; m.p. 270–272 °C (DMFA-CH$_3$COOH). IR (cm^{-1}): 3241.22 (NH), 1706.92 (C=O), 1681.85 (C=O), 1589.27 (C=C), 1572.87 (C=S). ^{1}H-NMR (300 MHz, DMSO-d$_6$, ppm) δ 11.75 (s, 1H, NH-CO), 9.16 (d, J = 1.9 Hz, 1H, H$_4$ pyridine), 8.77 (dd, J = 4.8, 1.3 Hz, 1H, H$_2$ pyridine), 8.36–8.31 (m, 1H, H$_6$ pyridine), 8.12 (s, 1H, CH=), 7.96 (s, 1H, H$_5$ pyridine), 7.91 (d, 1H, J = 7.9 Hz, H$_4$ indole), 7.58–7.47 (m, 2H, H$_2$ + H$_7$, indole), 7.32 (t, J = 7.5 Hz, 1H, H$_6$ indole), 7.26 (t, J = 7.4 Hz, 1H, H$_5$ indole), 4.00 (s, 3H, CH$_3$N). ^{13}C NMR (101 MHz, DMSO, ppm) δ 189.64, 163.34, 163.01, 153.40, 148.60, 136.99, 135.59, 134.68, 127.57, 127.30, 126.77, 123.97, 123.60, 122.10, 118.80, 111.08, 110.55, 109.95, 33.54. ESI-MS [m/z]:

[M + H]$^+$ = 395.0; [M − H]$^-$ = 394.0. Anal. Calcd. for C$_{19}$H$_{14}$N$_4$O$_2$S$_2$ (%): C, 57.85; H, 3.58; N, 14.20; S, 16.26 Found (%):C, 57.94; H, 3.51; N, 14.15; S, 16.35.

N-{(5Z)-5-[(5-Methoxy-1H-indol-3-yl)methylene]-4-oxo-2-thioxothiazolidin-3-yl}nicotinamide 5g. Yield 00%; m.p. 199–201 °C. IR (cm^{-1}): 3254.72 (NH), 1718.49 (C=O), 1681.85 (C=O), 1585.41 (C=C), 1576.73 (C=S). ^{1}H-NMR (300 MHz, DMSO-d$_6$, ppm) ^{1}H-NMR (300 MHz, DMSO-d$_6$, ppm) δ 12.17 (s, 1H, NH), 11.72 (s, 1H, NH-CO), 9.17 (s, 1H, H$_4$ pyridine), 8.77 (d, J = 3.0 Hz, 1H, H$_2$ pyridine), 8.35 (d, J = 7.5 Hz, 1H, H$_6$ pyridine), 8.19 (s, 1H, CH=), 7.74 (s, 1H, H$_5$ pyridine), 7.59–7.49 (m, 1H, H$_2$ indole), 7.46–7.30 (m, 2H, H$_4$ +H$_7$ indole), 6.83 (d, J = 8.5 Hz, 1H, H$_6$ indole), 3.86 (s, 3H, CH$_3$O). ^{13}C NMR (101 MHz, DMSO, ppm) δ 189.67, 163.30, 163.01, 155.51, 153.36, 148.61, 135.57, 131.33, 131.15, 128.76, 127.86, 126.82, 123.94, 113.69, 113.41, 111.12, 110.01, 100.64, 55.54. ESI-MS [m/z]: [M + H]$^+$ = 411.0; [M − H]$^-$ = 409.0. Anal. Calcd. for C$_{19}$H$_{14}$N$_4$O$_3$S$_2$ (%): C, 55.60; H, 3.44; N, 13.65; S, 15.62 Found (%): C, 55.49; H, 3.39; N, 13.58; S, 15.67.

N-[(5Z)-5-(1H-Indol-3-ylmethylene)-4-oxo-2-thioxothiazolidin-3-yl]isonicotinamide 5h. Yield 86%; m.p. > 275 °C Yield 86%; m.p. > 275 °C (DMFA-CH$_3$COOH). IR (cm^{-1}): 3196.86 (NH), 1718.49 (C=O), 1672.2 (C=O), 1594.09 (C=C), 1576.73 (C=S). ^{1}H-NMR (300 MHz, DMSO-d$_6$, ppm) δ 12.27 (s, 1H, NH), 11.79 (s, 1H, NH-CO), 8.78 (d, J = 5.8 Hz, 2H, H$_2$ +H$_6$, pyridine), 8.17 (s, 1H, CH=), 7.94–7.86 (m, 3H, H$_3$ +H$_5$, pyridine +H$_4$ indole), 7.82 (s, 1H, H$_7$ indole), 7.51 (d, J = 7.1 Hz, 1H, H$_2$ indole), 7.30–7.15 (m, 2H, H$_5$ +H$_6$, indole). ^{13}C NMR (101 MHz, DMSO, ppm) δ 189.53, 163.32, 162.94, 150.76, 137.94, 136.42, 131.46, 128.34, 126.77, 123.54, 121.76, 121.38, 118.66, 112.65, 110.99, 110.78. ESI-MS [m/z]: [M + H]$^+$ = 381.0; [M − H]$^-$ = 379.0. Anal. Calcd. for C$_{18}$H$_{12}$N$_4$O$_2$S$_2$ (%): C, 56.83; H, 3.18; N, 14.73; S, 16.86 Found (%):C, 56.89; H, 3.26; N, 14.65; S, 16.88.

N-{(5Z)-5-[(1-Methyl-1H-indol-3-yl)methylene]-4-oxo-2-thioxothiazolidin-3-yl}isonicotinamide 5i. Yield 95%; m.p. 269–271 °C (DMFA-CH$_3$COOH). IR (cm^{-1}): 3217.11 (NH), 1710.78 (C=O), 1674.13 (C=O), 1587.34 (C=C), 1570.95 (C=S).^{1}H-NMR (300 MHz, DMSO-d$_6$, ppm) δ 11.81 (s, 1H, NH-CO), 8.79 (d, J = 5.9 Hz, 2H, H$_2$ +H$_6$, pyridine), 8.13 (s, 1H, CH=), 7.99–7.86 (m, 4H, H$_3$ +H$_5$, pyridine + H$_4$ +H$_7$, indole), 7.51 (d, J = 7.9 Hz, 1H, H$_2$ indole), 7.37–7.20 (m, 2H, H$_5$ +H$_6$, indole), 4.00 (s, 3H, CH$_3$N). ^{13}C NMR (101 MHz, DMSO, ppm) δ 189.49, 163.32, 162.90, 150.78, 137.88, 137.00, 134.73, 127.68, 127.30, 123.61, 122.12, 121.38, 118.81, 111.09, 110.46, 109.95, 33.55. ESI-MS [m/z]: [M + H]$^+$ = 395.0; [M − H]$^-$ = 393.0. Anal. Calcd. for C$_{19}$H$_{14}$N$_4$O$_2$S$_2$ (%): C, 57.85; H, 3.58; N, 14.20; S, 16.26 Found (%):C, 57.78; H, 3.53; N, 14.28; S, 16.17.

N-{(5Z)-5-[(5-Methoxy-1H-indol-3-yl)methylene]-4-oxo-2-thioxothiazolidin-3-yl}isonicotinamide 5j. Yield 89%; m.p. 261–263 °C (CH$_3$COOH).). IR (cm^{-1}): 3199.75 (NH), 1706.92 (C=O), 1676.06 (C=O), 1588.3 (C=C, C=S). ^{1}H-NMR (300 MHz, DMSO-d$_6$, ppm) δ 12.20 (s, 1H, NH), 11.83 (s, 1H, NH-CO), 8.78 (d, J = 5.4 Hz, 2H, H$_2$ +H$_6$, pyridine), 8.20 (s, 1H, CH=), 7.90 (d, J = 5.4 Hz, 2H, H$_3$ +H$_5$, pyridine), 7.76 (d, J = 3.0 Hz, 1H, H$_4$ indole), 7.44–7.33 (m, 2H, H$_2$ +H$_7$, indole), 6.83 (dd, J = 8.9, 1.7 Hz, 1H, H$_6$ indole), 3.86 (s, 3H, CH$_3$O). ^{13}C NMR (101 MHz, DMSO, ppm) δ 189.50, 163.29, 162.91, 155.49, 150.78, 137.91, 131.39, 131.12, 128.89, 127.88, 121.39, 113.72, 113.42, 111.12, 109.87, 100.58, 55.51. ESI-MS [m/z]: [M + H]$^+$ = 411.0; [M − H]$^-$ = 409.0. Anal. Calcd. for C$_{19}$H$_{14}$N$_4$O$_3$S$_2$ (%): C, 55.60; H, 3.44; N, 13.65; S, 15.62 Found (%): C, 55.52; H, 3.47; N, 13.73; S, 15.55.

N-{(5Z)-5-[(6-Methoxy-1H-indol-3-yl)methylene]-4-oxo-2-thioxothiazolidin-3-yl}isonicotinamide 5k. Yield 89%; m.p. 275–277 °C (CH$_3$COOH). IR (cm^{-1}): 3550.78 (NH), 3346.34 (NH), 1725.24 (C=O), 1689.56 (C=O), 1596.98 (C=C), 1576.73 (C=S). ^{1}H-NMR (300 MHz, DMSO-d$_6$, ppm) δ 12.11 (s, 1H, NH), 11.85 (s, 1H, NH-CO), 8.78 (d, J = 5.3 Hz, 2H,H$_2$ +H$_6$, pyridine), 8.11 (s, 1H, CH=), 7.89 (d, J = 5.3 Hz, 2H, H$_3$ +H$_5$, pyridine), 7.74 (dd, J = 13.7, 5.6 Hz, 2H, H$_2$ +H$_4$, indole), 6.96 (s, 1H, H$_7$ indole), 6.83 (d, J = 8.6 Hz, 1H, H$_5$ indole), 3.84 (s, 3H, CH$_3$O). ^{13}C NMR (101 MHz, DMSO, ppm) δ 189.49, 163.30, 162.91, 156.97, 150.78, 137.88, 137.36, 130.66, 128.61, 121.38, 120.66, 119.52, 111.71, 111.17, 110.52, 95.46, 55.29. ESI-MS [m/z]: [M + H]$^+$ = 411.0; [M − H]$^-$ = 409.0. Anal. Calcd. for C$_{19}$H$_{14}$N$_4$O$_3$S$_2$ (%): C, 55.60; H, 3.44; N, 13.65; S, 15.62 Found (%): C, 55.73; H, 3.49; N, 13.57; S, 15.54.

(5Z)-5-(1H-Indol-3-ylmethylene)-3-morpholin-4-yl-2-thioxothiazolidin-4-one7a. Yield 86%; m.p. 273–275 °C (DMFA:CH$_3$COOH). IR (cm^{-1}): 3247.97 (NH), 1690.53 (C=O), 1594.09 (C=C), 1575.77 (C=S).^{1}H-NMR (300 MHz, DMSO-d$_6$, ppm) δ 12.10 (s, 1H, NH), 7.98 (s, 1H, CH=), 7.85 (d, J = 6.8 Hz, 1H, H$_4$ indole), 7.66 (d, J = 2.8 Hz, 1H, H$_7$ indole), 7.51–7.45 (m, 1H, H$_2$ indole), 7.27–7.13 (m, 2H, H$_5$ +H$_6$, indole), 3.81 (s, 6H, morpholine), 3.06 (s, 2H, morpholine). ^{13}C NMR (101 MHz, DMSO, ppm) δ 189.92, 165.21, 136.32, 130.51, 126.72, 126.03, 123.34, 121.50, 118.48, 112.53, 111.68, 110.95, 66.56, 50.14. ESI-MS [m/z]: [M + H]$^+$ = 346.2; [M − H]$^−$ = 344.2. Anal. Calcd. for C$_{16}$H$_{15}$N$_3$O$_2$S$_2$ (%): C, 55.63; H, 4.38; N, 12.16; S, 18.56 Found (%):C, 55.74; H, 4.32; N, 12.24; S, 18.49.

(5Z)-5-[(1-Methyl-1H-indol-3-yl)methylene]-3-morpholin-4-yl-2-thioxo-thiazolidin-4-one 7b was prepared according to [42].

(5Z)-5-[(5-Methoxy-1H-indol-3-yl)methylene]-3-morpholin-4-yl-2-thioxo-thiazolidin-4-one7c. Yield 82%; m.p. 250–252 °C (CH$_3$COOH). IR (cm^{-1}): 3163.11 (NH), 1690.53 (C=O), 1580.59 (C=C, C=S). ^{1}H-NMR (300 MHz, DMSO-d$_6$, ppm) δ 12.08 (s, 1H, NH), 7.99 (s, 1H, CH=), 7.61 (s, 1H, H$_4$ indole), 7.34 (d, J = 3.4 Hz, 2H, H$_2$ +H$_7$, indole), 6.81 (d, J = 8.7 Hz, 1H, H$_6$ indole), 4.05–3.57 (m, 9H, CH$_3$O, morpholine), 3.03 (s, 2H, morpholine). ^{13}C NMR (101 MHz, DMSO, ppm) δ 189.87, 165.20, 155.29, 131.04, 130.51, 127.75, 126.61, 113.52, 113.30, 111.04, 110.74, 100.34, 66.56, 55.46, 50.11. ESI-MS [m/z]: [M + H]$^+$ = 376.0; [M − H]$^−$ = 374.0. Anal. Calcd. for C$_{17}$H$_{17}$N$_3$O$_3$S$_2$ (%): C, 54.38; H, 4.56; N, 11.19; S, 17.08 Found (%):C, 54.31; H, 4.62; N, 11.04; S, 17.15.

3.3. Antibacterial Activity Evaluation

Bacterial strains utilized include Gram-negative: *Salmonella typhimurium* (ATCC 13311) *Pseudomonas aeruginosa* (ATCC 27853), *Escherichia coli* (ATCC 35210), *Enterobacter cloacae* (ATCC 35030) and Gram-positive bacteria: *Micrococcus flavus* (ATCC 10240), *Bacillus cereus* (isolated clinically), *Staphylococcus aureus* (ATCC 6538), and *Listeria monocytogenes* (NCTC 7973) bacteria. Pathogens were provided from the Mycological Laboratory, Institute for Biological Research "Siniša Stankovic" National institute of Republic of Serbia Belgrade. Resistant strains used were MRSA, *E. coli*, and *P. aeruginosa* [77,78].

For the determination of minimum inhibitory (MIC) and minimum bactericidal concentrations, the microdilution method, as previously described [77–79]. The minimum inhibitory (MIC) and minimum bactericidal (MBC) concentrations were determined by the modified microdilution method as previously reported [77–79]. Briefly, the fresh overnight culture of bacteria was adjusted to a concentration of 1×10^5 CFU/mL. The tested compounds were dissolved in 5% DMSO and serially diluted in tryptic soy broth (TSB) medium with bacterial inoculum (1.0×10^4 CFU per well). The microplates were incubated for 24 h at 37 °C. The MIC of the samples was detected following the addition of 40 μL of iodonitrotetrazolium chloride (INT) (0.2 mg/mL) and incubation at 37 °C for 30 min. The lowest concentration that produced a significant inhibition of the growth of the bacteria in comparison with the positive control was identified as the MIC. MBC was determined by serial sub-cultivation of 10 μL into microplates containing 100 μL of TSB. The lowest concentration that shows no growth after this sub-culturing was identified as the MBC, indicating 99.5% death of the original inoculum. Streptomycin and ampicillin were used as positive controls.

3.4. Antifungal Evaluation

The following fungi were used: Aspergillus niger (ATCC 6275), Aspergillus ochraceus (ATCC 12066), Aspergillus fumigatus (human isolate), Aspergillus versicolor (ATCC 11730), Penicillium funiculosum (ATCC 36839), Penicillium ochrochloron (ATCC 9112), Trichoderma viride (IAM 5061), Penicillium verrucosum var. cyclopium (food isolate). The organisms were obtained from the Mycological Laboratory, Department of Plant Physiology, Institute for Biological Research "Siniša Stankovic", National institute of Republic of Serbia, Belgrade, Serbia. All experiments were performed in duplicate and repeated three times, as previously described [80,81].

The fungal spores were washed from the surface of agar plates with sterile 0.85% saline containing 0.1% Tween 80 (*v/v*). The spore suspension was adjusted with sterile saline to a concentration of approximately 1.0×10^5 in a final volume of 100 μL per well. MIC determinations were performed by a serial dilution technique using 96-well microtiter plates. The examined compounds were serially diluted in broth Malt medium (MA), after which inoculum was added. The microplates were incubated for 72 h at 28 °C. The lowest concentrations without visible growth (at the binocular microscope) were defined as MICs. The fungicidal concentrations (MFCs) were determined by serial subcultivation of 2 μL of tested fractions dissolved in medium and inoculation into microtiter plates containing 100 μL of broth per well and further incubation 72 h at 28 °C. The lowest concentration with no visible growth was defined as MFC, indicating 99.5% killing of the original inoculum. The fungicides bifonazole and ketoconazole were used as positive controls.

3.5. Docking Studies

The program AutoDock 4.2® software was used for the docking simulation. The free energy of binding (ΔG) of *E. coli* DNA GyrB, Thymidylate kinase, *E. coli* MurA, *E. coli* primase, *E. coli* MurB, DNA topo IV, and CYP51 of *C. albicans,* in complex with the inhibitors were generated using this molecular docking program. The X-ray crystal structures data of all the enzymes used were obtained from the Protein Data Bank (PDB ID: 1KZN, AQGG, 1DDE, JV4T, 2Q85, 1S16, and 5V5Z respectively). All procedures were performed according to our previous paper [78].

3.6. Cytotoxicity

HEK 293 cells were cultured in DMEM medium, supplemented with 10% fetal calf serum (Sigma Chemical Co., St. Louis, MO, USA), 50 μg/mL streptomycin (Sigma Chemical Co.), and 50 units/mL penicillin (Sigma Chemical Co.) in 5% CO_2-containing humidified atmosphere at 37°C. Since compound solutions contained DMSO, control cultures containing only DMSO at the final concentration obtained when the appropriate volume of compound solution was added were performed.

MTT Assay for Determination of Cell Viability

MTT assay based on the colorimetric measurement of formazan formed after reducing MTT by cellular NAD(P)H-dependent oxidoreductases was used to examine the cytotoxic activity of the compounds. Briefly, the cells were seeded into 96-well plates in 100 μL of complete culture medium at a concentration of 5,000 substrate-dependent cells per well and left incubated overnight as described above. The formulations to be tested (100 μL aliquots) were added to the culture medium at different concentrations and left incubated for 72 h. The MTT assay was performed following the manufacturer's recommendations and assessed using an EL ×800 absorbance reader (BioTek Instruments; Winooski, VT, USA).

4. Conclusions

Eleven 5-[(R-1*H*-indol-3-yl)methylene]-4-oxo-2-thioxo-thiazolidin-3-ylcarbamides **5a-k** and three 5-[(R-1*H*-indol-3-yl) methylene] -3-morpholin-4-yl-2-thioxothiazolidin-4-ones **7a-c** were designed, synthesized and evaluated in silico and experimentally for their antimicrobial action against panel of Gram positive, Gram negative bacteria and fungi.

It should be mentioned that all compounds appeared to be more potent than ampicillin against all bacteria tested and then streptomycin against all bacteria except *B. cereus (isolated clinically M. flavus* (ATCC 10240), and *En. cloacae* (ATCC 35030). The most sensitive bacteria was found to be *S. aureus* (ATCC 6538), while *L. monocytogenes* (NCTC 7973) was the most resistant one. Compounds also appeared to be active against three resistant strains MRSA, *E. coli,* and *P. aeruginosa* showing better activity against MRSA than both reference drugs while against the other two resistant strains better than ampicillin.

Concerning antifungal action, the tested compounds exhibited very good activity against all the fungal species tested, being more active than ketoconazole and bifonazole. The most sensitive fungal strain appeared to be *T. viride* (IAM 5061), while the most resistant filamentous *A. fumigatus* (human isolate).

It can be observed that the growth of both Gram-negative and Gram-positive bacteria and fungi responded differently to the tested compounds, which indicates that different substituents may lead to different modes of action or that the metabolism of some bacteria/fungi was better able to overcome the effect of the compounds or adapt to it.

Docking analysis to DNA Gyrase, Thymidylate kinase and *E.coli* MurB indicated a probable involvement of MurB inhibition in the antibacterial mechanism of compounds tested while docking analysis to 14α-lanosterol demethylase (CYP51) and tetrahydrofolate reductase of *Candida albicans* indicated a likely implication of CYP51 reductase at the antifungal activity of the compounds and secondary involvement of dihydrofolate reductase inhibition at the mechanism of action of the most active compounds.

Since the most active compounds **5d**, **5g**, **5k**, **7c** demonstrated the low cytotoxicity against HEK-293 human embryonic kidney cell line and reasonable selectivity index, this chemical series looks promising for investigations as the antimicrobial agents.

Finally, compounds **5d** (Z)-N-(5-((1H-indol-3-yl)methylene)-4-oxo-2-thioxothiazolidin-3 -yl)-4-hydroxybenzamide and **5g** (Z)-N-(5-((5-methoxy-1H-indol-3-yl)methylene)-4-oxo-2- thioxothiazolidin-3-yl)nicotinamide as well as **7c** (Z)-5-((5-methoxy-1H-indol-3-yl)methylene)-3- morpholino-2-thioxothiazolidin-4-one can be considered as lead compounds for further development of more potent and safe antibacterial and antifungal agents.

Author Contributions: Conceptualization, A.G. and V.K.; methodology, V.H.; software, P.A. and P.P.; formal analysis, V.M.; investigation, M.I., M.K. and M.D.S; data curation, A.G., V.P., M.D.S. and P.E., original draft preparation, A.G. and P.P.; review & editing, A.G. and V.P.; supervision, A.G. and V.P. All authors have read and agreed to the published version of the manuscript.

Acknowledgments: Computational predictions of biological activity by AntiBac-Pred, AntiFun-Pred and AcuTox web-services (P.P. and V.P.) were performed in the framework of the Russian State Academies of Sciences Fundamental Research Program for 2013–2020.

References

1.   Michaud, C.M. Global Burden of Infectious Diseases. *Encycl. Microbiol.* **2009**, 444–454.

2.   Nii-Trebi, N.I. Emerging and neglected infectious diseases: Insights, advances, and challenges. *Biomed. Res. Int.* **2017**, *2017*, 5245021. [CrossRef] [PubMed]

3.   Mukherjee, S. Emerging Infectious Diseases: Epidemiological Perspective. *Indian J. Dermatol.* **2017**, *62*, 459–467.

4.   Ventola, C.L. The antibiotic resistance crisis: Part 1: Causes and threats. *Pharm. Ther.* **2015**, *40*, 277–283.

5.   Michael, C.A.; Dominey-Howes, D.; Labbate, M. The antimicrobial resistance crisis: Causes, consequences, and management. *Front. Public Health* **2014**, *16*, 145. [CrossRef]

6.   Rice, L.B. Federal funding for the study of antimicrobial resistance in nosocomial pathogens: No ESKAPE. *J. Infect. Dis.* **2008**, *197*, 1079–1081. [CrossRef]

7.   Holmes, A.H.; Moore, L.S.; Sundsfjord, A.; Steinbakk, M.; Regmi, S.; Karkey, A.; Guerin, P.J.; Piddock, L.J. Understanding the mechanisms and drivers of antimicrobial resistance. *Lancet* **2016**, *387*, 176–187. [CrossRef]

8.   Tripathi, A.C.; Gupta, S.J.; Fatima, G.N.; Sonar, P.K.; Verma, A.; Saraf, S.K. 4- Thiazolidinones: The Advances Continue . . . . *Eur. J. Med. Chem.* **2014**, *7*, 52–57. [CrossRef]

9. Kaminskyy, D.; Kryshchyshyn, A.; Lesyk, R. 5-Ene-4-thiazolidinones–An efficient tool in medicinal chemistry. *Eur. J. Med. Chem.* **2017**, *140*, 542–594. [CrossRef]

10. Kaminskyy, D.; Kryshchyshyn, A.; Lesyk, R. Recent developments with rhodanine as a scaffold for drug discovery. *Expert Opin. Drug Discov.* **2017**, *12*, 1233–1252.

11. Baell, B. Observations on screening-based research and some concerning trends in the literature. *Future Med. Chem.* **2010**, *2*, 1529–1546.

12. Mendgen, T.; Steuer, C.; Klein, C.D. Privileged scaffolds or promiscuous binders: A comparative study on rhodanines and related heterocycles in medicinal chemistry. *J. Med. Chem.* **2012**, *55*, 743–753. [CrossRef] [PubMed]

13. Morphy, R.; Rankovic, Z. Designed multiple ligands. An emerging drug discovery paradigm. *J. Med. Chem.* **2005**, *48*, 6523–6543. [CrossRef] [PubMed]

14. Fortin, S.; Bérubé, G. Advances in the development of hybrid anticancer drugs. *Expert Opin. Drug Discov.* **2013**, *8*, 1029–1047.

15. Kryshchyshyn, A.; Roman, O.; Lozynskyi, A.; Lesyk, R. Thiopyrano[2,3-d]thiazoles as new efficient scaffolds in medicinal chemistry. *Sci. Pharm.* **2018**, *86*, 26. [CrossRef] [PubMed]

16. Cong, N.T.; Nhan, H.T.; Van Hung, L.; Thang, T.D.; Kuo, P.C. Synthesis and antibacterial activity of analogs of 5-arylidene-3-(4-methylcoumarin-7-yloxyacetylamino)-2-thioxo-1,3-thiazoli-din-4-one. *Molecules* **2014**, *19*, 13577–13586. [CrossRef]

17. Song, M.-X.; Deng, X.-Q.; Li, Y.-R.; Zheng, C.-J.; Hong, L.; Piao, H.-R. Synthesis and biological evaluation of (E)-1-(substituted)-3-phenylprop-2-en-1-ones bearing rhodanines as potent anti-microbial agents. *J. Enzyme Inhib. Med. Chem.* **2014**, *29*, 647–653. [CrossRef]

18. Krátký, M.; Vinšová, J.; Stolaříková, J. Antimicrobial activity of rhodanine-3-acetic acid derivatives. *Bioorg. Med. Chem.* **2017**, *25*, 1839–1845. [CrossRef]

19. Horishny, V.; Kartsev, V.; Geronikaki, A.; Matiychuk, V.; Petrou, A.; Glamoclija, J.; Ciric, A.; Sokovic, M. 5-(1H-Indol-3-ylmethylene)-4-oxo-2-thioxothiazolidin-3-yl)alkancarboxylic Acids as Antimicrobial Agents: Synthesis, Biological Evaluation, and Molecular Docking Studies. *Molecules* **2020**, *25*, 1964. [CrossRef]

20. Incerti, M.; Vicini, P.; Geronikaki, A.; Eleftheriou, P.; Tsagkadouras, A.; Zoumpoulakis, P.; Fotakis, C.; Ćirić, A.; Glamočlija, J.; Soković, M. New N-(2-phenyl-4-oxo-1,3-thiazolidin-3-yl)-1,2-benzothiazole -3-carboxamides and Acetamides as Antimicrobial Agents. *Med. Chem. Commun.* **2017**, *8*, 2142–2154. [CrossRef]

21. Ozen, C.; Ceylan-Unlusoy, M.; Aliary, N.; Ozturk, M.; Bozdag-Dundar, O. Thiazolidinedione or Rhodanine: A Study on Synthesis and Anticancer Activity Comparison of Novel Thiazole Derivatives. *Pharm. Pharm. Sci.* **2017**, *20*, 415–427. [CrossRef]

22. Fu, H.; Hou, X.; Wang, L.; Dun, Y.; Yang, X.; Fang, H. Design, synthesis and biological evaluation of 3-aryl-rhodanine benzoic acids as anti-apoptotic protein Bcl-2 inhibitors. *Bioorg. Med. Chem. Lett.* **2015**, *25*, 5265–5269. [CrossRef] [PubMed]

23. Havrylyuk, D.; Zimenkovsky, B.; Lesyk, R. Synthesis and Anticancer Activity of Novel Nonfused Bicyclic Thiazolidinone Derivatives. *Phosphorus Sulfur* **2009**, *184*, 638–650. [CrossRef]

24. El-Miligy, M.; Hazzaa, A.; El-Messmary, H.; Nassra, R.A. El-Hawash, Soad, New hybrid molecules combining benzothiophene or benzofuran with rhodanine as dual COX-1/2 and 5-LOX inhibitors: Synthesis, biological evaluation and docking study. *Bioorg. Chem.* **2017**, *72*, 102–115. [CrossRef] [PubMed]

25. R. Atta-Allah, S.; Nassar, I.F.; El-Sayed, W.A. Design, synthesis and anti-inflammatoryvel 5-(Indol-3-yl)-thiazolidinone derivatives as COX-2 inhibitors. *J. Pharmacol. Ther. Res.* **2020**, *5*, 1–16.

26. Powers, J.P.; Piper, D.E.; Li, Y.; Mayorga, V.; Anzola, J.; Chen, J.M.; Jaen, J.C.; Lee, G.; Liu, J.; Peterson, M.G.; et al. SAR and mode of action of novel non-nucleoside inhibitors of hepatitis C NS5b RNA polymerase. *J. Med. Chem.* **2006**, *49*, 1034–1046. [CrossRef] [PubMed]

27. Ramkumar, K.; Yarovenko, V.N.; Nikitina, A.S.; Zavarzin, I.V.; Krayushkin, M.M.; Kovalenko, L.V.; Esqueda, A.; Odde, S.; Neamati, N. Design, synthesis and structure-activity studies of rhodanine derivatives as HIV-1 integrase inhibitors. *Molecules* **2010**, *15*, 3958–3992. [CrossRef]

28. Petrou, A.; Eleftheriou, P.; Geronikaki, A.; Akrivou, M.G.; Vizirianakis, I. Novel thiazolidin-4-ones as potential non-nucleoside inhibitors of HIV-1 reverse transcriptase. *Molecules* **2019**, *24*, 3821. [CrossRef]

29. Kryshchyshyn, A.; Kaminskyy, D.; Roman, O.; Kralovics, R.; Karpenko, O.; Lesyk, R. Synthesis and anti-leukemic activity of pyrrolidinedione-thiazolidinone hybrids. *Ukr Biochem. J.* **2020**, *92*, 108–119.

30. Havrylyuk, D.; Zimenkovsky, B.; Vasylenko, O.; Gzella, A.; Lesyk, R. Synthesis of new 4- thiazolidinone-, pyrazoline-, and isatin-based conjugates with promising antitumor activity. *J. Med. Chem.* **2012**, *55*, 8630–8641. [CrossRef]

31. Havrylyuk, D.; Roman, O.; Lesyk, R. Synthetic approaches, structure activity relationship and biological applications for pharmacologically attractive pyrazole/pyrazoline–thiazolidine– based hybrids. *Eur. J. Med. Chem.* **2016**, *113*, 145–166. [CrossRef]

32. Saini, T.; Kumar, S.; Narasimhan, B. Central nervous system activities of indole derivatives: An overview. *Cent. Nerv. Syst. Agents Med. Chem.* **2016**, *16*, 19–28. [CrossRef] [PubMed]

33. Singh, P.; Singh, O.M. Recent progress in biological activities of indole and indole alkaloids. *Mini Rev. Med. Chem.* **2018**, *18*, 9–25.

34. Kaur, J.; Utreja, D.; Jain, N.; Sharma, S. Recent Developments in the Synthesis and Antimicrobial Activity of Indole and Its Derivatives. *Curr. Org. Synth.* **2019**, *16*, 17–37. [CrossRef]

35. Bathula, C.; Tripathi, S.; Srinivasan, R.; Jha, K.K.; Ganguli, A.; Chakrabarti, G.; Singh, S.; Munshi, P.; Sen, S. Synthesis of novel 5-arylidenethiazolidinones with apoptotic properties via a three component reaction using piperidine as a bifunctional reagent. *Org. Biomol. Chem.* **2016**, *14*, 8053–8063. [CrossRef]

36. Sayed, M.; El-Dean, A.; Ahmed, M.; Hassanien, R. Synthesis of some heterocyclic compounds derived from indole as antimicrobial agents. *Synth. Commun.* **2018**, *48*, 413–421. [CrossRef]

37. Jain, P.; Utreja, D.; Sharma, P. An efficacious synthesis of N-1–, C-3–substituted indole derivatives and their antimicrobial studies. *J. Hetrocyclic Chem.* **2020**, *57*, 428–435. [CrossRef]

38. Shaikh, T.M.A.; Debebe, H. Synthesis and Evaluation of Antimicrobial Activities of Novel N-Substituted Indole Derivatives. *J. Chem.* **2020**, 1–9, Article ID 4358453, 9 pages.

39. Kumar, P.; Singh, S.; Rizki, M.; Pratama, F. Synthesis of some novel 1H-indole derivatives with antibacterial activity and antifungal activity. *Lett. Appl. NanoBioScience* **2020**, *9*, 961–967.

40. Liu, Z.; Tang, L.; Zhu, H.; Xu, T.; Qiu, C.; Zheng, S.; Gu, Y.; Feng, J.; Zhang, Y.; Liang, G. Design, Synthesis, and Structure−Activity Relationship Study of Novel Indole-2-carboxamide Derivatives as Anti-inflammatoryAgents for the Treatment of Sepsis. *J. Med. Chem.* **2016**, *59*, 4637–4650. [CrossRef]

41. Li, S.; Wang, Z.; Xiao, H.; Bian, Z.; Wang, J. Enantioselective synthesis of indole derivatives byRh/Pd relay catalysis and their anti-inflammatory evaluation. *Chem. Commun.* **2020**, *56*, 7573–7576. [CrossRef]

42. Abdellatif, K.R.A.; Elsaady, M.Y.; Amin, N.H.; Hefny, A.A. Design, Synthesis and biological evaluation of some novel indole derivatives as selective COX-2 inhibitors. *J. Appl. Pharm. Sci.* **2017**, *7*, 69–77.

43. Bhat, M.A.; Al-Omar, M.A.; Raish, M. Indole Derivatives as Cyclooxygenase Inhibitors: Synthesis, Biological Evaluation and Docking Studies. *Molecules* **2018**, *23*, 1250. [CrossRef] [PubMed]

44. Sidhu, J.S.; Singla, R.; Jaitak, V. Indole Derivatives as Anticancer Agents for Breast Cancer Therapy: A Review. *Anticancer Agents Med. Chem.* **2015**, *16*, 160–173. [CrossRef] [PubMed]

45. El-Sharief, A.M.S.; Ammar, Y.A.; Belal, A.; El-Sharief, M.A.S.; Mohamed, Y.A.; Ahmed, B.M.; Mehany, A.B.M.; Elhag Ali, G.A.M.; Ragab, A. Design, synthesis, molecular docking and biological activity evaluation of some novel indole derivatives as potent anticancer active agents and apoptosis inducers. *Bioorg. Chem.* **2019**, *85*, 399–412. [CrossRef]

46. Cascioferro, S.; Li Petri, G.; Parrino, B.; El Hassouni, B.; Carbone, D.; Arizza, V.; Perricone, U.; Padova, A.; Funel, N.; Peters, G.J.; et al. 3-(6-Phenylimidazo [2,1-b][1,3,4]thiadiazol-2-yl)-1H-Indole Derivatives as New Anticancer Agents in the Treatment of Pancreatic Ductal Adenocarcinoma. *Molecules* **2020**, *25*, 329. [CrossRef] [PubMed]

47. Zhang, M.-Z.; Chen, Q.; Yang, G.F. A review on recent developments of indole-containing antiviral agents. *J. Med. Chem.* **2015**, *89*, 421–441. [CrossRef] [PubMed]

48. Bardiot, D. Discovery of Indole Derivatives as Novel and Potent Dengue Virus Inhibitors. *J. Med. Chem.* **2018**, *61*, 8390–8401. [CrossRef]

49. Che, Z.; Tian, Y.; Liu, S.; Hu, M.; Che, G. Discovery of N-arylsulfonyl-3-acylindole benzoyl hydrazone derivatives as anti-HIV-1 agents. *Braz. J. Pharm. Sci* **2019**, *54*, e17543. [CrossRef]

50. Sanna, G.; Madeddu, S.; Giliberti, G.; Piras, S.; Struga, M.; Wrzosek, M.; Kubiak-Tomaszewska, G.; Koziol, A.E.; Savchenko, O.; Lis, T.; et al. Synthesis and Biological Evaluation of Novel Indole-Derived Thioureas. *Molecules* **2018**, *23*, 2554. [CrossRef]

51. Ramya, V.; Vembu, S.; Ariharasivakumar, G.; Gopalakrishnan, M. Synthesis, Characterisation, Molecular Docking, Anti-microbial and Anti-diabetic Screening of Substituted 4-indolylphenyl-6-arylpyrimidine-2-imine Derivatives. *Drug Res. (Stuttg)* **2017**, *67*, 515–526. [CrossRef]

52. Tymiak, A.A.; Rinehart, K.L.; Bakus, G.J. Constituents of morphologically similar sponges: Aplysina and Smenospongia species. *Tetrahedron* **1985**, *41*, 1039–1047. [CrossRef]

53. Djura, P.; Stierle, D.B.; Sullivan, B. Some metabolites of the marine sponges Smenospongia aurea and Smenospongia (ident.Polyfibrospongia) echina. *J. Org.Chem.* **1980**, *45*, 1435–1441. [CrossRef]

54. Fattorusso, E.; Lanzotti, V.; Magno, S.; Novellino, E. Tryptophan derivatives from a Mediterranean anthozoan, Astroides calycularis. *J. Nat. Prod.* **1985**, *48*, 924–927. [CrossRef]

55. Buyukbingol, E.; Suzen, S.; Klopman, G. Studies on the synthesis and structure–activity relationships of 5-(3'-indolyl)-2-thiohydantoin derivatives as aldose reductase enzyme inhibitors. *Farmaco* **1994**, *49*, 443–447. [PubMed]

56. Pogodin, P.V.; Lagunin, A.A.; Rudik, A.V.; Druzhilovskiy, D.S.; Filimonov, D.A.; Poroikov, V.V. AntiBac-Pred: A Web Application for Predicting Antibacterial Activity of Chemical Compounds. *J. Chem. Inf. Model.* **2019**, *59*, 4513–4518. [CrossRef] [PubMed]

57. Poroikov, V.; Filimonov, D.; Gloriozova, T.; Lagunin, A.; Druzhilovskiy, D.; Rudik, A.; Stolbov, L.; Dmitriev, A.; Tarasova, O.; Ivanov, S.; et al. Computer-aided prediction of biological activity spectra for organic compounds: The possibilities and limitations. *Russ. Chem. Bull.* **2019**, *68*, 2143–2154. [CrossRef]

58. Clarivate Analytics Integrity. Available online: https://integrity.clarivate.com/integrity/ (accessed on 21 July 2020).

59. Antifungal Activity Predictor. Available online: http://www.way2drug.com/micf (accessed on 21 July 2020).

60. Filimonov, D.A.; Zakharov, A.V.; Lagunin, A.A.; Poroikov, V.V. QNA-based 'Star Track' QSAR approach. *SAR QSAR Env. Res.* **2009**, *20*, 679–709. [CrossRef]

61. Lagunin, A.; Zakharov, A.; Filimonov, D.; Poroikov, V. QSAR Modelling of Rat Acute Toxicity on the Basis of PASS Prediction. *Mol. Inform.* **2011**, *30*, 241–250. [CrossRef]

62. Bruno, G.; Costantino, L.; Curinga, C.; Maccari, R.; Monforte, F.; Nicolo, F.; Ottana, R.; Vigorita, M.G. Synthesis and Aldose Reductase Inhibitory Activity of5-Arylidene-2,4-thiazolidinediones. *Bioorg. Med. Chem.* **2002**, *10*, 1077–1084. [CrossRef]

63. Abdeen, S.; Kunkle, T.; Salim, N.; Ray, A.-M.; Mammadova, N.; Summers, C.; Stevens, M.; Ambrose, A.J.; Park, Y.; Schultz, P.G.; et al. Sulfonamido-2-arylbenzoxazole GroEL/ES Inhibitors as Potent Antibacterials against Methicillin-Resistant Staphylococcus aureus (MRSA). *J. Med. Chem.* **2018**, *61*, 7345–7357. [CrossRef]

64. Menozzi, G.; Merello, L.; Fossa, P.; Ranise, A.; Mosti, L.; Bondavalli, F.; Loddo, R.; Murgioni, C.; Mascia, V.; La Colla, P.; et al. Synthesis, antimicrobial activity and molecular modeling studies of halogenated 4-[1H-imidazol-1-yl(phenyl)methyl]-1,5-diphenyl-1H-pyrazoles. *Bioorg. Med. Chem.* **2004**, *12*, 5465–5483. [CrossRef] [PubMed]

65. Vieira, F.T.; de Lima, G.M.; Maia, J.R.; Speziali, N.L.; Ardisson, J.D.; Rodrigues, L.; Correa, A., Jr.; Romero, O.B. Synthesis, characterization and biocidal activity of new organotin complexes of 2-(3-oxocyclohex-1-enyl)benzoic acid. *Eur. J. Med. Chem.* **2010**, *45*, 883–889. [CrossRef] [PubMed]

66. Gjorgjieva, M.; Tomasic̆, T.; Barancokova, M.; Katsamakas, S.; Ilas, J.; Tammela, P.; Masic̆, L.P.; Kikelj, D. Discovery of Benzothiazole Scaffold-Based DNA Gyrase B Inhibitors. *J. Med. Chem.* **2016**, *59*, 8941–8954. [CrossRef] [PubMed]

67. Parvathy, N.G.; Manju, P.; Mukesh, M.; Thomas, L. Design, synthesis and molecular docking studies of benzothiazole derivatives as anti microbial agents. *Int. J. Pharm. Pharm. Sci.* **2013**, *5*, 101–106.

68. Ren, Y.; Zhang, L.; Zhou, C.H.; Geng, R.X. Recent Development of Benzotriazole-based Medicinal Drugs. *Med. Chem.* **2014**, *4*, 640–662. [CrossRef]

69. Andres, C.J.; Bronson, J.J.; D'Andrea, S.V.; Walsh, A.W. 4-thiazolidinones: Novel inhibitors of the bacterial enzyme MurB. *Bioorg. Med. Chem. Lett.* **2000**, *10*, 715–717. [CrossRef]

70. Ahmed, S.; Zayed, M.F.; El-Messery, S.M.; Al-Agamy, M.H.; Abdel-Rahman, H.M. Design, Synthesis, Antimicrobial Evaluation and Molecular Modeling Study of 1,2,4-Triazole-Based 4-Thiazolidinones. *Molecules* **2016**, *21*, 568. [CrossRef]

71. Pitta, E.; Tsolaki, E.; Geronikaki, A.; Petrovic, J.; Glamočlija, J.; Sokovic, M.; Crespan, E.; Maga, G.; Bhunia, S.S.; Saxena, A.K. 4-Thiazolidinone derivatives as potent antimicrobial agents: Microwave-assisted synthesis, biological evaluation and docking studies. *MedChemComm* **2015**, *6*, 319–326. [CrossRef]

72. Karanth,   S.;   Narayana,   B.;   Kodandoor,   S.C.;   Sarojini,   B.K.
    2-{[(4-Hydroxy-3,5-dimethoxyphenyl)methylidene]hydrazinylidene}-4-oxo-1,3-thiazolidin-5-yl Acetic Acid.
    Molbank **2018**, *2018*, 2-9 M1009. [CrossRef]

73. Stana, A.; Vodnar, D.C.; Tamaian, R.; Pîrnău, A.; Vlase, L.; Ionuț, I.; Oniga, O.; Tiperciuc, B. Design, Synthesis
    and Antifungal Activity Evaluation of New Thiazolin-4-ones as Potential Lanosterol 14α-Demethylase
    Inhibitors. *Int. J. Mol. Sci.* **2017**, *18*, 177. [CrossRef]

74. Incerti, M.; Vicini, P.; Geronikaki, A.; Eleftheriou, P.; Tsagkadouras, A.; Zoumpoulakis, P.; Fotakis, C.; Ćirić, A.;
    Glamočlija, J.; Soković, M. New N-(2-phenyl-4-oxo-1,3-thiazolidin-3-yl)-1,2-benzothiazole-3-carboxamides
    and acetamides asantimicrobial agents. *Med. Chem. Commun.* **2017**, *8*, 2142. [CrossRef] [PubMed]

75. Can, N.O.; Çevik, U.A.; Sağlık, B.N.; Levent, S.; Korkut, B.; Özkay, Y.; Kaplancıklı, Z.A.; Koparal, A.S.
    Synthesis, Molecular Docking Studies, and Antifungal Activity Evaluation of New Benzimidazole-Triazoles
    as Potential Lanosterol 14α-Demethylase Inhibitors. *J. Chem.* **2017**, 1–15, Article ID 9387102, 15 pages.
    [CrossRef]

76. Benson, T.E.; Walsh, C.T.; Massey, V. Kinetic characterization of wild-type and S229A mutant MurB: Evidence
    for the role of Ser 229 as a general acid. *Biochemistry* **1997**, *36*, 796–805. [CrossRef] [PubMed]

77. Kartsev, V.; Lichitsky, B.; Geronikaki, A.; Petrou, A.; Smiljkovic, M.; Kostic, M.; Radanovic, O.; Soković, M.
    Design, synthesis and antimicrobial activity of usnic acid derivatives. *MedChemComm* **2018**, *9*, 870–882.
    [CrossRef]

78. Fesatidou, M.; Zagaliotis, P.; Camoutsis, C.; Petrou, A.; Eleftheriou, P.; Tratrtat, C.; Haroun, M.; Geronikaki, A.;
    Ciric, A.; Sokovic, M. 5-Adamantan thiadiazole-based thiazolidinones as antimicrobial agents. Design,
    synthesis, molecular docking and evaluation. *Bioorg. Med. Chem.* **2018**, *26*, 4664–4676. [CrossRef]

79. Kostić, M.; Smiljković, M.; Petrović, J.; Glamočilija, J.; Barros, L.; Ferreira, I.C.F.R.; Ćirić, A.; Soković, M.
    Chemical, nutritive composition and a wide range of bioactive properties of honey mushroom Armillaria
    mellea (Vahl: Fr.) Kummer. *Food Function* **2017**, *8*, 3239–3249. [CrossRef]

80. Kritsi, E.; Matsoukas, M.T.; Potamitis, C.; Detsi, A.; Ivanov, M.; Sokovic, M.; Zoumpoulakis, P. Novel Hit
    Compounds as Putative Antifungals: The Case of Aspergillus fumigatus. *Molecules* **2019**, *24*, 3853. [CrossRef]

81. Aleksić, M.; Stanisavljević, D.; Smiljković, M.; Vasiljević, P.; Stevanović, M.; Soković, M.; Stojković, D.
    Pyrimethanil: Between efficient fungicide against Aspergillus rot on cherry tomato and cytotoxic agent on
    human cell lines. *Ann. App. Bio.* **2019**, *175*, 228–235. [CrossRef]

9

Potential of Cell-Free Supernatant from *Lactobacillus plantarum* NIBR97, Including Novel Bacteriocins, as a Natural Alternative to Chemical Disinfectants

Sam Woong Kim [1](ID), Song I. Kang [1](ID), Da Hye Shin [1](ID), Se Yun Oh [1](ID), Chae Won Lee [2],
Yoonyong Yang [2], Youn Kyoung Son [2], Hee-Sun Yang [2], Byoung-Hee Lee [2], Hee-Jung An [3],
In Sil Jeong [4],* and Woo Young Bang [2],*(ID)

[1] Gene Analysis Center, Gyeongnam National University of Science & Technology, Jinju 52725, Korea;
    swkim@gntech.ac.kr (S.W.K.); mole160104@naver.com (S.I.K.); nini1114@naver.com (D.H.S.);
    ks-sy0809@naver.com (S.Y.O.)
[2] National Institute of Biological Resources (NIBR), Environmental Research Complex, Incheon 22689, Korea;
    chaewon326@korea.kr (C.W.L.); tazemenia@korea.kr (Y.Y.); sophy004@korea.kr (Y.K.S.);
    moeicy@korea.kr (H.-S.Y.); dpt510@korea.kr (B.-H.L.)
[3] Department of Pathology, CHA Bundang Medical Center, CHA University, Seongnam 13496, Korea;
    hjahn@cha.ac.kr
[4] Center for Immune Cell Research, CHA Advanced Research Institute, Seongnam 13488, Korea
*   Correspondence: insiljeong@gmail.com (I.S.J.); wybang@korea.kr (W.Y.B.)

Abstract: The recent pandemic of coronavirus disease 2019 (COVID-19) has increased demand for chemical disinfectants, which can be potentially hazardous to users. Here, we suggest that the cell-free supernatant from *Lactobacillus plantarum* NIBR97, including novel bacteriocins, has potential as a natural alternative to chemical disinfectants. It exhibits significant antibacterial activities against a broad range of pathogens, and was observed by scanning electron microscopy (SEM) to cause cellular lysis through pore formation in bacterial membranes, implying that its antibacterial activity may be mediated by peptides or proteins and supported by proteinase K treatment. It also showed significant antiviral activities against HIV-based lentivirus and influenza A/H3N2, causing lentiviral lysis through envelope collapse. Furthermore, whole-genome sequencing revealed that NIBR97 has diverse antimicrobial peptides, and among them are five novel bacteriocins, designated as plantaricin 1 to 5. Plantaricin 3 and 5 in particular showed both antibacterial and antiviral activities. SEM revealed that plantaricin 3 causes direct damage to both bacterial membranes and viral envelopes, while plantaricin 5 damaged only bacterial membranes, implying different antiviral mechanisms. Our data suggest that the cell-free supernatant from *L. plantarum* NIBR97, including novel bacteriocins, is potentially useful as a natural alternative to chemical disinfectants.

Keywords: AMP; antimicrobial activity; antiviral activity; bacteriocin; COVID-19; disinfectant; *Lactobacillus plantarum*; plantaricin

---

1. Introduction

Severe acute respiratory syndrome coronavirus 2 (SARS-CoV-2), responsible for the global pandemic of coronavirus disease 2019 (COVID-19), is the foremost concern among recent global health issues [1]. For prevention of this infection, disinfectants have been widely used—mainly because SARS-CoV-2, like other coronaviruses and enveloped viruses, is surrounded by a fragile outer lipid envelope, which makes it more susceptible to disinfectants than non-enveloped viruses such as rotavirus, norovirus, and poliovirus [2]. Accordingly, the pandemic of COVID-19 has led to a large surge in demand for disinfectants, especially chemical disinfectants such as alcohol- or chlorine-based formulas for the disinfection of hands or environmental surfaces [3–5]. Although chemical disinfectants are considered very effective, they could be hazardous to users if they are not properly handled; for example, alcohol-based disinfectants are flammable and can be harmful to humans if they enter the body [3]. For this reason, there is increasing interest in disinfectants based on natural products.

Lactic acid bacteria, traditionally used in fermented foods, have been considered as interesting resources to contribute to developing a safe alternative to biocides, which are potentially hazardous to humans, because they produce diverse antimicrobial substances and are seldom hazardous to humans [6,7]; most are approved by the U.S. Food and Drug Administration as GRAS (Generally Recognized as Safe). As typical antimicrobial substances, they secrete lactic acid with bacteriocins and antimicrobial peptides (AMPs), which are produced by most microbes [6,7].

In particular, bacteriocins, such as nisin, sakacin, plantaricin, and leucocin from lactic acid bacteria have been reported to have antibacterial activity against foodborne bacteria, such as *Escherichia coli*, *Salmonella enterica*, and *Listeria monocytogenes*, and thus many studies have highlighted their application as natural alternatives to artificial preservatives and antibiotics [6,8–10]. In addition, several bacteriocins have shown antiviral activities against pathogenic viruses such as poliovirus, herpes simplex virus, and influenza viruses [10–12]. Accordingly, the cell-free supernatant, including the bacteriocins and lactic acid, has potential as a natural alternative to chemical disinfectants, although there have been no attempts to apply it as a disinfectant as of yet. To the best of our knowledge, this report is the first that addresses these issues.

In this study, we first suggest that the cell-free supernatant from *Lactobacillus plantarum* NIBR97, a lactic acid bacterium isolated from kimchi, a Korean fermented food, could potentially be useful for disinfection against both pathogenic bacteria and viruses, mediated by bacteriocins as well as lactic acid. Through the genomic analysis of the NIBR97 strain, we discovered novel bacteriocins functioning as antibacterial and antiviral peptides. Our study will provide important information that will guide new strategies to replace chemical disinfectants with natural substances.

2. Results

2.1. Antibacterial Activity of Cell-Free Supernatant from L. plantarum NIBR97

Lactobacillus plantarum NIBR97 were screened from kimchi as a strain with superior antibacterial activity, and its cell-free supernatant was further used for the examination of antibacterial activity, as shown in Figure 1. The minimum inhibitory concentrations (MIC50 and MIC90) were determined as 30.04 and 67.43 μg total proteins/mL against *Salmonella enterica* Serovar Enteritidis (*S.* Enteritidis), respectively, which indicates significantly higher antibacterial activity than the three *Lactobacillus plantarum* strains, KCTC33131, KCTC21004, and KCTC13093, with higher MIC50 and MIC90 values than NIBR97 (Figures 1A and S1A). The cell-free supernatant also showed MIC50s and MIC90s against *Salmonella* Gallinarum, *Edwardsiella tarda*, *Pasteurella multocida*, and *Streptococcus iniae* (Figures 1B and S1B), implying antibacterial activity against broad pathogenic bacteria. In addition, when *Escherichia coli* and *Staphylococcus aureus* were treated with the cell-free supernatant for 5 min, they showed a reduction of at least 99.9% ($\geq 3 \log_{10}$) of the total count in the original inoculum (Figure 1C), indicating bactericidal activity and potential as a disinfectant.

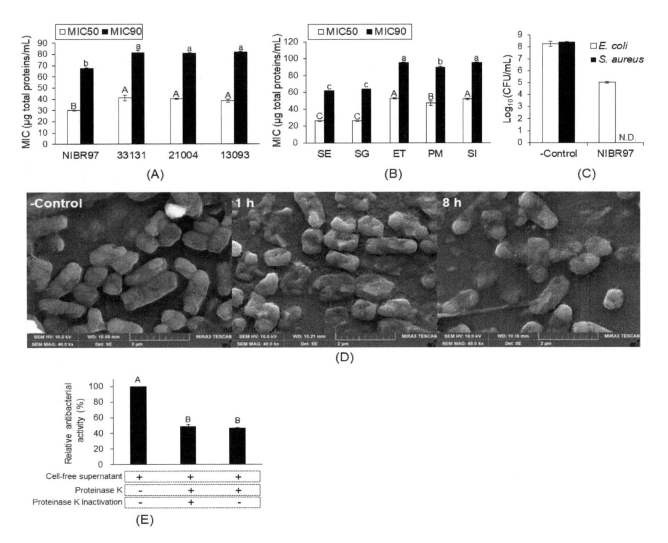

Figure 1. Antibacterial activity of cell-free supernatant from *Lactobacillus plantarum* NIBR97. Antibacterial activities of the cell-free supernatant from the *L. plantarum* strains NIBR97, KCTC33131, KCTC21004, and KCTC13093 were examined against *Salmonella* Enteritidis, whose MIC50s and MIC90s were determined (**A**). The MIC50s and MIC90s of the cell-free supernatant were determined against *Salmonella* Gallinarum (SG), *Edwardsiella tarda* (ET), *Pasteurella multocida* (PM), and *Streptococcus iniae* (SI), as well as *S.* Enteritidis (SE) (**B**). For bactericidal activity, *Escherichia coli* and *Staphylococcus aureus* were treated with the cell-free supernatant (126.6 μg total proteins/mL) for 5 min, and then were counted to determine the titer (Log$_{10}$ (colony-forming unit (CFU)/mL) and reduction rate (%) (**C**). For scanning electron microscopy, *S.* Enteritidis was treated without (control) or with the cell-free supernatant (70.8 μg total proteins/mL, MIC against *S.* Enteritidis) for 1 h and 8 h (**D**). The red arrows indicate the pores forming in the *Salmonella* membrane. (**E**) To investigate the effect of protease on the antibacterial activity of the cell-free supernatant, we added the proteinase K (100 μg/mL) to the cell-free supernatant at 70.8 μg total proteins/mL and the treated sample was used to examine its antibacterial activity against *S.* Enteritidis. In (**E**), the plus (+) mark indicates the treatment of cell-free supernatant or proteinase K, whereas the minus (−) mark does no treatment, and the proteinase K was inactivated at 80 °C for 10 min (+) or not (−). The different letters (A, B, C, a, b and c) in the graphs ((**A**), (**B**), (**C**) and (**E**)) represent significant differences ($p < 0.05$) and in (**A**) and (**B**), the capital (A, B and C) and small letters (a, b c) indicate the significant differences in MIC50 and MIC90 data, respectively.

In order to prove the antibacterial activity against pathogenic bacteria with the cell-free supernatant from *L. plantarum* NIBR97, we observed the *S.* Enteritidis treated with the cell-free supernatant using scanning electron microscopy (SEM). As shown in Figure 1D, the SEM images revealed that the cell-free supernatant effectively caused the Salmonella death via pore formation by cellular penetrating peptides, as is the case for typical AMPs [13]. Furthermore, when the cell-free supernatant was treated with proteinase K, its antibacterial activity against *S*. Enteritidis decreased by about 50% compared with the control without the proteinase K treatment (Figure 1E). Therefore, we suggest that proteins or peptides play major roles for the antibacterial activities of cell-free supernatant from *L. plantarum* NIBR97.

2.2. Antiviral Activity of Cell-Free Supernatant from L. plantarum NIBR97

To assess its antiviral activity, the cell-free supernatant from *L. plantarum* NIBR97 was exposed to green fluorescent protein (GFP)-labeled lentiviruses, based on human immunodeficiency virus (HIV), which causes acquired immunodeficiency syndrome (AIDS), for 5 min and 24 h, as shown in Figure 2. When the GFP-labeled lentiviruses, treated with the cell-free supernatant, infected the HEK-293T cells (human host cells), they were observed by fluorescence microscopy to decrease dose- and time-dependently within the host cells (Figure 2A, the GFP images) without any cytotoxic effect on the human host cells (Figure 2A, the Bright images). SEM also confirmed its antiviral activity by showing that the cell-free supernatant effectively causes lentiviral lysis through the collapse of envelopes after 5 min (Figure 2B). In addition, when the human influenza A virus subtype H3N2 (A/H3N2) was treated with the cell-free supernatant, it showed a reduction of at least 99.5% of the total count of its original inoculums, which increased until 99.999% with treatment time (Table 1). These results indicate that the cell-free supernatant from *L. plantarum* NIBR97 has superior antiviral activity, as well as potential as a disinfectant.

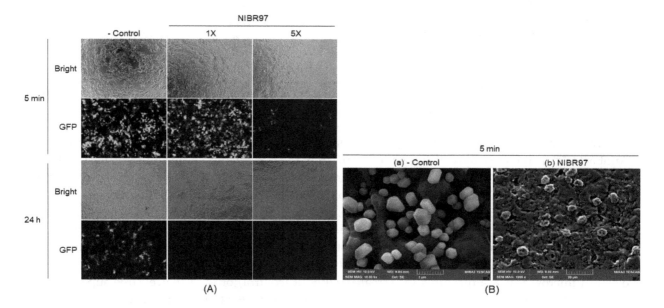

Figure 2. Antiviral activity of cell-free supernatant from *L. plantarum* NIBR97. (**A**) For fluorescence microscopy, we treated GFP-labeled lentiviruses with the cell-free supernatant for 5 min and 24 h, and then were infected in HEK-293T human host cells. The 1× and 5× correspond to the concentrations treated to the lentiviruses, 79.15 and 395.75 μg total proteins/mL, respectively. The bright-field images (Bright) indicate the HEK-293T cells, and the green signals in the fluorescent images (GFP) represent the GFP-labeled lentiviruses. (**B**) For scanning electron microscopy, the GFP-labeled lentiviruses were treated without (**a**) or with the cell-free supernatant (395.75 μg total proteins/mL) (**b**) for 5 min.

Table 1. Disinfection activity of the cell-free supernatant from *L. plantarum* NIBR97 against A/H3N2.

Treatments [1]	10 min [1]		30 min [1]		18 h [1]	
	Titer [2]	Reduction [3]	Titer [2]	Reduction [3]	Titer [2]	Reduction [3]
Water	5.66	0	5.45	0	5.34	0.21
NIBR97	3.27	99.594	<0.51	>99.999	<0.51	>99.999

[1] The A/H3N2 viruses were treated with water, a negative control, or the cell-free supernatant (NIBR97) for 10 min, 30 min, and 18 h; [2] and [3] indicate the viral titer ($\log_{10}$CCID50) and reduction (%), respectively.

2.3. Discovery of Novel Bacteriocins by the Genomic Analysis of L. plantarum NIBR97

Analysis of the whole-genome sequence for the *L. plantarum* NIBR97 was carried out by the PacBio RS II (Pacific Biosciences, Menlo Park, CA, USA) sequencing platform to identify the AMPs from the NIBR97. The NIBR97 genome identified from de novo assembly was composed of a single circular bacterial chromosome and four plasmids, containing 2927 predicted open reading frames (ORFs), 68 tRNAs, and 16 rRNAs (Table 2 and Figure S2). Among the ORFs, 10 were identified to encode homologous proteins with known AMPs via an NCBI (National Center for Biotechnology Information) homology BLAST (Basic Local Alignment Search Tool) (Table S1). Furthermore, their expression in *L. plantarum* NIBR97 was confirmed by the transcriptomic data (Table S2). In detail, the five ORFs—orf02155, orf02163, orf02164, orf02421, and orf00645—were found to have 100% identities with plantaricin N, F, and E, as well as bacteriophage holing and lysozyme, known previously as AMPs from the *Lactobacillus* genus (Table S1). Five ORFs—orf00467, orf01336, orf01363, orf01599, and orf01790—which were previously uncharacterized until now, were discovered in this study to consist of amino acid sequences with high positives (>60%) with AMPs undiscovered in *L. plantarum* strains: grammistin Pp3, indolicidin, bactofencin A, hymenochirin-5B, and latarcin-2a, (Table S1). Thus, we herein designated the AMPs as novel bacteriocins called plantaricin (Pln) 1, 2, 3, 4, and 5 (Table S1). Interestingly, their structural models revealed that the three plantaricins—Pln 1, 4 and 5—form helix structures, and the two plantaricins—Pln 2 and 3—form random coil structures (Figure 3), similar to typical AMPs [14,15], implying that they may have antibacterial activities.

2.4. Antibacterial and Antiviral Activities of Plantaricins from L. plantarum NIBR97

To confirm whether the five Plns function as AMPs, we assessed their synthetic peptides for antibacterial activity against *Salmonella* Typhimurium (Figure S3). Among them, Pln 5 exhibited the highest antimicrobial activity, showing the lowest MIC50 compared with others, whereas Pln 4 showed the lowest antimicrobial activity (Figure S3). In addition, the Pln 3 and 5 were identified to inhibit the growth of *Salmonella* Enteritidis (Figure 4A) and were observed by SEM to effectively cause cellular lysis by damaging the membrane of *S.* Enteritidis via pore formation (Figure 4B), as did the cell-free supernatant from *L. plantarum* NIBR97 (Figure 1D).

Table 2. Summary of the de novo genome assembly of *L. plantarum* NIBR97.

Items	Contig 1	Contig 2	Contig 3	Contig 4	Contig 5
Form	A circular chromosome	A circular plasmid	A circular plasmid	A linear plasmid	A linear plasmid
Length [1]	3,022,780	61,378	32,520	7394	6876
GC [2]	44.74	39.22	39.59	34.33	35.67
ORF [3]	2816	60	32	10	9
rRNA [4]	16	0	0	0	0
tRNA [5]	68	0	0	0	0

[1] and [2] indicate the length (bp, base pair) and GC (guanine-cytosine) contents (%) of contig in the form, respectively; [3], [4], and [5] represent the number of predicted open reading frames (ORFs), rRNA, and tRNA, respectively.

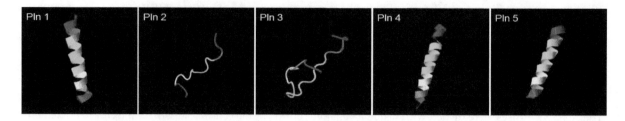

Figure 3. Structural models of plantaricins. Pln 1, 2, 3, 4, and 5 comprise the amino acid sequences VLGSLIGSVGIGVLSSLAARYK, IYPEKQPEEPVRR, KKSRRCQVYNNGMPTGMYTSC, PIVREPFKAMAVGIILAVMSGLLVT, and KAKKRFLRNRLSQQARKARTK, respectively. Pln 1, 4, and 5 form helix structures, and Pln 2 and 3 form random coil structures. The structures of Pln 1, 2, 3, 4, and 5 were predicted by the automated I-TASSER server (https://zhanglab.ccmb.med.umich.edu/I-TASSER/).

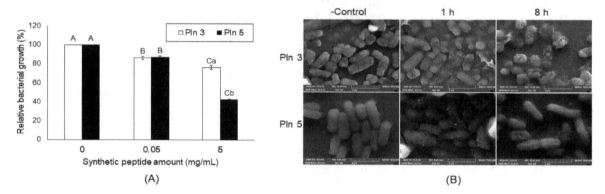

Figure 4. Antibacterial activity of plantaricin 3 and 5 against *S.* Enteritidis. Pln 3 and 5 were synthesized according to the amino acid sequences in Figure 3, and further examined for their antibacterial activity against *S.* Enteritidis (**A**). The y-axis and different letters (A, B, C, a and b) in the graphs represent the relative bacterial growth (%) and significant differences ($p < 0.05$), respectively. In (**A**), the capital (A, B and C) and small letters (a and b) indicate the significant differences between different concentrations (0-5 mg/mL) and the ones between Pln 3 and 5, respectively. (**B**) For scanning electron microscopy, *S.* Enteritidis was treated without or with synthetic Pln 3 or 5 (5 mg/mL) for 1 h and 8 h. The red arrows indicate the pores forming in the *Salmonella* membrane.

The synthetic Pln 3 and 5 were further examined for antiviral activity against GFP-labeled lentiviruses. The synthetic peptides exhibited a cytotoxicity on the human host cells when the lentiviruses were treated with 5 µg/µL of synthetic peptides, but not with ≈2.5 µg/µL of synthetic peptides (Figure 5, the Bright images). The fluorescence microscopy revealed that the lentiviruses decreased considerably within the host cells when they were treated with the Pln 3 or 5 for 24 h, but not for 5 min (Figure 5, the GFP images). This suggests that Pln 3 and 5 can considerably suppress viral infection in host cells. Interestingly, SEM revealed that Pln 3 effectively caused lentiviral lysis through the collapse of the envelopes (Figure 6), as the cell-free supernatant did (Figure 2B), whereas Pln 5 did not (Figure 6). This implies that Pln 3 and 5 may exert their antiviral role through different mechanisms.

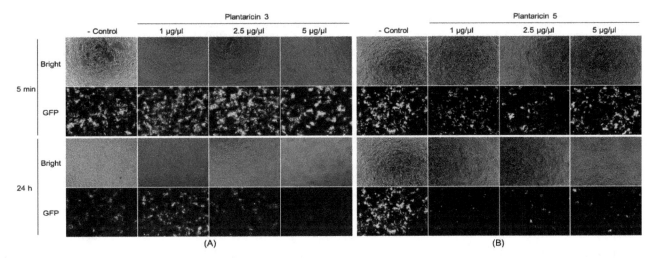

Figure 5. Fluorescence micrographs of HEK-293T cells infected with GFP-labeled lentiviruses treated with synthetic Pln 3 and 5. The lentiviruses were treated without (control) or with the synthetic peptides (1 to 5 µg/µL) Pln 3 (**A**) and 5 (**B**) for 5 min or 24 h, and then the HEK-293T human host cells were infected. The bright-field images (Bright) indicate the HEK-293T cells, and the green signals in the fluorescent images (GFP) represent the GFP-labeled lentiviruses.

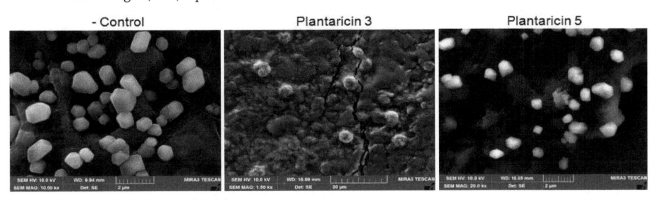

Figure 6. Scanning electron micrographs of the GFP-labeled lentiviruses treated with synthetic Pln 3 and 5. The lentiviruses were treated without or with the synthetic peptides at 5 µg/µL for 24 h.

3. Discussion

Lactobacillus plantarum is one of the most widespread lactic acid bacteria species and is largely used for the production of fermented products of animal and plant origin [16]. Moreover, some strains are known to produce several natural antibacterial substances, such as bacteriocins, organic acids (mainly lactic and acetic acid), and hydrogen peroxide [17,18], and thus many studies have highlighted their application as preservatives and antibiotics [6,8–10]. Here, we investigated their potential as a natural alternative to chemical disinfectants.

In this study, the NIBR97 strain was screened from kimchi, a Korean fermented food, and its cell-free supernatant was identified to have higher antibacterial activity against *Salmonella* bacteria than other *L. plantarum* strains (Figure 1A), as well as possessing antibacterial activities against a broad range of pathogenic bacteria (Figure 1B). It exhibited significant disinfection activities against the human pathogens influenza A virus H3N2, *Escherichia coli*, and *Staphylococcus aureus*, reducing them by at least 99.9% of the total count of their original inoculums within 30 min (Figure 1C and Table 1). These results indicate that the cell-free supernatant from *L. plantarum* NIBR97 has potential as a natural disinfectant, and thus further investigations were performed to identify the antimicrobial substances, such as AMPs, in the NIBR97 strain.

AMPs are small peptides composed of 10 to 40 amino acids, which cause microbial membrane modification via either pore formation by cell-penetrating property through a barrel stave or a toroidal pore mechanism, or through a non-pore carpet-like mechanism [13,19]. Our scanning electron micrographs of *S*. Enteritidis showed clearly that the cell-free supernatant from the NIBR97 formed a pore on the *Salmonella* surface (Figure 1D), as do typical AMPs [13]. Proteinase K treatment of the cell-free supernatant led to a considerable decrease in its antibacterial activity against both *S*. Enteritidis and *S*. Gallinarum (Figure 1E). Thus, these results confirm that the antibacterial activities of the cell-free supernatant from the NIBR97 are mediated mainly by its proteins or peptides, functioning as AMPs. The scanning electron micrographs of GFP-labeled lentivirus showed that the cell-free supernatant causes lentiviral lysis through envelope collapse (Figure 2A), but it was unclear whether the AMPs were involved in the envelope collapse of the virus.

Finally, to identify AMPs from the NIBR97 strains, we performed whole-genome sequencing, which revealed that the 10 ORFs encoded AMPs, including known forms (plantaricin E, F, N; bacteriophage holin; lysozyme) and novel forms (Pln 1 to 5 (Table S1)). In the case of the known AMPs, plantaricin E, F, and N are bacteriocins produced in *Lactobacillus plantarum* C11 [20]; holin, produced by bacteriophages, triggers and controls the degradation of the cell wall of the host bacteria [21]; and lysozyme functions as 1,4-beta-N-acetylmuramidase, an antimicrobial enzyme, and has been found mainly in *Lactobacillus rhamnosus* strains [22]. Interestingly, five ORFs were discovered as novel bacteriocins in this study (Figure 3) and were designated as Pln 1, 2, 3, 4, and 5. They were further confirmed as being expressed in the NIBR97 strain through transcriptomic sequencing (Table S2), and even their synthetic peptides exhibited antibacterial activity against *Salmonella* Typhimurium (Figure S3). The synthetic Pln 3 and 5 also inhibited the growth of *S*. Enteritidis and effectively caused cellular lysis through damage to the *Salmonella* membrane via pore formation (Figure 4), suggesting that they function as AMPs. However, the synthetic Plns showed overall lower antibacterial activities than antibiotics such as octenidine when their MICs were compared with each other (Figure S3) [23]. This is presumably because the Plns were not synthesized on the basis of complete amino acid sequences for the optimal antibacterial activity but were done on the basis of minimal sequences for the activity; thus, it is further necessary to identify the mature peptide sequence responsible for the optimal antibacterial activity, following the signal peptide cleavage. Moreover, Pln 3 and 5 were identified to suppress lentiviral infection in human host cells (Figure 5). Collectively, these results suggest that the cell-free supernatant from *L. plantarum* NIBR97 may include AMPs, such as Pln 3 and 5, exhibiting antibacterial and antiviral activities. However, Pln 3 and 5 were observed by SEM to act differentially in the suppression of viral infection; Pln 3 had a significant effect on the viral shape through the collapse of the viral envelope, which suggests that it may cause direct damage to the envelope. In contrast, Pln 5 had little effect on it (Figure 6), which implies that it may interfere with the interaction between viruses and host cells [24,25].

Noticeably, Pln 3 and 5 suppressed viral infection when used against lentivirus for 24 h, but not for 5 min (Figure 5), which indicates that long exposure is required for their antiviral role. Although the Plns exhibited low antibacterial activities as mentioned above, during long expose (i.e., 24 h), they may also contribute significantly to the antibacterial activities of cell-free supernatant, together with other AMPs discovered by genomic analysis of NIBR97, which is strongly supported by the proteinase K treatment leading to a considerable decrease (>50%) in antibacterial activity of the cell-free supernatant (Figure 1E). Furthermore, this is confirmed by Figure S4—the cell-free supernatant from the *E. coli* Top10 strain (Invitrogen, Carlsbad, CA, USA), harboring each *Pln* gene cloned, showed significant antibacterial activities against both Gram-negative and Gram-positive bacteria, whereas very little antibacterial activity was detected in the negative control, that is, treatment with the cell-free supernatant from the strain without the *Pln* genes (Figure S4). Meanwhile, the disinfection activity of the cell-free supernatant during short exposures (i.e., within 30 min), as shown in Figure 1C and Table 1, was presumably because the lactic acid may have functioned as a disinfectant during the short exposure. This is supported by the data, showing that the cell-free supernatant contained considerable lactic acids ($\approx$2%) when the NIBR97 strain was cultured in the de Man, Rogosa and Sharpe (MRS) medium, consisting of 5% solutes and 95% water, for 24 h (Figure S5), and by a previous report stating that they induce sudden severe acid stress, leading to a shock of oxidative stress and resulting in the destabilization of the bacterial membrane [26]. Therefore, the cell-free supernatant may exert its role as a disinfectant, mainly through lactic acid during short exposure (i.e., within 30 min), while it does so through an integrated effect between the lactic acid and the various AMPs during long exposure (i.e., 24 h).

4. Materials and Methods

4.1. Materials

As susceptible bacteria to AMPs, S. Enteritidis, S. Gallinarum, *Edwardsiella tarda*, *Pasteurella multocida*, and *Streptococcus iniae* were obtained from Dr. Jin Hur (Chonbuk National University, Iksan, Korea) and Dr. Tae Sung Jung (Gyeongsang National University, Jinju, Korea). The *Lactobacillus plantarum* strains KCTC33131, KCTC21004, and KCTC13093, as well as the susceptible bacteria *Escherichia coli* ATCC 10536 and *Staphylococcus aureus* ATCC 6538, were purchased from KCTC (Korean Collection for Type of Cultures, Daejeon, Korea). The human influenza A/H3N2 was provided by the Korea Centers for Disease Control and Prevention (KCDC, Chungcheongbuk-do, Korea). The plasmids for lentiviral packaging (two packaging vectors, pRSV-Rev and pCgpV, and an envelope vector, pCMV-VSV-G) and for a positive control of transduction (pSIH1-H1-siLUC-copGFP) were purchased from Cellbiolab (San Diego, CA, USA) and System Biosciences (Palo Alto, CA, USA), respectively. The five synthetic peptides—plantaricin 1 to 5—were purchased from Cosmogenetech Inc. (Seoul, Korea).

4.2. Analysis of the Minimal Inhibitory Concentration (MIC50 and MIC90)

L. plantarum NIBR97 was incubated at 37 °C for 24 h in an MRS liquid medium (10 g/L peptone, 8 g/L meat extract, 4 g/L yeast extract, 20 g/L d(+)-glucose, 2 g/L dipotassium hydrogen phosphate, 5 g/L sodium acetate trihydrate, 2 g/L triammonium citrate, 0.2 g/L magnesium sulfate heptahydrate, and 0.05 g/L manganous sulfate tetrahydrate). The cultural broth was centrifuged for 20 min at $2000 \times g$, and the centrifugal supernatant was collected and then sterilized by a 0.22 μm filtration. The sterilized fluid was either applied directly for the examination of antimicrobial activity or fractionated and stored at −80 °C until use. The assessment of antimicrobial activity on a microtiter plate was performed by some modification of the dilution assay of Wiegand et al. [27]. The MIC50 and MIC90 were expressed as total proteins equivalent (μg) per volume (mL) of the sample, and the effect of proteinase K treatment was examined by a previously described procedure [28].

4.3. Measurement of Bactericidal Activity

The susceptible bacterial strains *Escherichia coli* ATCC 10536 and *Staphylococcus aureus* ATCC 6538 were adjusted into 1.5 to 5.0×10^8 CFU/mL after pre-culture, and 10% sucrose was used as an interfering agent, 0.25 M KH_2PO_4 (pH 7.2) was used as a neutralizing agent, and 20 mg/mL proteinase K was used to degrade the AMPs. For the bactericidal activity assay, we mixed 100 μL of prepared susceptible bacterial solution, 100 μL 10% sucrose, and 800 μL cell-free supernatant (126.6 μg total proteins/mL) from *L. plantarum* NIBR97 and reacted the mixture at 20 °C for 5 min. An aliquot (100 μL) of the reaction solution was mixed with 800 μL 0.25 M KH_2PO_4 (pH 7.2), 5 μL proteinase K, and 100 μL distilled water, and then reacted at 20 °C for 5 min. The surviving cells were counted by serial dilution of the treated solution and incubation on an Luria-Bertani (LB) plate.

4.4. Scanning Electron Microscopy (SEM)

The S. Enteritidis was treated with the cell-free supernatant (70.8 μg total proteins/mL, MIC against S. Enteritidis) from *L. plantarum* culture or the synthetic peptides, Pln 3 (1 μg/μL) or Pln 5 (1 μg/μL), for 0, 1, and 8 h, and the lentivirus was assessed with the cell-free supernatant (15.8 μg total proteins/mL) for 5 min and with the synthetic peptides Pln 3 (5 μg/μL) or Pln 5 (5 μg/μL) for 24 h. The treated bacteria and viruses were observed by a scanning electron microscope according to previously described procedures [28].

4.5. Antiviral Analysis Against Influenza A/H3N2

For the antiviral test, we co-incubated 0.1 mL of the A/H3N2 soup (2–4×10^5 viruses/μL) with 0.9 mL of the cell-free supernatant (142.5 μg total proteins/mL) for 10 min, 30 min, and 18 h at 25 °C. After the co-incubation, the cell-free supernatant-A/H3N2 mixture was 10-fold serially diluted to infect Madin–Darby canine kidney (MDCK) cells (3×10^4 cells per well) and, thereafter, the cell culture infectious dose (CCID50) and the viral reduction were determined by cytopathic effect (CPE) and plaque assays, as previously described [29].

4.6. Antiviral Analysis Against GFP-Labeled Lentivirus

For the production of GFP-labeled lentivirus, we transfected 5 μg of pRSV-Rev, 5 μg of pCMV-VSV-G, 5 μg of pCgpV, and 15 μg of pSIH1-H1-siLUC-copGFP plasmids into HEK-293T cells (6×10^6 cells per well) using lipofectamine 2000 (Invitrogen, Carlsbad, CA, USA). The lentiviral supernatants were harvested 72 h after transfection, filtered through Millex-GP 0.45 μm filters (Millipore, Schwalbach, Germany), and concentrated using Retro-Concentin Retroviral Concentration Reagent (System Biosciences, Palo Alto, CA, USA). The titer of lentiviruses was measured with a QuickTiter Lentivirus Titer Kit (Cellbiolabs, San Diego, CA, USA) and stored at −80 °C.

For the anti-viral test, we co-incubated 2 μL of lentivirus soup (2.8×10^6 lentiviruses/μL) with 2 μL of test sample for 5 min and 24 h at 25 °C. After the co-incubation, 2 μL from the total 4 μL of the test sample–lentivirus mixture was infected in HEK-293T cells (1×10^4 cells per well). Expression of the copGFP protein was observed at day 3 after infection with a Zeiss 510 fluorescence microscope (Carl Zeiss Co., Oberkochen, Germany).

4.7. Analysis of the Genome

Genomic analysis of *L. plantarum* NIBR97 was performed by previously described procedures. In detail, genomic DNA from the NIBR97 was extracted and sequenced by previously described procedures [28]. De novo assembly and putative gene coding sequences (CDSs) from the assembled contigs was performed by the hierarchical genome assembly process (HGAP, Version 3) workflow [30] and the bacterial genome was checked by MUMmer 3.5 [31], identifying that the genome comprises a single circular DNA chromosome of 3,022,780 bp with four plasmids by trimming one of the self-similar ends for manual genome closure (Table 2). Putative gene coding sequences (CDSs) from the assembled contigs were identified by Glimmer v3.02 [32], and the obtained ORFs were examined by Blastall alignment (http://www.ncbi.nlm.nih.gov/books/NBK1762). Gene ontology annotations of the ORFs were assigned by Blast2GO software [33]. In addition, ribosomal RNAs and transfer RNAs were separated by RNAmmer 1.2 and tRNAscan-SE 1.4 [34,35]. Finally, the whole-genome sequence data were deposited as Sequence Read Archive (SRA) data in GenBank (SRA no., SRR12344691; BioProject no., PRJNA647132).

4.8. Statistical Analysis

The mean values were separated by the probability difference option according to significant differences. The results are exhibited as least square means with standard deviations. Duncan's multiple range tests (MRT) were applied for verification of significant differences ($p < 0.05$) between sample types. All the analyses were performed by the SAS statistical software package (version 9.1, SAS Inst., Inc., Cary, NC, USA), for which differences were considered significant at $p < 0.05$.

5. Conclusions

Together, our data showed that the cell-free supernatant from *L. plantarum* NIBR97, producing novel bacteriocins, has superior antibacterial and antiviral activities during both short and long exposures, which suggests that it is potentially useful as a natural material to completely or partially replace chemical disinfectants.

Supplementary Materials:
Figure S1. Antibacterial activity of cell-free supernatant from *L. plantarum* NIBR97. Figure S2. Overall features of the *L. plantarum* NIBR97 genome (contig 1) and plasmids (contig 2 to 5). Figure S3. Antibacterial activity of synthetic plantaricins identified from the *L. plantarum* NIBR97 genome. Figure S4 Antibacterial activity of the cell-free supernatant from *E. coli.* Top10 strain, harboring each *Pln* gene. Figure S5. The content of lactic acid in the cell-free supernatant from *L. plantarum* NIBR97. Table S1. Identification of ORFs predicted as antimicrobial peptides (AMPs) from the genome assembly data of *L. plantarum* NIBR97. Table S2. Transcriptomic analysis results of AMPs from *L. plantarum* NIBR97.

Author Contributions: W.Y.B., I.S.J., and S.W.K. conceived and designed the experiments; S.I.K., D.H.S., S.Y.O., Y.Y., and S.W.K. performed the experiments; C.W.L., Y.K.S., H.-S.Y., and B.-H.L. analyzed the data; S.W.K., B.-H.L., H.-J.A., I.S.J., and W.Y.B contributed reagents/materials/analysis tools; I.S.J. and W.Y.B. wrote the paper. All authors have read and agreed to the published version of the manuscript.

Acknowledgments: The *S. Gallinarum*, pathogenic *E. coli*, and *S. iniae* that are susceptible to AMPs were obtained from Jin Hur (Chonbuk National University, Iksan, Republic of Korea) and Tae Sung Jung (Gyeongsang National University, Jinju, Republic of Korea).

References

1. World Health Organization. *Coronavirus Disease (COVID-19): Situation Report, 150*; World Health Organization: Geneva, Switzerland, 2020.

2. World Health Organization. *Cleaning and Disinfection of Environmental Surfaces in the Context of COVID-19: Interim Guidance*; World Health Organization: Geneva, Switzerland, 2020.

3. Atolani, O.; Baker, M.T.; Adeyemi, O.S.; Olanrewaju, I.R.; Hamid, A.A.; Ameen, O.M.; Oguntoye, S.O.; Usman, L.A. COVID-19: Critical discussion on the applications and implications of chemicals in sanitizers and disinfectants. *EXCLI J.* **2020**, *19*, 785. [PubMed]

4. Pradhan, D.; Biswasroy, P.; Ghosh, G.; Rath, G. A review of current interventions for COVID-19 prevention. *Arch. Med. Res.* **2020**, *51*, 363–374. [CrossRef]

5. Berardi, A.; Perinelli, D.R.; Merchant, H.A.; Bisharat, L.; Basheti, I.A.; Bonacucina, G.; Cespi, M.; Palmieri, G.F. Hand sanitisers amid CoViD-19: A critical review of alcohol-based products on the market and formulation approaches to respond to increasing demand. *Int. J. Pharm.* **2020**, *584*, 119431. [CrossRef] [PubMed]

6. Ibrahim, O.O. Classification of Antimicrobial Peptides Bacteriocins, and the Nature of Some Bacteriocins with Potential Applications in Food Safety and Bio-Pharmaceuticals. *EC Microbiol.* **2019**, *15*, 591–608.

7. Stanojević-Nikolić, S.; Dimić, G.; Mojović, L.; Pejin, J.; Djukić-Vuković, A.; Kocić-Tanackov, S. Antimicrobial activity of lactic acid against pathogen and spoilage microorganisms. *J. Food Process. Preserv.* **2016**, *40*, 990–998. [CrossRef]

8. Vieco-Saiz, N.; Belguesmia, Y.; Raspoet, R.; Auclair, E.; Gancel, F.; Kempf, I.; Drider, D. Benefits and inputs from lactic acid bacteria and their bacteriocins as alternatives to antibiotic growth promoters during food-animal production. *Front. Microbiol.* **2019**, *10*, 57. [CrossRef]

9. Ahmad, V.; Khan, M.S.; Jamal, Q.M.S.; Alzohairy, M.A.; Al Karaawi, M.A.; Siddiqui, M.U. Antimicrobial potential of bacteriocins: In therapy, agriculture and food preservation. *Int. J. Antimicrob. Agents* **2017**, *49*, 1–11. [CrossRef]

10. Hashim, H.; Sikandar, S.; Khan, M.A.; Qurashi, A.W. Bacteriocin: The avenues of innovation towards applied microbiology. *Pure Appl. Biol. (PAB)* **2019**, *8*, 460–478. [CrossRef]

11. Cerqueira, J.; Dimitrov, S.; Silva, A.; Augusto, L. Inhibition of Herpes simplex virus 1 and Poliovirus (PV-1) by bacteriocins from Lactococcus lactis subsp. lactis and Enterococcus durans strains isolated from goat milk. *Int. J. Antimicrob. Agents* **2018**, *51*, 33–37.

12. Ermolenko, E.; Desheva, Y.; Kolobov, A.; Kotyleva, M.; Sychev, I.; Suvorov, A. Anti–Influenza Activity of Enterocin B In vitro and Protective Effect of Bacteriocinogenic Enterococcal Probiotic Strain on Influenza Infection in Mouse Model. *Probiotics Antimicrob. Proteins* **2019**, *11*, 705–712. [CrossRef]

13. Park, S.-C.; Park, Y.; Hahm, K.-S. The role of antimicrobial peptides in preventing multidrug-resistant bacterial infections and biofilm formation. *Int. J. Mol. Sci.* **2011**, *12*, 5971–5992. [CrossRef] [PubMed]

14. Jenssen, H.; Hamill, P.; Hancock, R.E. Peptide antimicrobial agents. *Clin. Microbiol. Rev.* **2006**, *19*, 491–511. [CrossRef] [PubMed]

15. O'Connor, P.M.; O'Shea, E.F.; Cotter, P.D.; Hill, C.; Ross, R.P. The potency of the broad spectrum bacteriocin, bactofencin A, against staphylococci is highly dependent on primary structure, N-terminal charge and disulphide formation. *Sci. Rep.* **2018**, *8*, 1–8.

16. Vescovo, M.; Bottazzi, V.; Torriani, S.; Dellaglio, F. Basic characteristics, ecology and application of Lactobacillus plantarum [in the production of fermented foods of animal and plant origin]: A review. *Ann. Microbiol. Enzimol. (Italy)* **1993**, *43*, 261–284.

17. Tremonte, P.; Pannella, G.; Succi, M.; Tipaldi, L.; Sturchio, M.; Coppola, R.; Luongo, D.; Sorrentino, E. Antimicrobial activity of Lactobacillus plantarum strains isolated from different environments: A preliminary study. *Int. Food Res. J.* **2017**, *24*, 852–859.

18. Dinev, T.; Beev, G.; Tzanova, M.; Denev, S.; Dermendzhieva, D.; Stoyanova, A. Antimicrobial activity of Lactobacillus plantarum against pathogenic and food spoilage microorganisms: A review. *Bulg. J. Vet. Med.* **2018**, *21*, 253–268. [CrossRef]

19. Fjell, C.D.; Hiss, J.A.; Hancock, R.E.; Schneider, G. Designing antimicrobial peptides: Form follows function. *Nat. Rev. Drug Discov.* **2012**, *11*, 37–51. [CrossRef]

20. Diep, D.B.; Håvarstein, L.S.; Nes, I.F. Characterization of the locus responsible for the bacteriocin production in Lactobacillus plantarum C11. *J. Bacteriol.* **1996**, *178*, 4472–4483. [CrossRef]

21. Young, R. Bacteriophage holins: Deadly diversity. *J. Mol. Microbiol. Biotechnol.* **2002**, *4*, 21–36.

22. Nissilä, E.; Douillard, F.P.; Ritari, J.; Paulin, L.; Järvinen, H.M.; Rasinkangas, P.; Haapasalo, K.; Meri, S.; Jarva, H.; De Vos, W.M. Genotypic and phenotypic diversity of Lactobacillus rhamnosus clinical isolates, their comparison with strain GG and their recognition by complement system. *PLoS ONE* **2017**, *12*, e0176739.

23. Karpiński, T.M. Efficacy of octenidine against Pseudomonas aeruginosa strains. *Eur. J. Biolog. Res.* **2019**, *9*, 135–140.

24. Hsieh, I.-N.; Hartshorn, K.L. The role of antimicrobial peptides in influenza virus infection and their potential as antiviral and immunomodulatory therapy. *Pharmaceuticals* **2016**, *9*, 53. [CrossRef] [PubMed]

25. Ahmed, A.; Siman-Tov, G.; Hall, G.; Bhalla, N.; Narayanan, A. Human antimicrobial peptides as therapeutics for viral infections. *Viruses* **2019**, *11*, 704. [CrossRef] [PubMed]

26. Desriac, N.; Broussolle, V.; Postollec, F.; Mathot, A.-G.; Sohier, D.; Coroller, L.; Leguerinel, I. Bacillus cereus cell response upon exposure to acid environment: Toward the identification of potential biomarkers. *Front. Microbiol.* **2013**, *4*, 284. [CrossRef] [PubMed]

27. Wiegand, I.; Hilpert, K.; Hancock, R.E. Agar and broth dilution methods to determine the minimal inhibitory concentration (MIC) of antimicrobial substances. *Nat. Protoc.* **2008**, *3*, 163. [CrossRef] [PubMed]

28. Kim, S.W.; Ha, Y.J.; Bang, K.H.; Lee, S.; Yeo, J.-H.; Yang, H.-S.; Kim, T.-W.; Lee, K.P.; Bang, W.Y. Potential of Bacteriocins from Lactobacillus taiwanensis for Producing Bacterial Ghosts as a Next Generation Vaccine. *Toxins* **2020**, *12*, 432. [CrossRef]

29. Jang, Y.; Shin, J.S.; Lee, J.-Y.; Shin, H.; Kim, S.J.; Kim, M. In Vitro and In Vivo Antiviral Activity of Nylidrin by Targeting the Hemagglutinin 2-Mediated Membrane Fusion of Influenza A Virus. *Viruses* **2020**, *12*, 581. [CrossRef] [PubMed]

30. Chin, C.-S.; Alexander, D.H.; Marks, P.; Klammer, A.A.; Drake, J.; Heiner, C.; Clum, A.; Copeland, A.; Huddleston, J.; Eichler, E.E. Nonhybrid, finished microbial genome assemblies from long-read SMRT sequencing data. *Nat. Methods* **2013**, *10*, 563–569. [CrossRef] [PubMed]

31. Kurtz, S.; Phillippy, A.; Delcher, A.L.; Smoot, M.; Shumway, M.; Antonescu, C.; Salzberg, S.L. Versatile and open software for comparing large genomes. *Genome Biolog.* **2004**, *5*, R12. [CrossRef]

32. Delcher, A.L.; Bratke, K.A.; Powers, E.C.; Salzberg, S.L. Identifying bacterial genes and endosymbiont DNA with Glimmer. *Bioinformatics* **2007**, *23*, 673–679. [CrossRef]

33. Conesa, A.; Götz, S.; García-Gómez, J.M.; Terol, J.; Talón, M.; Robles, M. Blast2GO: A universal tool for annotation, visualization and analysis in functional genomics research. *Bioinformatics* **2005**, *21*, 3674–3676. [CrossRef] [PubMed]

34. Lagesen, K.; Hallin, P.; Rødland, E.; Stærfeldt, H.; Rognes, T.; Ussery, D. RNammer: Consistent annotation of rRNA genes in genomic sequences. *Nucleic Acids Res.* **2007**, *35*, 3100–3108. [CrossRef] [PubMed]

35. Lowe, T.M.; Eddy, S.R. tRNAscan-SE: A program for improved detection of transfer RNA genes in genomic sequence. *Nucleic Acids Res.* **1997**, *25*, 955–964. [CrossRef] [PubMed]

Bromo-Cyclobutenaminones as New Covalent UDP-*N*-Acetylglucosamine Enolpyruvyl Transferase (MurA) Inhibitors

David J. Hamilton [1,2], **Péter Ábrányi-Balogh** [2]⦿, **Aaron Keeley** [2]⦿, **László Petri** [2], **Martina Hrast** [3]⦿, **Tímea Imre** [4], **Maikel Wijtmans** [1], **Stanislav Gobec** [3], **Iwan J. P. de Esch** [1] and **György Miklós Keserű** [2,*]

[1] Division of Medicinal Chemistry, Amsterdam Institute of Molecular and Life Sciences (AIMMS), Faculty of Science, Vrije Universiteit Amsterdam, De Boelelaan 1108, 1081 HZ Amsterdam, The Netherlands; d.j.hamilton@vu.nl (D.J.H.); m.wijtmans@vu.nl (M.W.); i.de.esch@vu.nl (I.J.P.d.E.)

[2] Medicinal Chemistry Research Group, Research Centre for Natural Sciences, Magyar tudósok krt 2, H-1117 Budapest, Hungary; abranyi-balogh.peter@ttk.hu (P.Á.-B.); aaron.keeley@ttk.hu (A.K.); petri.laszlo@ttk.hu (L.P.)

[3] Faculty of Pharmacy, University of Ljubljana, Aškerčeva 7, SI-1000 Ljubljana, Slovenia; martina.hrast@ffa.uni-lj.si (M.H.); Stanislav.Gobec@ffa.uni-lj.si (S.G.)

[4] MS Metabolomics Research Group, Research Centre for Natural Sciences, Magyar tudósok krt 2, H-1117 Budapest, Hungary; imre.timea@ttk.hu

* Correspondence: keseru.gyorgy@ttk.hu

Abstract: Drug discovery programs against the antibacterial target UDP-*N*-acetylglucosamine enolpyruvyl transferase (MurA) have already resulted in covalent inhibitors having small three- and five-membered heterocyclic rings. In the current study, the reactivity of four-membered rings was carefully modulated to obtain a novel family of covalent MurA inhibitors. Screening a small library of cyclobutenone derivatives led to the identification of bromo-cyclobutenaminones as new electrophilic warheads. The electrophilic reactivity and cysteine specificity have been determined in a glutathione (GSH) and an oligopeptide assay, respectively. Investigating the structure-activity relationship for MurA suggests a crucial role for the bromine atom in the ligand. In addition, MS/MS experiments have proven the covalent labelling of MurA at Cys115 and the observed loss of the bromine atom suggests a net nucleophilic substitution as the covalent reaction. This new set of compounds might be considered as a viable chemical starting point for the discovery of new MurA inhibitors.

Keywords: covalent inhibitor; MurA; cyclobutenaminone; antibacterial; irreversible

1. Introduction

MurA (UDP-*N*-acetylglucosamine enolpyruvyl transferase) is a key enzyme in the peptidoglycan biosynthesis that catalyzes the transfer of phosphoenolpyruvate (PEP) to UDP-*N*-acetylglucosamine (UNAG) [1]. Targeting the catalytic site of MurA leads to the inactivation of the enzyme that increases the osmotic vulnerability of bacteria [2]. MurA is a preferred antibacterial target, as there is no human orthologue for the enzyme. Known MurA inhibitors contain a three- (**1,3**), five-(**2,4–9**) or occasionally six-membered (**10**) heterocycle equipped with a halogen atom leaving group (**6,10**), or an epoxide ring (**1,3**) that are prone to nucleophilic substitution. Other inhibitors contain a double bond (**2,4,5,7–9**) that is available for Michael addition (Figure 1) [3–6].

Our attention was drawn to the cyclobutenone scaffold, as it also harbors a ring with electrophilic character. Cyclobutenones have received relatively little attention in the literature [7–12], and cyclobutyl compounds, in general, are underrepresented in most (fragment) screening libraries [13]. The ring strain of the cyclobutenone unit suggests a substantial reactivity as an electrophile [10,12,14]. Given the foreseen use as covalent fragments, the reactivity and stability in biological assays need to be balanced. Therefore, the electrophilic reactivity was carefully modulated by incorporating an amine functionality in the electrophilic core, giving cyclobutenaminones. As an additional advantage, appending the amine group to the core provides further chemical handles for growing any hit fragments. Last, cyclobutenaminones contain a double bond enabling the incorporation of, e.g., halogen atoms, that can target nucleophilic amino acid side chains, especially that of cysteines.

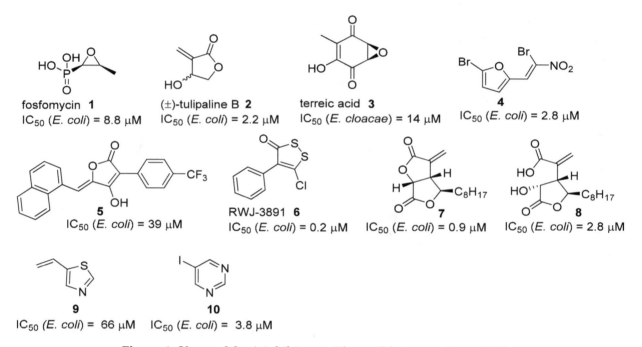

fosfomycin **1**
IC$_{50}$ (*E. coli*) = 8.8 μM

(±)-tulipaline B **2**
IC$_{50}$ (*E. coli*) = 2.2 μM

terreic acid **3**
IC$_{50}$ (*E. cloacae*) = 14 μM

4
IC$_{50}$ (*E. coli*) = 2.8 μM

5
IC$_{50}$ (*E. coli*) = 39 μM

RWJ-3891 **6**
IC$_{50}$ (*E. coli*) = 0.2 μM

7
IC$_{50}$ (*E. coli*) = 0.9 μM

8
IC$_{50}$ (*E. coli*) = 2.8 μM

9
IC$_{50}$ (*E. coli*) = 66 μM

10
IC$_{50}$ (*E. coli*) = 3.8 μM

Figure 1. Known MurA inhibitors with small heterocyclic scaffolds.

In continuation of our interests in finding new MurA inhibitors and in the use of the cyclobutyl motif in drug discovery [6,15–17], here we describe cyclobutenaminone derivatives with carefully-modulated electrophilic character as new warheads for covalently targeting the Cys115 residue in the active site of MurA.

2. Results and Discussion

The synthesis of a small set of cyclobutenaminones was accomplished using a strategy based on that from Brand et al. (Scheme 1) [18]. The sequence began with ethoxyacetylene (**11**), which underwent a [2+2] cycloaddition [18–21] with the in situ generated ketene formed via the base-mediated HCl elimination from isobutyryl chloride. The two methyl groups were incorporated so as to restrict the nucleophilic character of enaminones (**14a–e**) to but one position in, e.g., the electrophilic bromination. The sequence furnished ethoxyenone (**12**) in moderate yield, which was transformed by acidic hydrolysis to 2,2-dimethylcyclobutane-1,3-dione (**13**) in high yield [18–21]. Next, dione **13** was condensed with various amines in the presence of AcOH as catalyst at 65 °C to generate the desired enaminones (**14a–e**) in moderate yields [18,22]. Bromination of all enaminones was achieved via electrophilic substitution using Br$_2$ and base at 0 °C to produce bromoenaminones **15a–e** [18,22]. Selected compounds were subjected to *N*-acylation via deprotonation of the secondary enaminone in tetrahydrofurane (THF) at –78 °C by sodium bis(trimethylsilyl)amide (NaHDMS), followed by subsequent trapping by the relevant acid chloride. Conceivably, the acylation of **14a** to **16a** could also take place at the nucleophilic vinylic position. However, the correct regiochemistry was proven by 2D NMR experiments. The acylations resulted in the corresponding *N*-acyl-cyclobutenaminones (**16a** and **17a–b**) in good yields.

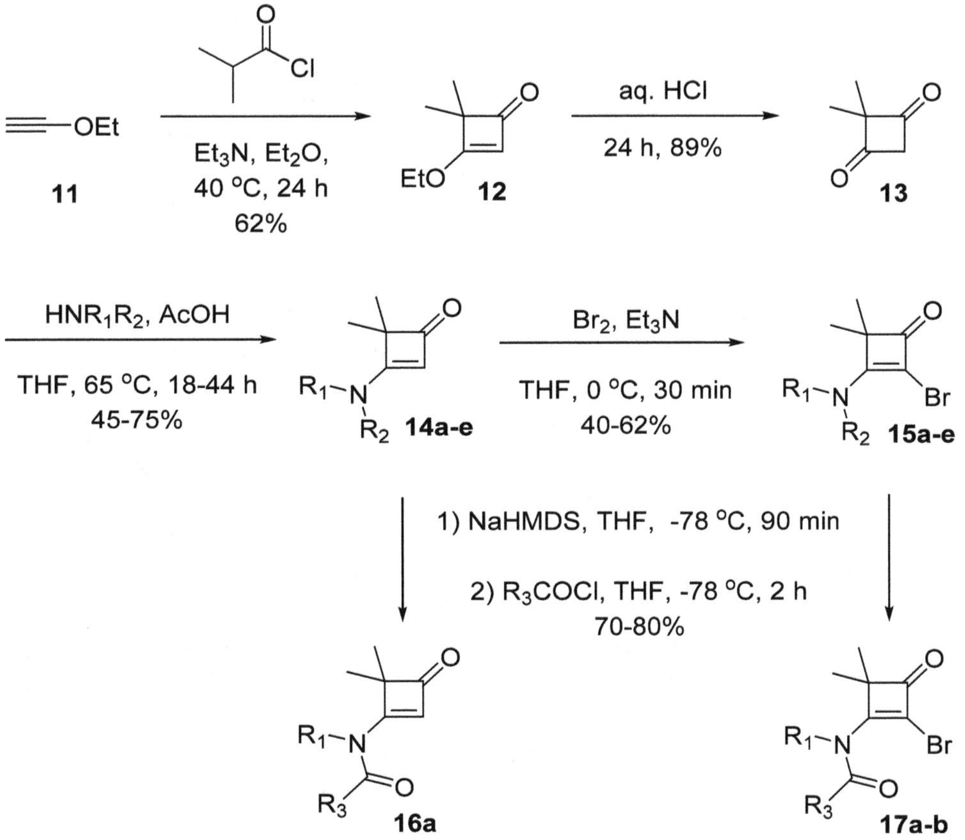

Scheme 1. General synthesis route to various (bromo)enaminones and subsequent N-acylation of secondary enaminones. Table 1 shows the different substituents introduced (R$_1$, R$_2$), while R$_3$ = Me or Ph.

Table 1. Structures and biological activity of synthesized compounds.

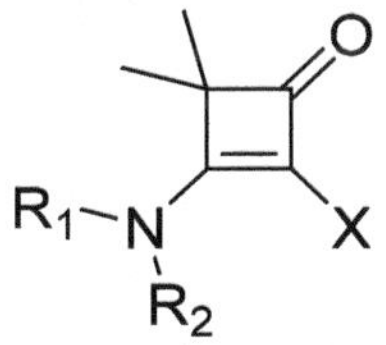

Compound	R$_1$	R$_2$	X	RA[a] [%] at 500 μM and IC$_{50}$ [μM]
14a	Me	H	H	93 ± 4
14b	Me	Me	H	99 ± 1
14c	Et	Et	H	96 ± 2
14d	Me	PMB [b]	H	99 ± 3
14e	Me	F$_3$CCH$_2$	H	98 ± 7
16a	Me	PhCO	H	99 ± 8
12	-	-	-	98 ± 2
15a	Me	H	Br	100 ± 7
15b	Me	Me	Br	91 ± 5
15c	Et	Et	Br	88 ± 6
15d	Me	PMB[b]	Br	13 ± 1, IC$_{50}$ = 363 ± 11
15e	Me	F$_3$CCH$_2$	Br	84 ± 4
17a	Me	PhCO	Br	12 ± 3, IC$_{50}$ = 138 ± 9
17b	Me	MeCO	Br	8 ± 2, IC$_{50}$ = 128 ± 10
fosfomycin	-	-	-	8.8 [3]

[a] RA% refers to the remaining activity in the MurA (*E. coli*) biochemical assay with a fragment concentration of 500 μM with 30 min preincubation at 37 °C; [b] PMB: 4-methoxy-benzyl.

A library of thirteen fragments was prepared, containing nonbrominated (six) and brominated (seven) cyclobutenaminones, all of which are novel to the best of our knowledge (Table 1). This library was then screened against MurA from *E. coli* in order to identify possible starting points for the future development of covalent MurA inhibitors. The screening showed that the cyclobutenaminones with a vinylic proton (**14a–d**) do not give any substantial inhibition. Indeed, the amine substituent selected for balancing reactivity and stability (vide supra) will likely deactivate the double bond by its electron-donating character. We postulated that *N*-trifluoroethylation or *N*-acylation of the nitrogen atom might reactivate the system towards nucleophiles by withdrawing electron density from the conjugated system, but the results on **14e** and **16a** did not support this postulate. As an intermediate in the synthetic route, ethoxycyclobutenone (**12**) was also tested as the ethoxy unit could serve as an improved leaving group, but to no avail. Next, bromination of the vinylic position was explored for activation, bearing in mind that this modification has been successfully applied already in Diels-Alder reactions for improving reactivity [23]. Gratifyingly, several brominated cyclobutenaminones (**15d**, **17a–b**) inhibit MurA from *E. coli* at the 500 μM screening concentration (RA < 15%). Compounds containing amines alkylated with small substituents (**15a–c**) do not show any affinity to the protein, but the incorporation of the 4-methoxybenzyl group (**15d**) increases the affinity to IC_{50} = 363 μM. Turning attention to electron withdrawing groups once again, it was found that *N*-trifluoroethylation has no effect (**15e**), but the *N*-acetyl- and *N*-benzoyl-methylamino derivatives (**17a** and **17b**) substantially inhibit MurA activity. The time-dependent IC_{50} values of these compounds after 30 min are 138 μM and 128 μM, respectively—a substantial effect for such small fragments, with the latter possessing only thirteen heavy atoms. The time dependency of the IC_{50} values (see Supplementary Table S1) and the enhanced electrophilicity caused by the electron-withdrawing substituents suggest a covalent mechanism of action, which was confirmed by proving the labeling on Cys115 by MS/MS measurements for both compounds (Scheme 2E,F, Supplementary Figure S1). The MIC (Minimal Inhibitory Concentrations) values for the antimicrobial action of all compounds were determined against *S. aureus* (ATCC 29213) and *E. coli* (ATCC 25922) bacterial strains. These values were > 625 μM, implying that although MurA inhibition is clearly related to antibiotic action, more finetuning on these structures is needed on the path to a potential new class of antibiotics.

In order to characterize this new electrophilic chemotype, the cysteine reactivity of compound **17a** was evaluated in a GSH (glutathione)-based cysteine surrogate assay (Scheme 2A,B) [15]. The reaction of **17a** with GSH gives an adduct in the HPLC-MS-based assay (M + H$^+$ = 535 Da], suggesting loss of the Br atom, and the conjugation reaction could be characterized with a rate constant of k_{GSH} = 0.0128 (M min)$^{-1}$. Next, the selectivity of **17a** was explored using a nonapeptide assay (Scheme 2C,D) [15]. The KGDYHFPIC nonapeptide contains a cysteine but also other nucleophilic residues i.e., lysine, tyrosine, aspartate, proline, and histidine. As such, the nonapeptide can help to assess the selectivity between different biologically-relevant nucleophiles. In the case of **17a**, only the thiol group of the oligopeptide reacts with the warhead, indicating a high degree of cysteine specificity. To evaluate if the warhead is not too reactive for standard assay conditions, the aqueous stability of the compound (**17a**) was also investigated in PBS buffer (pH 7.4) [15]. The stability proves to be appropriate for biological investigations, as the $t_{1/2}$ value for the aqueous degradation was determined to be 36.5 h at room temperature. The stability and bioavailability of these structures is also supported by the fact that interestingly, the rather unique bromocyclobutenaminone core has been incorporated both in the α4β1/α4β7 integrin antagonist prodrug, Zaurategrast [24,25], which progressed to phase II clinical trials [26], as well as in related compounds [22].

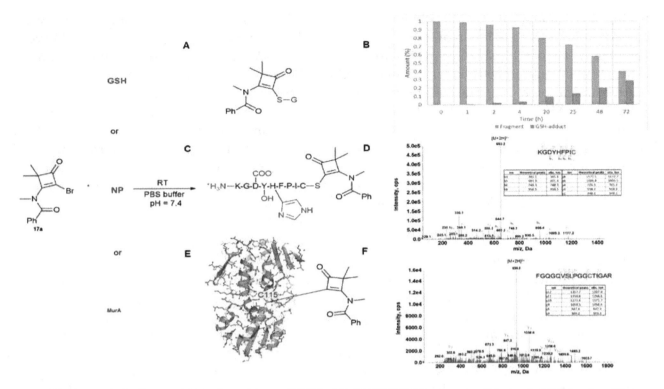

Scheme 2. Labelling of (**A**) glutathione (GSH), (**C**) KGDHFPIC nonapeptide and (**E**) MurA with fragment **17a** together with (**B**) the measured consumption of the fragment (blue columns) and the increasing amount of the GSH-adduct (orange columns) in the GSH-assay, (**D**) the MS/MS spectrum of the Cys-labelled nonapeptide indicating the Cys-labelling together with the theoretical and observed ion peaks and (**F**) the MS/MS spectrum of the digested MurA fragment (amino acids 104–120) labelled on Cys115 together with the theoretical and observed ion peaks. For E the 1UAE X-ray structure has been used [27].

3. Materials and Methods

3.1. Synthesis and Characterisation of Compounds

All starting materials were obtained from commercial suppliers (primarily being Sigma-Aldrich (Swijndrecht, The Netherlands), Fluorochem (Hadfield, Derbyshire, UK) and CombiBlocks (San Diego, CA, USA)) and used without purification. Anhydrous Et_2O, dichloromethane (DCM), acetonitrile (MeCN) and tetrahydrofurane (THF) were obtained by passing through an activated alumina column prior to use. All other solvents used were used as received unless otherwise stated. All reactions were carried out under a nitrogen atmosphere unless mentioned otherwise. TLC analyses were performed using Merck F_{254} (Merck KGaA, Darmstadt, Germany or VWR International B.V., Amsterdam, The Netherlands) aluminum-backed silica gel plates and visualized with 254 nm UV light or a potassium permanganate stain. Flash column chromatography was executed using Silicycle Siliaflash F_{60} silica gel (SiliCycle Inc., Quebec City, QC, Canada or Screening Devices, Amersfoort, The Netherlands) or by means of a Teledyne Isco CombiFlash (Teledyne Isco Inc., Lincoln, NE, USA or Beun de Ronde, Abcoude, The Netherlands) or a Biotage Isolera equipment using Biotage SNAP columns (Biotage AB, Uppsala, Sweden). All HRMS spectra were recorded on a Bruker micrOTOF mass spectrometer (Bruker Corp., Billerica, MA, USA) using ESI in positive-ion mode. All NMR spectra were recorded on either a Bruker Avance 300, Bruker Avance 500, or Bruker Avance 600 spectrometer (Bruker Corp., Billerica, MA, USA or Fällanden, Switzerland). The peak multiplicities are defined as follows: s, singlet; bs, broad singlet; d, doublet; t, triplet; q, quartet; p, pentet; dd, doublet of doublets; dt, doublet of triplets; td, a triplet of doublets; m, multiplet; app, apparent. The spectra were referenced to the internal solvent peak as follows: $CDCl_3$ (^1H = 7.26 ppm, ^{13}C = 77.16 ppm), DMSO-d6 (^1H = 2.50 ppm, ^{13}C = 39.52 ppm). IUPAC names were adapted from ChemDraw Professional 16.0 (PerkinElmer). Purities were measured

Antibiotic Drug Discovery and Development

with the aid of analytical LC−MS using a Shimadzu LC-20AD liquid chromatography pump system (Shimadzu Corp., Kyoto, Japan or 's Hertogenbosch, The Netherlands) with a Shimadzu SPDM20A diode array detector (Shimadzu Corp., Kyoto, Japan) with the MS detection performed with a Shimadzu LC-MS-2010EV mass spectrometer (Shimadzu Corp., Kyoto, Japan) operating in both positive and negative ionization mode. The column used was an XBridge (C18) 5 μm column (50 mm × 4.6 mm) (Waters Corp., Milford, MA, USA or Phenomenex, Utrecht, The Netherlands). The following solutions are used for the eluents. Solvent A: H_2O (+0.1% HCOOH) and solvent B: MeCN (+0.1% HCOOH). The eluent program used is as follows: flow rate: 1.0 mL/min, start 95% A in a linear gradient to 10% A over 4.5 min, hold 1.5 min at 10% A, in 0.5 min in a linear gradient to 95% A, hold 1.5 min at 95% A, total run time: 8.0 min. Compound purities were calculated as the percentage peak area of the analysed compound by UV detection at 254 nm.

3.2. GSH Reactivity and Aqueous Stability Assay

The assay was adapted from our former publication [15].

For the glutathione assay, 500 μM solution of the fragment (PBS buffer pH 7.4, 10% MeCN, 250 μL) with 200 μM solution of indoprofen (Merck KGaA, Darmstadt, Germany) as internal standard was added to 10 mM glutathione (Merck KGaA, Darmstadt, Germany) solution (dissolved in PBS buffer, 250 μL) in a 1:1 ratio. The final concentration was 250 μM fragment, 100 μM indoprofen, 5 mM glutathione and 5% MeCN (500 μL). The final mixture was analyzed by HPLC-MS (Shimadzu LCMS-2020) after 0, 1, 2, 4, 20, 25, 48, 72 h time intervals. Degradation kinetics were also investigated respectively using the previously described method, applying pure PBS buffer instead of the glutathione solution. In this experiment, the final concentration of the mixture was 250 μM fragment, 100 μM indoprofen and 5% MeCN. The AUC (area under the curve) values were determined via integration of HPLC spectra then corrected using the internal standard. The fragment AUC values were applied for ordinary least squares (OLS) linear regression and for computing the important parameters (kinetic rate constant, half-life time) a programmed excel (Visual Basic for Applications) was utilized. The data are expressed as means of duplicate determinations, and the standard deviations were within 10% of the given values.

The calculation of the kinetic rate constant for the degradation and corrected GSH-reactivity is as follows:

The reaction half-life for pseudo-first-order reactions is $t_{1/2} = \ln2/k$, where k is the reaction rate. In the case of competing reactions (reaction with GSH and degradation), the effective rate for the consumption of the starting compound is $k_{eff} = k_{deg} + k_{GSH}$. When measuring half-lives experimentally, the $t_{1/2(eff)} = \ln2/(k_{eff}) = \ln2/(k_{deg} + k_{GSH})$. In our case, the corrected k_{deg} and k_{eff} (regarding blank and GSH-containing samples, respectively) can be calculated by linear regression of the data points of the kinetic measurements. The corrected k_{GSH} is calculated by $k_{eff} - k_{deg}$, and finally, the half-life time is determined using the equation $t_{1/2(GSH)} = \ln2/k_{GSH}$.

3.3. Oligopeptide Selectivity Assay

The assay was adapted from our former publication [15].

For the nonapeptide assay, a 2 mM solution of the fragment (PBS buffer pH 7.4 with 20% MeCN) was added to 200 μM nonapeptide solution (PBS buffer pH 7.4) in a 1:1 ratio. The final assay mixture contained 1 mM fragment, 100 μM peptide and 10% MeCN. Based on the GSH reactivity, the applied incubation time was 24 h.

3.4. LC-MS/MS Measurement and Data Analysis of the Nonapeptide Reactivity Assay

A Sciex 6500 QTRAP triple quadrupole—linear ion trap mass spectrometer, equipped with a Turbo V Source in electrospray mode (AB Sciex Pte. Ltd., Framingham, MA, USA) and an Agilent 1100 Binary Pump HPLC system (Agilent Technologies, Waldbronn, Germany) equipped with an autosampler was used for LC-MS/MS analysis. Data acquisition and processing were performed using Analyst software version 1.6.2 (AB Sciex Pte. Ltd., Framingham, MA, USA). Chromatographic separation was achieved by Purospher STAR RP-18 endcapped (50 mm × 2.1 mm, 3μm) LiChocart® 55-2 HPLC Cartridge (Merck KGaA, Darmstadt, Germany). The sample was eluted with gradient elution using solvent A (0.1% HCOOH in water) and solvent B (0.1% HCOOH in MeCN). Flow rate was set to 0.5 mL/min. The initial condition was 5% B for 2 min, followed by a linear gradient to 95% B for 6 min, followed by holding at 95% B 6–8 min; and from 8 to 8.5 min back to the initial condition with 5% eluent B and held for 14.5 min. The column temperature was kept at room temperature and the injection volume was 10 μL. Nitrogen was used as the nebulizer gas (GS1), heater gas (GS2), and curtain gas with the optimum values set at 35, 45 and 45 (arbitrary units). The source temperature was 450 °C and the ion spray voltage set at 5000 V. The declustering potential value was set to 150 V. Information Dependent Acquisition (IDA) LC-MS/MS experiment was used to determine if the fragment binding was specific to thiol residues or not. An enhanced MS scan was applied as the survey scan and enhanced product ion (EPI) was the dependent scan. The collision energy in EPI experiments was set to 30 eV with a collision energy spread (CES) of 10 V. The identification of the binding position of the fragments to the nonapeptide was performed using GPMAW 4.2. software.

3.5. Tryptic Digestion of MurA

The tryptic digestion method was adapted from our former publication [15].

Briefly, 50 μL of MurA (42 μM) and 10 μL 0.2% (w/v) RapiGest SF (Waters Corp., Milford, MA, USA) solution buffered with 50 mM ammonium bicarbonate (NH_4HCO_3) were mixed (pH = 7.8). 4.5 μL of 45 mM DTT (~200 nmol) in 100 mM NH_4HCO_3 was added and the mixture kept at 37.5 °C for 30 min. After cooling the sample to room temperature, 7.5 μL of 100 mM iodoacetamide (750 nmol) in 100 mM NH_4HCO_3 was added and the mixture placed in the dark at room temperature for 30 min. The reduced and alkylated protein was then digested by 10 μL (1 mg mL^{-1}) trypsin (the enzyme-to-protein ratio was 1:10) (Sigma, St Louis, MO, USA). The sample was incubated at 37 °C overnight. To degrade the surfactant, 7 μL of HCOOH (500 mM) solution was added to the digested HDAC8 sample to obtain the final 40 mM (pH ≈ 2) solution which was incubated at 37 °C for 45 min. For LC-MS analysis, the acid-treated sample was centrifuged for 5 min at 13,000 rpm.

3.6. LC-MS/MS Measurements on Digested MurA

A QTRAP 6500 triple quadruple—linear ion trap mass spectrometer, equipped with a Turbo V source in electrospray mode (AB Sciex Pte. Ltd., Framingham, MA, USA) and an Agilent 1100 Binary Pump HPLC system (Agilent Technologies, Waldbronn, Germany) equipped with an autosampler was used for LC-MS/MS analysis. Data acquisition and processing were performed using Analyst software version 1.6.2 (AB Sciex Pte. Ltd., Framingham, MA, USA). Chromatographic separation was achieved by using the Discovery® BIO Wide Pore C-18-5 (250 mm × 2.1 mm, 5 μm). The sample was eluted with a gradient of solvent A (0.1% HCOOH in water) and solvent B (0.1% HCOOH in MeCN). The flow rate was set to 0.2 mL min^{-1}. The initial conditions for separation were 5% B for 7 min, followed by a linear gradient to 90% B for 53 min, followed by 90% B for 3 min; over 2 min back to the initial conditions with 5% eluent B retained for 10 min. The injection volume was 10 μL (300 pmol on the column).

An Information-Dependent Acquisiton (IDA) LC-MS/MS experiment was used to identify the modified tryptic MurA peptide fragments. Enhanced MS scan (EMS) was applied as the survey scan and an enhanced product ion (EPI) was the dependent scan. The collision energy in EPI experiments was set to rolling collision energy mode, where the actual value was set on the basis of the mass and charge state of the selected ion. Further IDA criteria: ions greater than: 400.00 m/z, which exceeds 106 counts, exclude former target ions for 30 s after 2 occurrence(s). In EMS and in EPI mode, the scan rate was 1000 Da/s as well. Nitrogen was used as the nebulizer gas (GS1), heater gas (GS2), and curtain gas with the optimum values set at 50, 40 and 40 (arbitrary units). The source temperature was 350 °C and the ion spray voltage was set at 5000 V. The declustering potential value was set to 150 V.

GPMAW 4.2. software was used to analyse a large number of MS-MS spectra and identify the modified tryptic MurA peptides.

3.7. MurA Assay

$MurA_{EC}$ protein was recombinant, expressed in *E. coli.* [28] The inhibition of MurA was monitored with the colorimetric malachite green method in which orthophosphate generated during the reaction is measured. MurA enzyme (*E. coli*) was pre-incubated with the substrate UNAG and compound for 30 min at 37 °C. The reaction was started by the addition of the second substrate PEP, resulting in a mixture with a final volume of 50 μL. The mixtures contained: 50 mM Hepes, pH 7.8, 0.005% Triton X-114, 200 μM UNAG, 100 μM PEP, purified MurA (diluted in 50 mM Hepes, pH 7.8) and 500 μM of each tested compound dissolved in DMSO. All compounds were soluble in the assay mixtures containing 5% DMSO (*v/v*). After incubation for 15 min at 37 °C, the enzyme reaction was terminated by adding Biomol® reagent (100μL) and the absorbance was measured at 650 nm after 5 min. All of the experiments were run in duplicate. Remaining activities (RAs) were calculated with respect to similar assays without the tested compounds and with 5% DMSO. The IC_{50} values, the concentration of the compound at which the remaining activity was 50%, were determined by measuring the remaining activities at seven different compound concentrations. The data are expressed as means of duplicate determinations, and the standard deviations were within 10% of the given values. A time-dependent inhibition assay was also performed. The IC_{50} values were determined at 0, 15 and 30 min of pre-incubation.

3.8. Antimicrobial Testing (MIC Determination)

Antimicrobial testing was carried out by the broth microdilution method in 96-well plate format following the CLSI guidelines and European Committee for Antimicrobial Susceptibility Testing recommendations. Bacterial suspension of specific bacterial strain, equivalent to 0.5 McFarland turbidity standard, was diluted with cation-adjusted Mueller Hinton broth to obtain a final inoculum of 10^5 CFU/mL. Compounds dissolved in DMSO and inoculum were mixed together and incubated for 20–24 h at 37 °C. After incubation the minimal inhibitory concentration (MIC) values were determined by visual inspection as the lowest dilution of compounds showing no turbidity. The MICs were determined against *S. aureus* (ATCC 29213) and *E. coli* (ATCC 25922) bacterial strains. Tetracycline was used as a positive control on every assay plate, showing a MIC of 0.5 μg/mL and 1 μg/mL for *S. aureus* and *E. coli*, respectively.

3.9. Chemical Syntheses

3-Ethoxy-4,4-dimethylcyclobut-2-en-1-one (12)

To a stirred solution of isobutyryl chloride (10.7 mL, 102 mmol) and ethoxyacetylene **11** (50.0 mL, 205 mmol, 40% wt in hexanes) in Et_2O (128 mL), Et_3N (21.4 mL, 154 mmol) was added slowly over 5 min. The mixture was stirred at rt for 30 min before being heated at 40 °C for 24 h. The mixture was then allowed to cool. The precipitate was filtered and the filtrate was concentrated in vacuo. The crude product was purified over silica gel with a gradient of 10–40% EtOAc/cHex to afford the title compound **2** (8.90 g, 62% yield) as a yellow oil.

^{1}H NMR (500 MHz, Chloroform-*d*) δ 4.78 (s, 1H), 4.21 (q, *J* = 7.1 Hz, 2H), 1.45 (t, *J* = 7.1 Hz, 3H), 1.24 (s, 6H). ^{13}C NMR (126 MHz, Chloroform-*d*) δ 194.1, 190.4, 102.4, 69.4, 60.1, 19.7, 14.3. LC-MS: RT = 3.33 min, 99+% (254 nm), *m/z* [M + H]$^+$ = 141. HRMS calculated for $C_8H_{13}O_2^+$ [M + H]$^+$ = 141.0910, found 141.0923.

2,2-Dimethylcyclobutane-1,3-dione (13)

To a flask containing enol ether **12** (8.40 g, 59.9 mmol) was added HCl (2.0 M in H_2O, 45.0 mL, 90.0 mmol) in one portion and the mixture was stirred vigorously at rt for 24 h. The product was extracted with DCM (3×). The organic layers were combined, dried over $MgSO_4$, and concentrated in vacuo to afford the title compound **3** (6.20 g, 92% yield) as a flaky brown solid.

^1H NMR (600 MHz, Chloroform-d) δ 3.92 (s, 2H), 1.28 (s, 6H). ^{13}C NMR (151 MHz, Chloroform-d) δ 207.0, 73.0, 60.4, 17.6. LC-MS: RT = 1.78 min, 98% (254 nm), m/z $[M + H]^+$ = 113. HRMS calculated for $C_6H_9O_2^+$ $[M + H]^+$ = 113.0597, found 113.0603.

3.10. General Procedure A: Enaminone Formation

To a solution of dione **13** (1.0 eq) in THF (0.50 M) was added amine (1.1 eq), AcOH (1.1 eq) and a spatula of Na_2SO_4. The reaction mixture was stirred at 65 °C for the indicated time. The reaction mixture was allowed to cool to rt. The solids were filtered and the filtrate concentrated in vacuo. The residue was taken up in EtOAc and washed with satd. aq. Na_2CO_3 and brine. The organic layer was dried over Na_2SO_4, filtered and concentrated *in vacuo*. The crude product was purified over silica gel using the indicated gradient of MeOH/DCM to afford the product enaminone.

3-(Methylamino)-4,4-dimethylcyclobut-2-en-1-one (14a)

This compound was prepared according to General Procedure **A** using dione **13** (388 mg, 3.46 mmol), $MeNH_2$ (2.0 M in THF, 1.90 mL, 3.81 mmol) and a reaction time of 40 h. Purification over silica gel using a gradient of 0–10% MeOH/DCM afforded the title compound **14a** (350 mg, 81%) as a pale brown solid.

Rotamers are observed in ratio ca. 1.0:0.1 in Chloroform-d. Only peaks corresponding to the major rotamer are reported. ^1H NMR (500 MHz, Chloroform-d) δ 5.63 (br s, 1H), 4.59 (s, 1H), 2.99 (d, J = 5.0 Hz, 3H), 1.24 (s, 6H). ^{13}C NMR (126 MHz, Chloroform-d) δ 192.2, 178.8, 95.7, 58.5, 31.8, 20.3. LC-MS: RT = 3.20 min, 99+% (254 nm), m/z $[M + H]^+$ = 126. HRMS calculated for $C_7H_{12}NO^+$ $[M + H]^+$ = 126.0913, found 126.0912.

3-(Dimethylamino)-4,4-dimethylcyclobut-2-en-1-one (14b)

This compound was prepared according to General Procedure **A** using dione **13** (200 mg, 1.78 mmol), Me_2NH (2.0 M in THF, 0.20 mL, 1.96 mmol) and a reaction time of 40 h. Purification over silica gel using a gradient of 0–10% MeOH/DCM afforded the title compound **14b** (191 mg, 77% yield) as a brown crystalline solid.

Rotamers are observed in ratio 1.0:1.0 in Chloroform-d. All peaks for both rotamers are reported. ^1H NMR (500 MHz, Chloroform-d) δ 4.53 (s, 1H), 3.07 (s, 3H), 2.99 (s, 3H), 1.32 (s, 6H). ^{13}C NMR (126 MHz, Chloroform-d) δ 190.9, 178.4, 96.0, 58.2, 40.1, 39.4, 21.2. LC-MS: RT = 2.34 min, 99 + % (254 nm), m/z $[M + H]^+$ = 140. HRMS calculated for $C_8H_{14}NO^+$ $[M + H]^+$ = 140.1064, found 140.1066.

3-(Diethylamino)-4,4-dimethylcyclobut-2-en-1-one (14c)

This compound was prepared according to General Procedure **A** using dione **13** (200 mg, 1.78 mmol), Et_2NH (0.20 mL, 1.96 mmol) and a reaction time of 40 h, followed by an additional portion of Et_2NH (0.10 mL, 0.89 mmol) and stirring for a further 5 h. Purification over silica gel using a gradient of 0–10% MeOH/DCM afforded the title compound **14c** (175 mg, 59% yield) as a brown oil.

Rotamers are observed in ratio 1.0:1.0 in Chloroform-d. All peaks for both rotamers are reported. ^1H NMR (500 MHz, Chloroform-d) δ 4.54 (s, 1H), 3.34 (q, J = 7.2 Hz, 2H), 3.27 (q, J = 7.2 Hz, 2H), 1.33 (s, 6H), 1.25 (t, J = 7.2 Hz, 3H), 1.22 (t, J = 7.2 Hz, 3H). ^{13}C NMR (126 MHz, Chloroform-d) δ 190.9, 177.5, 95.6, 58.4, 44.6, 44.1, 21.4, 14.2, 12.3. LC-MS: RT = 3.06 min, 99+% (254 nm), m/z $[M+H]^+$ = 168. HRMS calculated for $C_{10}H_{18}NO^+$ $[M + H]^+$ = 168.1377, found 168.1382.

3-((4-Methoxybenzyl)(methyl)amino)-4,4-dimethylcyclobut-2-en-1-one (14d)

This compound was prepared according to General Procedure **A** using dione 13 (200 mg, 1.78 mmol), (4-methoxybenzyl)-*N*-methylamine (0.29 mL, 1.96 mmol) and a reaction time of 40 h. Purification over silica gel using a gradient of 0–10% MeOH/DCM afforded the title compound **14d** (330 mg, 75% yield) as a viscous brown oil.

Rotamers are observed in ratio 1.0:1.0 in Chloroform-d. All peaks for both rotamers are reported. ^{1}H NMR (600 MHz, Chloroform-d) δ 7.18–7.12 (m, 2H), 6.93–6.88 (m, 2H), 4.70 (s, 1H), 4.59 (s, 1H), 4.42 (s, 2H), 4.29 (s, 2H), 3.82 (s, 3H), 3.81 (s, 3H), 2.95 (s, 3H), 2.80 (s, 3H), 1.38 (s, 6H), 1.34 (s, 6H). ^{13}C NMR (151 MHz, Chloroform-d) δ 190.9, 190.8, 178.4, 178.3, 159.6, 129.1, 128.7, 126.9, 126.7, 114.5, 114.4, 96.2, 95.9, 58.4, 58.3, 56.2, 55.4, 55.4, 55.3, 36.6, 36.3, 21.4, 21.1. LC-MS: RT = 3.62 min, 99+% (254 nm), m/z [M + H]$^+$ = 246. HRMS calculated for $C_{15}H_{20}NO_2^+$ [M + H]$^+$ = 246.1489, found 246.1489.

4,4-Dimethyl-3-(methyl(2,2,2-trifluoroethyl)amino)cyclobut-2-en-1-one (14e)

This compound was prepared according to General Procedure **A** using dione **13** (140 mg, 1.25 mmol), (2,2,2-trifluoroethyl)-methylamine (0.14 mL, 1.37 mmol) and a reaction time of 16 h. Purification over silica gel using a gradient of 0–10% MeOH/DCM afforded the title compound **14e** (197 mg, 76% yield) as a brown oil.

Rotamers are observed in ratio 1.0:0.8 in Chloroform-d. All peaks for both rotamers are reported. ^{1}H NMR (500 MHz, Chloroform-d) δ 4.67 (s, 1H), δ 4.70 (s, 1H), 3.80 (q, J = 8.6 Hz, 2H), 3.75 (q, J = 9.0 Hz, 2H), 3.20 (s, 3H), 3.09–3.10 (m, 3H), 1.35 (s, 6H), 1.32 (s, 6H). ^{13}C NMR (151 MHz, Chloroform-d) δ 190.63, 179.51, 179.47, 124.47 (q, J = 281.9 Hz), 123.70 (q, J = 281.9 Hz), 99.72, 99.03, 54.29 (q, J = 34.1 Hz), 53.51 (q, J = 34.1 Hz), 39.06, 21.19, 21.08. LC-MS: RT = 3.30 min, 99+% (254 nm), m/z [M + H]$^+$ = 208. HRMS calculated for $C_9H_{13}F_3NO^+$ [M + H]$^+$ = 208.0944, found 208.0947.

3.11. General Procedure B: Bromination

A solution of enaminone (1.0 eq) and Et$_3$N (2.0 eq) in THF (0.10 M) at 0 °C was treated dropwise with a solution of Br$_2$ (1.1 eq) in THF (2.0 mL). The reaction mixture was stirred at 0 °C for the indicated time. The mixture was diluted with EtOAc and washed with satd. aq. NaHCO$_3$ and brine. The organic layer was dried over MgSO$_4$, filtered and concentrated *in vacuo*. The crude product was purified over silica gel using the indicated gradient of MeOH/EtOAc followed by reversed-phase chromatography on C18 silica gel using the indicated gradient of MeCN/H$_2$O to afford the product bromoenaminone.

2-Bromo-4,4-dimethyl-3-(methylamino)cyclobut-2-en-1-one (15a)

This compound was prepared according to General Procedure B using enaminone **14a** (80 mg, 0.64 mmol) and a reaction time of 1 h. Purification over silica gel using a gradient of 0–10% MeOH/EtOAc and over reversed-phase C18 silica gel using a gradient of 0–100% MeCN/H$_2$O (+0.1% HCOOH) afforded the title compound **15a** (81 mg, 62% yield) as a pale yellow solid.

Rotamers are observed in ratio 1.0:0.6 in Chloroform-d. All peaks for both rotamers are reported. ^{1}H NMR (600 MHz, Chloroform-d) δ 5.97 (br s, 1H), 5.55 (br s, 1H), 3.30 (d, J = 5.2 Hz, 3H), 3.12 (d, J = 5.2 Hz, 3H), 1.38 (s, 6H), 1.24 (s, 6H). ^{13}C NMR (151 MHz, Chloroform-d) δ 187.8, 185.9, 177.6, 175.5, 72.8, 70.5, 59.1, 58.7, 31.6, 31.4, 20.8, 19.9. LC-MS: RT = 2.80 min, 99+% (254 nm), m/z [M + H]$^+$ = 204 (light isotope). HRMS calculated for $C_7H_{11}NOBr^+$ [M + H]$^+$ = 205.9998 (heavy isotope), found 205.9997.

2-Bromo-4,4-dimethyl-3-(methylamino)cyclobut-2-en-1-one (15b)

This compound was prepared according to General Procedure B using enaminone **14b** (80 mg, 0.58 mmol) and a reaction time of 1 h. Purification over silica gel using a gradient of 0–10% MeOH/EtOAc and over reversed-phase C18 silica gel using a gradient of 0–100% MeCN/H$_2$O (+0.1% HCOOH) afforded the title compound **15b** (59 mg, 47% yield) as a pale yellow solid.

Rotamers are observed in ratio 1.0:1.0 in Chloroform-d. All peaks for both rotamers are reported. ^{1}H NMR (600 MHz, Chloroform-d) δ 3.35 (s, 3H), 3.07 (s, 3H), 1.32 (s, 6H). ^{13}C NMR (151 MHz, Chloroform-d) δ 186.5, 174.5, 70.3, 58.7, 40.7, 39.6, 20.9. LC-MS: RT = 3.06 min, 99+% (254 nm), m/z [M + H]$^+$ = 218 (light isotope). HRMS calculated for $C_8H_{13}NOBr^+$ [M + H]$^+$ = 218.0175 (light isotope), found 218.0182.

2-Bromo-3-(diethylamino)-4,4-dimethylcyclobut-2-en-1-one (**15c**)

This compound was prepared according to General Procedure B using enaminone **14c** (80 mg, 0.48 mmol) and a reaction time of 1 h. Purification over silica gel using a gradient of 0–10% MeOH/EtOAc and over reversed-phase C18 silica gel using a gradient of 0–100% MeCN/H$_2$O (+0.1% HCOOH) afforded the title compound **15c** (49 mg, 42% yield) as a colourless oil.

Rotamers are observed in ratio 1.0:1.0 in Chloroform-*d*. All peaks for both rotamers are reported. ^{1}H NMR (600 MHz, Chloroform-*d*) δ 3.64 (q, *J* = 7.2 Hz, 1H), 3.35 (q, *J* = 7.2 Hz, 1H), 1.30 (t, *J* = 7.2 Hz, 3H), 1.28 (t, *J* = 7.2 Hz, 3H). ^{13}C NMR (151 MHz, Chloroform-*d*) δ 186.6, 173.9, 69.7, 58.8, 45.7, 43.0, 21.1, 14.4, 14.2. LC-MS: RT = 3.78 min, 97% (254 nm), *m/z* [M + H]$^+$ = 248 (heavy isotope). HRMS calculated for C$_{10}$H$_{17}$NOBr$^+$ [M + H]$^+$ = 246.0488 (light isotope), found 246.0488.

2-Bromo-3-((4-methoxybenzyl)(methyl)amino)-4,4-dimethylcyclobut-2-en-1-one (**15d**)

This compound was prepared according to General Procedure B using enaminone **14d** (100 mg, 0.41 mmol) and a reaction time of 2 h. Purification over silica gel using a gradient of 0–10% MeOH/EtOAc and over reversed-phase C18 silica gel using a gradient of 0–100% MeCN/H$_2$O (+0.1% HCOOH) afforded the title compound **15d** (51 mg, 39% yield) as a pale yellow oil.

Rotamers are observed in ratio 1:0.6 in Chloroform-*d*. All peaks for both rotamers are reported. ^{1}H NMR (600 MHz, Chloroform-*d*) δ 7.25–7.22 (m, 2H), 7.17–7.14 (m, 2H), 6.95–6.91 (m, 4H), 4.75 (s, 2H), 4.41 (s, 2H), 3.82 (s, 3H), 3.82 (s, 3H), 3.16 (s, 3H), 2.95 (s, 3H), 1.39 (s, 6H), 1.35 (s, 6H). ^{13}C NMR (151 MHz, Chloroform-*d*) δ 186.71, 186.68, 174.72, 174.28, 159.90, 159.82, 129.52, 128.88, 127.15, 125.90, 114.70, 114.60, 70.51, 70.45, 58.96, 58.93, 56.64, 55.50, 55.47, 54.65, 37.43, 36.27, 21.23, 20.94. LC-MS: RT = 4.24 min, 99+% (254 nm), *m/z* [M + H]$^+$ = 324 (light isotope). HRMS calculated for C$_{15}$H$_{19}$NO$_2$Br$^+$ [M + H]$^+$ = 326.0573 (heavy isotope), found 326.0573.

2-Bromo-4,4-dimethyl-3-(methyl(2,2,2-trifluoroethyl)amino)cyclobut-2-en-1-one (**15e**)

This compound was prepared according to General Procedure B using enaminone **14e** (80 mg, 0.39 mmol) and a reaction time of 1 h. Purification over silica gel using a gradient of 0–10% MeOH/EtOAc and over reversed-phase C18 silica gel using a gradient of 0–100% MeCN/H$_2$O (+0.1% HCOOH) afforded the title compound **15e** (32% yield) as a pale yellow solid.

Rotamers are observed in ratio 1:0.4 in Chloroform-*d*. All peaks for both rotamers are reported. ^{1}H NMR (600 MHz, Chloroform-*d*) δ 4.27 (q, *J* = 8.3 Hz, 2H), 3.79 (q, *J* = 8.3 Hz, 2H), 3.46 (s, 3H), 3.22 (s, 3H), 1.37 (s, 6H), 1.34 (s, 6H). ^{13}C NMR (151 MHz, Chloroform-*d*) δ 186.51, 175.87, 175.66, 123.95 (q, *J* = 282.1 Hz), 123.51 (q, *J* = 282.1 Hz), 74.86, 74.20, 59.70, 59.61, 54.57 (q, *J* = 34.0 Hz), 52.41 (q, *J* = 34.0 Hz), 40.05, 39.13, 20.93, 20.84. LC-MS: RT = 3.86 min, 99+% (254 nm), *m/z* [M + H]$^+$ = 286 (light isotope). HRMS calculated for C$_9$H$_{12}$NOF$_2$Br$^+$ [M + H]$^+$ = 286.0049 (light isotope), found 286.0044.

3.12. General Procedure C: Enaminone N-Acylation

To a solution of enaminone (1.0 eq) in THF (0.025 M) at −78 °C was added NaN(SiMe$_3$)$_2$ (1.0 M in THF, 1.5 eq) dropwise. The mixture was stirred at this temperature for 90 min before dropwise addition of the acid chloride (1.2 eq). The reaction mixture was stirred for a further 2 h at −78 °C. Brine was added slowly at this temperature whilst stirring vigorously and the mixture was allowed to warm to rt. The volatiles were removed in vacuo and the residue was partitioned between EtOAc and water. The organic layer was washed with brine, dried over Na$_2$SO$_4$, and concentrated *in vacuo*. The crude product was purified over silica gel to afford the product *N*-acyl-enaminone.

N-(4,4-dimethyl-3-oxocyclobut-1-en-1-yl)-*N*-methylbenzamide (**16a**)

This compound was prepared according to General Procedure C using enaminone **14a** (80 mg, 0.64 mmol) and BzCl (0.09 mL, 0.77 mmol). Purification over silica gel using a gradient of 20–80% EtOAc/cHex afforded the title compound **16a** (72% yield) as a white solid.

No significant rotamers are observed in NMR spectra. ^{1}H NMR (500 MHz, Chloroform-d) δ 7.56–7.52 (m, 3H), 7.49–7.45 (m, 2H), 4.83 (s, 1H), 3.35 (s, 3H), 1.41 (s, 6H). ^{13}C NMR (151 MHz, Chloroform-d) δ 194.2, 175.9, 171.1, 134.1, 132.0, 129.0, 127.9, 111.8, 62.7, 36.7, 21.4. LC-MS: RT = 3.85 min, 99% (254 nm), m/z [M + H]$^+$ = 230. HRMS calculated for $C_{14}H_{16}NO_2^+$ [M + H]$^+$ = 230.1176 found 230.1171.

The regiochemistry of the acylation (i.e., acylation of N atom and not of vinyl position) was proven by 2D NMR (HSQC + HMBC)—the singlet signal counting for 1H has an associated ^{13}C signal in HSQC and thus the vinyl position remains unsubstituted in the product.

N-(2-bromo-4,4-dimethyl-3-oxocyclobut-1-en-1-yl)-N-methylbenzamide (17a)

This compound was prepared according to General Procedure C using bromoenaminone **15a** (80 mg, 0.39 mmol) and BzCl (0.06 mL, 0.47 mmol). Purification over silica gel using a gradient of 20–70% EtOAc/cHex afforded the title compound **17a** (86 mg, 71% yield) as a white solid.

No significant rotamers are observed in NMR spectra. ^{1}H NMR (600 MHz, Chloroform-d) δ 7.62–7.54 (m, 3H), 7.53–7.46 (m, 2H), 3.61 (s, 3H), 1.43 (s, 6H). ^{13}C NMR (151 MHz, Chloroform-d) δ 191.4, 174.6, 170.1, 133.5, 132.5, 129.1, 128.5, 87.8, 63.5, 39.0, 21.2. LC-MS: RT = 4.55 min, 99+% (254 nm), m/z [M + H]$^+$ = 308 (light isotope). HRMS calculated for $C_{14}H_{15}BrNO_2^+$ [M + H]$^+$ = 310.0260 (heavy isotope), found 310.0254.

N-(2-bromo-4,4-dimethyl-3-oxocyclobut-1-en-1-yl)-N-methylacetamide (17b)

This compound was prepared according to General Procedure C using bromoenaminone **15a** (6 mg, 0.03 mmol) and AcCl (0.002 mL, 0.03 mmol). Extraction with DCM (5 mL) and water (2 × 1 mL) afforded the title compound **17b** (5.9 mg, 80% yield) as a white solid.

No significant rotamers are observed in NMR spectra. ^{1}H NMR (500 MHz, DMSO-$d6$) δ 3.19 (s, 3H), 1.90 (s, 3H), 1.11 (s, 6H). ^{13}C NMR (125 MHz, DMSO-$d6$) δ 186.3, 184.9, 175.3, 68.7, 40.9, 30.5, 20.8, 20.1. LC-MS: RT 1.53 min, 97% (254 nm), m/z [M + H]$^+$ = 246 (heavy isotope). HRMS calculated for deacetylated $C_7H_{11}BrNO^+$ [M-acetyl + H]$^+$ = 204.0018 (light isotope), found 204.0018.

4. Conclusions

A new electrophilic warhead chemotype, the bromocyclobutenaminone scaffold, was designed as a thiol-labelling agent. It was shown that the incorporation of the bromine atom in the cyclobutenaminone core, sometimes in conjunction with an electron withdrawing group on the nitrogen atom, turns the inactive fragments into novel and useful covalent probes. The investigation of a set of compounds against MurA protein from *E. coli* led to the identification of fragments with moderate inhibitory activity. These compounds represent promising starting points for hit optimization studies and fragment growing might lead to new and potent MurA inhibitors.

Author Contributions: Conceptualization, S.G., I.J.P.d.E. and G.M.K.; methodology, P.Á.-B., M.W.; investigation, D.J.H., A.K., L.P., M.H. and T.I.; writing—original draft preparation, P.Á.-B., D.J.H. and M.W., writing—review and editing, P.Á.-B., D.J.H., M.W., S.G., I.J.P.d.E. and G.M.K. All authors have read and agreed to the published version of the manuscript.

Acknowledgments: We thank Hélène Barreteau for *E. coli* MurA plasmid and Hans Custers for HRMS measurements. The authors are grateful for Krisztina Németh and Pál Szabó for contributing to the analytical experiments.

References

1.	Bugg, T.D.H.; Walsh, C.T. Intracellular steps of bacterial cell wall peptidoglycan biosynthesis: Enzymology, antibiotics, and antibiotic resistance. *Nat. Prod. Rep.* **1992**, *9*, 199–215. [CrossRef] [PubMed]
2.	Blake, K.L.; O'Neill, A.J.; Mengin-Lecreulx, D.; Henderson, P.J.F.; Bostock, J.M.; Dunsmore, C.J.; Simmons, K.J.; Fishwick, C.W.G.; Leeds, J.A.; Chopra, I. The nature of Staphylococcus aureus MurA and MurZ and approaches for detection of peptidoglycan biosynthesis inhibitors. *Mol. Microbiol.* **2009**, *72*, 335–343.

[CrossRef] [PubMed]

3.	Hrast, M.; Sosič, I.; Šink, R.; Gobec, S. Inhibitors of the peptidoglycan biosynthesis enzymes MurA-F. *Bioorg. Chem.* **2014**, *55*, 2–15. [CrossRef] [PubMed]

4.	Chang, C.-M.; Chern, J.; Chen, M.-Y.; Huang, K.-F.; Chen, H.-H.; Yang, Y.-L.; Wu, S.-H. Avenaciolides: Potential MurA-Targeted Inhibitors against Peptidoglycan Biosynthesis in Methicillin-Resistant Staphylococcus aureus (MRSA). *J. Am. Chem. Soc.* **2015**, *137*, 267–275. [CrossRef]

5.	Baum, E.Z.; Montenegro, D.A.; Licata, L.; Turchi, I.; Webb, G.C.; Foleno, B.D.; Bush, K. Identification and Characterization of New Inhibitors of the Escherichia coli MurA Enzyme. *Antimicrob. Agents Chemother.* **2001**, *45*, 3182–3188. [CrossRef] [PubMed]

6.	Keeley, A.; Ábrányi-Balogh, P.; Hrast, M.; Imre, T.; Ilas, J.; Gobec, S.; Keserű, G.M. Heterocyclic electrophiles as new MurA inhibitors. *Arch. Pharm. Chem. Life. Sci.* **2018**, *351*, e1800184. [CrossRef]

7.	Li, X.; Danishefsky, S.J. Cyclobutenone as a Highly Reactive Dienophile: Expanding Upon Diels−Alder Paradigms. *J. Am. Chem. Soc.* **2010**, *132*, 11004–11005. [CrossRef]

8.	Paton, R.S.; Kim, S.; Ross, A.G.; Danishefsky, S.J.; Houk, K.N. Experimental Diels-Alder reactivities of cycloalkenones and cyclic dienes explained through transition-state distortion energies. *Angew. Chem. Int. Ed.* **2011**, *50*, 10366–10368. [CrossRef]

9.	Ammann, A.A.; Rey, M.; Dreiding, A.S. Cyclobut-2-enones from Alkynes via Dichlorocyclobut-2-enones. *Helv. Chim. Acta* **1987**, *70*, 321–328. [CrossRef]

10.	Huisgen, R.; Mayr, H. Reactions of cyclobutenones with nucleophilic reagents via vinylketen intermediates. *J. Chem. Soc. Chem. Commun.* **1976**, 55–56. [CrossRef]

11.	Danheiser, R.L.; Savariar, S. A general method for the reductive dechlorination of 4,4-dichlorocyclobutenones. *Tetrahedron Lett.* **1987**, *28*, 3299–3302. [CrossRef]

12.	Lumbroso, A.; Catak, S.; Sulzer-Mossé, S.; De Mesmaeker, A. Efficient access to functionalized cyclobutanone derivatives using cyclobuteniminium salts as highly reactive Michael acceptors. *Tetrahedron Lett.* **2015**, *56*, 2397–2401. [CrossRef]

13.	Graaf, C.; Vischer, H.F.; de Kloe, G.E.; Kooistra, A.J.; Nijmeijer, S.; Kuijer, M.; Verheij, M.H.P.; England, P.J.; van Muijlwijk-Koezen, J.E.; Leurs, R.; et al. Small and colorful stones make beautiful mosaics: Fragment-based chemogenomics. *Drug Discov. Today* **2013**, *18*, 323–330. [CrossRef]

14.	Khatik, G.L.; Kumar, R.; Chakraborti, A.K. Catalyst-Free Conjugated Addition of Thiols to α,β-Unsaturated Carbonyl Compounds in Water. *Org. Lett.* **2006**, *8*, 2433–2436. [CrossRef]

15.	Ábrányi-Balogh, P.; Petri, L.; Imre, T.; Szijj, P.; Scarpino, A.; Hrast, M.; Mitrović, A.; Fonovič, U.P.; Németh, K.; Barreteau, H.; et al. A road map for prioritizing warheads for cysteine targeting covalent inhibitors. *Eur. J. Med. Chem.* **2018**, *160*, 94–107. [CrossRef]

16.	Mihalovits, L.M.; Ferenczy, G.G.; Keserű, G.M. Catalytic Mechanism and Covalent Inhibition of UDP-N-Acetylglucosamine Enolpyruvyl Transferase (MurA): Implications to the Design of Novel Antibacterials. *J. Chem. Inf. Model.* **2019**, *59*, 5161–5173. [CrossRef]

17.	Wijtmans, M.; Denonne, F.; Célanire, S.; Gillard, M.; Hulscher, S.; Delaunoy, C.; Vanhoutvin, N.; Bakker, R.A.; Defays, S.; Gérard, J.; et al. Histamine H3 receptor ligands with a 3-cyclobutoxy motif: A novel and versatile constraint of the classical 3-propoxy linker. *Med. Chem. Commun.* **2010**, *1*, 39–44. [CrossRef]

18.	Brand, S.; de Candole, B.C.; Brown, J.A. Efficient Synthesis of 3-Aminocyclobut-2-en-1-ones: Squaramide Surrogates as Potent VLA-4 Antagonists. *Org. Lett.* **2003**, *5*, 2343–2346. [CrossRef]

19.	Wasserman, H.H.; Piper, J.U.; Dehmlow, E.V. Cyclobutenone derivatives from ethoxyacetylene. *J. Org. Chem.* **1973**, *38*, 1451–1455. [CrossRef]

20.	Hasek, R.H.; Gott, P.G.; Martin, J.C. Ketenes III. Cycloaddition of ketenes to acetylenic ethers. *J. Org. Chem.* **1964**, *29*, 2510–2513. [CrossRef]

21.	McCarney, C.C.; Ward, R.S.; Roberts, D.W. Reactions of ketenes with ethoxyalkynes: Synthesis of 2,2,4-trialkylcyclobutane-1,3-diones. *Tetrahedron* **1976**, *32*, 1189–1192. [CrossRef]

22.	Philips, D.J.; Davenport, R.J.; Demaude, T.A.; Galleway, F.P.; Jones, M.W.; Knerr, L.; Perry, B.G.; Ratcliffe, A.J. Imidazopyriridines as VLA-4 integrin antagonists. *Bioorg. Med. Chem. Lett.* **2008**, *18*, 4146–4149. [CrossRef]

23.	Ross, A.G.; Townsend, S.D.; Danishefsky, S.J. Halocycloalkenones as Diels−Alder Dienophiles. Applications to Generating Useful Structural Patterns. *J. Org. Chem.* **2013**, *78*, 204–210. [CrossRef] [PubMed]

24.	Placebo Controlled Study in Subjects With Relapsing Forms of MS to Evaluate the Safety, Tolerability and Effects of CDP323. Available online: https://clinicaltrials.gov/ct2/show/NCT00484536 (accessed on 1 October 2020).

25. Chanteux, H.; Rosa, M.; Delatour, C.; Prakash, C.; Smith, S.; Nicolas, J.-M. In Vitro Hydrolysis and Transesterification of CDP323, an α4ß1/α4ß7 Integrin Antagonist Ester Prodrug. *Drug Metab. Dispos.* **2014**, *42*, 153–161. [CrossRef] [PubMed]

26. Schule, A.; Ates, C.; Palacio, M.; Stofferis, J.; Delatinne, J.-P.; Martin, B.; Lloyd, S. Monitoring and Control of Genotoxic Impurity Acetamide in the Synthesis of Zaurategrast Sulfate. *Org. Proc. Res. Dev.* **2010**, *14*, 1008–1014. [CrossRef]

27. Skarzynski, T.; Mistry, A.; Wonacott, A.; Hutchinson, S.E.; Kelly, V.A.; Duncan, K. Structure of UDP-N-acetylglucosamine enolpyruvyl transferase, an enzyme essential for the synthesis of bacterial peptidoglycan, complexed with substrate UDP-N-acetylglucosamine and the drug fosfomycin. *Structure* **1996**, *4*, 1465–1474. [CrossRef]

28. Rožman, K.; Lešnik, S.; Brus, B.; Hrast, M.; Sova, M.; Patin, D.; Barreteau, H.; Konc, J.; Janežič, D.; Gobec, S. Discovery of new MurA inhibitors using induced-fit simulation and docking. *Bioorg. Med. Chem. Lett.* **2017**, *27*, 944–949. [CrossRef] [PubMed]

11

Bactericidal and In Vitro Cytotoxicity of *Moringa oleifera* Seed Extract and Its Elemental Analysis Using Laser-Induced Breakdown Spectroscopy

Reem K. Aldakheel [1,2], Suriya Rehman [3,*] , Munirah A. Almessiere [1] , Firdos A. Khan [4] ,
Mohammed A. Gondal [5,*] , Ahmed Mostafa [6] and Abdulhadi Baykal [7]

[1] Department of Biophysics, Institute for Research & Medical Consultations (IRMC), Imam Abdulrahman Bin Faisal University, Dammam 31441, Saudi Arabia; reem.k.dakheel@gmail.com (R.K.A.); malmessiere@iau.edu.sa (M.A.A.)

[2] Department of Physics, College of Science, Imam Abdulrahman Bin Faisal University, Dammam 31441, Saudi Arabia

[3] Department of Epidemic Diseases Research, Institute for Research & Medical Consultations (IRMC), Imam Abdulrahman Bin Faisal University, Dammam 31441, Saudi Arabia

[4] Department of Stem Cell Research, Institute for Research & Medical Consultations (IRMC), Imam Abdulrahman Bin Faisal University, Dammam 31441, Saudi Arabia; fakhan@iau.edu.sa

[5] Department of Physics, Laser Research Group, King Fahd University of Petroleum & Minerals, Box 372, Dhahran 31261, Saudi Arabia

[6] Department of Pharmaceutical Chemistry, College of Clinical Pharmacy, Imam Abdulrahman Bin Faisal University, Dammam 31441, Saudi Arabia; ammostafa@iau.edu.sa

[7] Department of Nanomedicine Research, Institute for Research & Medical Consultations (IRMC), Imam Abdulrahman Bin Faisal University, Dammam 31441, Saudi Arabia; abaykal@iau.edu.sa

[*] Correspondence: surrehman@iau.edu.sa or suriyamir@gmail.com (S.R.); magondal@kfupm.edu.sa (M.A.G.)

Abstract: In the current study, we present the correlation between the capability of laser-induced breakdown spectroscopy (LIBS) to monitor the elemental compositions of plants and their biological effects. The selected plant, *Moringa oleifera*, is known to harbor various minerals and vitamins useful for human health and is a potential source for pharmaceutical interventions. From this standpoint, we assessed the antibacterial and in vitro cytotoxicity of the bioactive components present in *Moringa oleifera* seed (MOS) extract. Detailed elemental analyses of pellets of MOSs were performed via LIBS. Furthermore, the LIBS outcome was validated using gas chromatography–mass spectrometry (GC-MS). The LIBS signal was recorded, and the presence of the essential elements (Na, Ca, Se, K, Mg, Zn, P, S, Fe and Mn) in the MOSs were examined. The bactericidal efficacy of the alcoholic MOS extract was examined against *Escherichia coli (E. coli)* and *Staphylococcus aureus (S. aureus)* by agar well diffusion (AWD) assays and scanning electron microscopy (SEM), which depicted greater inhibition against Gram-positive bacteria. The validity and DNA nuclear morphology of human colorectal carcinoma cells (HCT-116) cells were evaluated via an MTT assay and DAPI staining. The MTT assay results manifested a profoundly inhibitory action of MOS extract on HCT116 cell growth. Additionally, MOS extracts produced inhibitory action in colon cancer cells (HCT-116), whereas no inhibitory action was seen using the same concentrations of MOS extract on HEK-293 cells (non-cancerous cells), suggesting that MOS extracts could be non-cytotoxic to normal cells. The antibacterial and anticancer potency of these MOS extracts could be due to the presence of various bioactive chemical complexes, such as ethyl ester and D-allose and hexadecenoic, oleic and palmitic acids, making them an ideal candidate for pharmaceutical research and applications.

Keywords: antibacterial; anticancer; GC-MS; LIBS; *Moringa oleifera*; seed extract

1. Introduction

Traditional herbalists throughout the globe have emphasized the role of plants used as remedies to treat different diseases, like inflammation and bacterial infections [1]. Enormous research is being carried out, where plants are being tested for active compounds that have antibacterial, antifungal and anticancer activities [2,3]. One such plant is *Moringa oleifera* Lam. (MOL), which originates mainly from Africa, Asia and South America [4,5]. The moringa leaves and fruits are considered as vegetables in the Philippines, Thailand, India and Pakistan [6]. Recently, sundry countries (Mexico, Caribbean islands, Hawaii and Cambodia) have begun planting it for its plentiful health benefits and nutritional value in addition to its medicinal importance [7,8]. *Moringa* fruits and leaves have various biological applications in addition to being enriched with vitamins, minerals, and proteins. The WHO recommends using MOL as a food because of its superior nutritional values for human health [6]. It is a well-known fact that *Moringa* plants (leaves and fruits) were grown as for skin sanitation, an energy source and also to relieve tension [8,9]. Innumerable reports have discovered that MOL has numerous significant merits, such as antioxidant, antimicrobial, anticancer, anti-inflammatory, antiulcer, antihypertensive, anti-urolithic, anti-asthmatic, antidiabetic, analgesic, anti-aging, diuretic, cardiovascular, hepatoprotective, hypoglycemic and immunomodulatory characteristics [10–13]. The hypotensive, antibacterial and anticancer efficacies of the MOL leaves and fruits are due to the presence of sundry distinctive chemical compounds (benzyl glucosinolate, niazimicin, benzyl iso-thiocyanate complexes and pterygospermin) in their structure [11]. Several methods have been improved to extract the initial contents from MOL plants for the production of food supplements and medicines (with natural organic components) and the determination of their other health benefits. Extraction procedures based on pressurized liquid, ultrasound, microwaves and supercritical fluid have been introduced [14–17].

Nevertheless, all extraction mechanisms experience several restrictions in terms of using a large amount of harmful organic solvents, sample production proceedings and cost [13]. To get better results, LIBS has emerged as an efficient approach for the identification and quantification of elemental compositions from different medicinal plant extractions. Over the past decade, the LIBS method has broadly been exploited for analyzing chemical elements existing in diverse kinds of specimens. This analytical method has distinguishing properties, like cost effectiveness, real-time measurement, sensitivity, rapidity and in situ elemental analysis [18–20]. Additionally, this type of analysis is easy, eco-friendly and is less complicated when preparing the sample. It is known that intensive sample treatments frequently produce erroneous results due to the presence of contaminants and loss-related effects. Thus, the LIBS technique can accurately disclose the identity of various medicinal plants in a scientific manner. In addition, most edible plants consist of proteins, vitamins and minerals, which possess immense benefits to health [21,22].

The purpose of the study is to analyze the presence of different elements in *Moringa oleifera* seed (MOS) extracts by using the LIBS approach and to examine the biological activities of MOS extracts by evaluating the antibacterial and anticancer potencies.

2. Results

2.1. Qualitative Analysis of MOS Using LIBS

The laser-induced breakdown spectroscopy (LIBS) spectra (Figure 1) of the MOS extract were recorded in the range of 200 to 800 nm. For the detection of the major elements, the spectra were recorded from different spots of the pellets and by scanning at a 50 nm wavelength range each time. In order to reduce the background noise and to enhance the LIBS signal intensity, LIBS parameters, including the delay times (delay between the incident laser pulse and the recording of spectra), the number of accumulations and laser energies, were optimized prior to the application of the LIBS setup for MOS sample analysis. The recorded LIBS spectra of the MOSs comprised various significant spectral peaks of the atomic and ionic lines (with varying intensities) related to the abundance of elements present in the tested MOS samples. Based on the NIST database, the recorded spectral lines were identified and classified in terms of the characteristic elements present in the MOSs, suggesting their significant role towards antibacterial and anticancer activities. Clearly, the measured LIBS spectra (Figure 1) exhibited the presence of vital elements such as Ca, K, Mg, P, S, Fe, Mn, Zn, Na and Se in MOS samples.

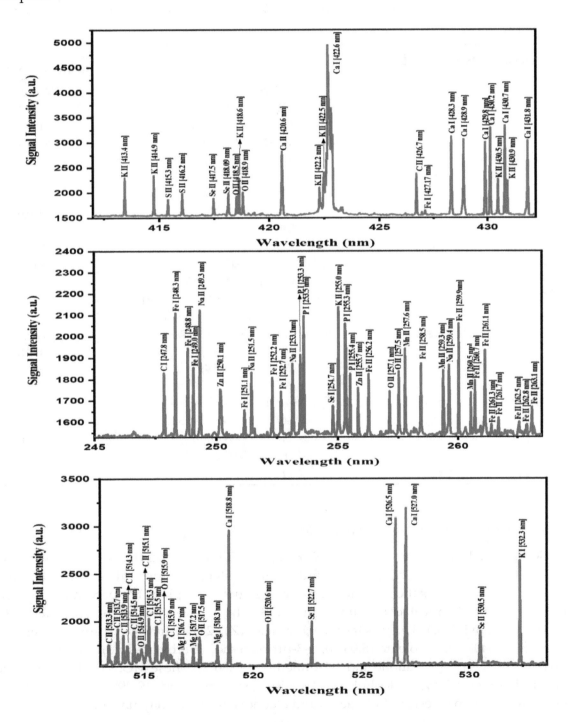

Figure 1. LIBS emission line spectra of various elements recorded in the wavelength range of 245–537 nm of MOS. The signature lines for different vital minerals present in MOSs are indicated in the figure.

Table 1 presents the LIBS signal intensities of the spectral transition lines corresponding to various detected elements in MOSs. In accordance with the Boltzmann distribution, the intensities of the LIBS spectral lines have a direct relationship with the elemental contents (concentration) present in MOSs [23,24]. This correlation was attained by considering the intensity ratio of the detected elemental lines with that of the C line taken as the reference (247.8 nm). The achieved intensity ratios of the elements Ca, K, Mg, P, S, Fe, Mn, Zn, Na and Se were in the ranges of 2.7–1.7, 1.2–1.4, 0.9, 1.1, 1.1, 1.1–0.9, 1.0, 0.9, 1.2 and 1.1, respectively, which were consistent with those reported in the literature [16].

Table 1. The detection of spectral lines of the different elements present in *MOS* by using our LIBS system.

Name of Element	Wavelength (nm)	Transition Configuration	LIBS Signal Intensity (arbitrary unit(a.u.))
Ca	422.6	$3p^6\,4s^2\,^1S_0 \rightarrow 3p^6\,4s\,4p\,^1P^\circ_1$	4960.9
	518.8	$3p^6\,4s\,4p\,^1P^\circ_1 \rightarrow 3p^6\,4s\,5d\,^1D_2$	2967.1
	527.0	$3p^6\,3d\,4s\,^3D_3 \rightarrow > 3p^6\,3d\,4p\,^3P^\circ_2$	3196.3
Fe	248.3	$3d^6\,4s^2\,^5D_4 \rightarrow 3d^6\,(^5D)\,4s\,4p\,(^1P^\circ)\,^5F^\circ_5$	2114.1
	252.2	$3d^6\,4s^2\,^5D_4 \rightarrow 3d^6\,(^5D)\,4s\,4p\,(^1P^\circ)\,^5D^\circ_4$	1810.1
	259.9	$3d^6\,(^5D)\,4s\,^6D_{9/2} \rightarrow 3d^6\,(^5D)\,4p\,^6D^\circ_{9/2}$	2061.9
K	414.9	$3p^5\,3d^3P^\circ_0 \rightarrow 3p^5\,4p\,^3D_1$	2347.6
	430.5	$3p^5\,3d^3P^\circ_2 \rightarrow 3p^5\,4p\,^1D_2$	2270.9
	532.3	$3p^6\,4p^2P^\circ_{1/2} \rightarrow 3p^6\,8s\,^2S_{1/2}$	2639.7
Mg	518.3	$3s\,3p\,^3P^\circ_2 \rightarrow 3s\,4s\,^3S_1$	1753.5
Mn	259.3	$3d^5\,(^6S)\,4s\,^7S_3 \rightarrow 3d^5\,(^6S)\,4p\,(^7P^\circ_3)$	1843.9
Na	249.3	$2s^2\,2p^5\,3s\,^1P^\circ_1 \rightarrow 2s^2\,2p^5\,3p\,^1S_0$	2128.4
	251.5	$2s^2\,2p^5\,3p\,^3S_1 \rightarrow 2s^2\,2p^5\,(^2P^\circ_{1/2})\,3d\,^2[\rightarrow]^\circ_2$	1834.7
P	253.5	$3s^2\,3p^3\,^2P^\circ_{3/2} \rightarrow 3s^2\,3p^2\,(^3P)\,4s\,^2P_{3/2}$	2100.0
	255.3	$3s^2\,3p^3\,^2P^\circ_{1/2} \rightarrow 3s^2\,3p^2\,(^3P)\,4s\,^2P_{1/2}$	2032.1
S	416.2	$3s^2\,3p^2\,(^3P)\,4p\,^4D^\circ_{7/2} \rightarrow 3s^2\,3p^2\,(^3P)\,4d\,^4F_{9/2}$	1987.8
Se	418.09	$4s^2\,4p^2\,(^3P)\,5p\,^4D^\circ_{7/2} \rightarrow 4s^2\,4p^2\,(^3P)\,5d\,^4F_{9/2}$	1969.7
	522.7	$4s^2\,4p^2\,(^3P)\,5s\,^4P_{5/2} \rightarrow 4s^2\,4p^2\,(^3P)\,5p\,^4D^\circ_{7/2}$	2002.0
Zn	250.1	$3d^{10}\,4p\,^2P^\circ_{1/2} \rightarrow 3d^{10}\,5s\,^2S_{1/2}$	1751.4
	255.7	$3d^{10}\,4p\,^2P^\circ_{3/2} \rightarrow 3d^{10}\,5s\,^2S_{1/2}$	1762.3
C	426.7	$2s^2\,3d\,^2D_{5/2} \rightarrow 2s^2\,4f\,^2F^\circ_{7/2}$	2379.0
	247.8	$2s^2\,2p^2\,^1S_0 \rightarrow 2s^2\,2p\,3s\,^1P^\circ_1$	1831.6
O	418.9	$2s^2\,2p^2\,(^1D)\,3p\,^2F^\circ_{7/2} \rightarrow 2s^2\,2p^2\,(^1D)\,3d\,^2G_{9/2}$	2003.4

2.2. Volatile Content Analyses of MOS using GC-MS

The GC-MS analyses of the *Moringa oleifera* seed (MOS) showed the presence of 114 volatile complexes with diverse chemical groups: fatty acids, esters, ketones, alcohols, aldehydes, and hydrocarbons. Table 2 shows the retention times and Figure 2 displays the percentage composition of all the identified chemical compounds in MOS. The main types were oleic acid (22.53%), 2-3-di-hydroxy-propyl (13.48%), 9-octa-decenoic acid (Z), 2-3-di-hydroxy-propyl ester (11.35%), docosenamide (6.04%), ethyl oleate (6.03%), 1-3-propanediol, 2-ethyl-2-(hydroxyl-methyl) (5.52%), oleic anhydride (3.96%), 2-propanone and 1-1-dimethoxy (3.86%). These MOSs contain fatty acids and their ester derivatives (65.45%), alcohols (9.4%), nitrogen compounds (9.09%), ketones (5.34%) and aldehydes (2.88%). To form esters, fatty acids and alcohols in plants may undergo esterification.

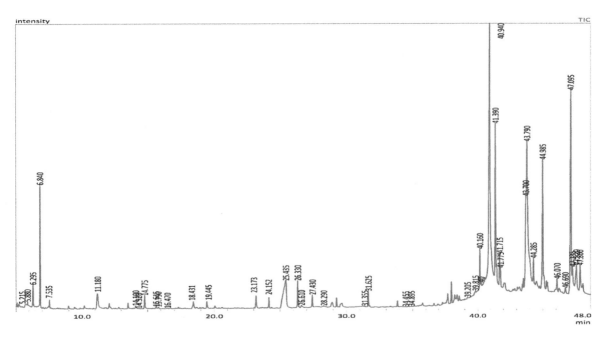

Figure 2. GC-MS chromatograph of MOS.

Table 2. Volatile compounds identified in MOS using GC-MS analysis.

No.	Compounds	RT	Peak area (%)
	Esters		
1	Propanoic acid, 2-oxo-, methyl ester	6.293	0.76
2	Acetic acid, ethoxyhydroxy-, ethyl ester	7.043	0.04
3	Diethoxymethyl acetate	12.827	0.09
4	2-Propenoic acid, 2-methyl-, 2-hydroxypropyl ester	13.134	0.02
5	6,9,12-Octadecatrienoic acid, phenylmethyl ester, (Z,Z,Z)-	17.797	0.01
6	Cyclopentanecarboxylic acid, 4-tridecyl ester	19.179	0.03
7	1-Cyclohexene-1-carboxylic acid, 2,6,6-trimethyl-, methyl ester	20.058	0.13
8	Hexanoic acid, 4-hexadecyl ester	28.291	0.07
9	Phthalic acid, diethyl ester	29.568	0.14
10	2-Propenoic acid, pentadecyl ester	31.625	0.59
11	Acetic acid, 3,7,11,15-tetramethyl-hexadecyl ester	33.627	0.02
12	Phthalic acid, dibutyl ester	35.692	0.07
13	Phthalic acid, diisobutyl ester	35.760	0.15
14	Palmitoleic acid, methyl ester	36.285	0.03
15	Pentadecanoic acid, 13-methyl-, methyl ester	36.642	0.09
16	9-Hexadecenoic acid, ethyl ester	37.652	0.15
17	Hexadecanoic acid, ethyl ester (Ethyl palmitate)	37.993	0.78
18	Heptadecanoic acid, ethyl ester	38.416	0.46
19	Propanoic acid, 3-mercapto-, dodecyl ester	38.588	0.25
20	9-Octadecenoic acid, methyl ester, (E)- (Methyl elaidate)	40.159	1.52
21	Oleic acid, methyl ester (Methyl oleate)	40.255	0.15
22	l-(+)-Ascorbic acid 2,6-dihexadecanoate	40.561	0.10
23	Ethyl oleate	41.389	6.03
24	Octadecanoic acid, ethyl ester (Ethyl stearate)	41.774	0.53
25	9-octadecenyl ester (Oleyl oleate)	43.516	0.34
26	2,3-dihydroxypropyl elaidate	43.794	13.48
27	9-Octadecenoic acid, 1,2,3-propanetriyl ester	44.287	0.90
28	Docosanoic acid, ethyl ester	45.273	0.37
29	Oleoyl chloride	46.066	0.65
30	9-Octadecenoic acid (Z)-, 2,3-dihydroxypropyl ester	47.099	11.35
31	Glycidol stearate	47.522	1.76
32	Hexadecanoic acid, 2-hydroxy-1-(hydroxymethyl)ethyl ester	47.803	1.57

Table 2. *Cont.*

No.	Compounds	RT	Peak area (%)
	Alcohols		
33	1,4-Cyclohexanediol, trans-	7.224	0.02
34	1,2-Propanediol, 3-methoxy-	7.430	0.05
35	Ethanol, 2,2-diethoxy-	7.535	0.31
36	1,2,4-Butanetriol	9.496	0.04
37	Glycerin	11.180	1.35
38	1-Butanol, 4-(ethylthio)-	11.742	0.02
39	Methoxyacetaldehyde diethyl acetal	11.883	0.02
40	1-Dodecanol	18.431	0.48
41	1-Tetradecanol	24.152	0.42
42	1,3-Propanediol, 2-ethyl-2-(hydroxymethyl)-	25.444	5.52
43	1-Tridecanol	26.331	1.06
44	3-Hexadecanol	31.348	0.05
45	3-Heptadecanol	35.561	0.06
	Aldehydes		
46	Butanal, 3-hydroxy-	8.375	0.00
47	Heptanal	10.006	0.02
48	Octanal	12.567	0.04
49	Nonanal	15.790	0.09
50	2-Methyl-oct-2-enedial	20.611	0.04
51	Undecanal	23.521	0.02
52	Tridecanal	34.455	0.01
53	10-Octadecenal	37.418	0.09
54	9-Octadecenamide	37.551	0.09
55	cis-9-Hexadecenal	38.241	0.55
56	cis-13-Octadecenal	47.228	1.92
	Ketones		
57	2-Propanone, 1,1-dimethoxy-	6.841	3.86
58	2-Butanone	8.151	0.03
59	Dihydroxyacetone	8.969	0.14
60	1,2-Cyclopentanedione	10.172	0.14
61	2-Propanone, 1-(1,3-dioxolan-2-yl)-	10.867	0.04
62	1,3-Dioxol-2-one,4,5-dimethyl-	13.528	0.28
63	2-Heptanol, 5-ethyl-	14.306	0.01
64	2-Methyl-4-octanone	16.466	0.03
65	2-Pentanone, 3,4-epoxy-	18.925	0.03
66	1-Oxa-spiro[4.5]deca-6,9-diene-2,8-dione	37.006	0.05
67	Z-11-Pentadecenol	39.209	0.05
68	Cyclopentadecanone, 2-hydroxy-	39.822	0.13
69	Cyclopentadecanone	43.430	0.21
70	2-Tetradecanone	46.691	0.34
	Acids		
71	Acetic acid, (acetyloxy)-	5.884	0.18
72	Butanoic acid, 3-hydroxy-	10.594	0.03
73	Octanoic acid	17.421	0.03
74	Nonanoic acid	20.363	0.02
75	n-Hexadecanoic acid (Palmitic acid)	37.305	0.05
76	Oleic acid	40.943	22.53
	Furans and lactones		
77	Furfural	7.624	0.02
78	2(5H)-Furanone	9.840	0.04
79	2-Hydroxy-gamma-butyrolactone	12.081	0.23

Table 2. *Cont.*

No.	Compounds	RT	Peak area (%)
80	2,5-Dimethyl-4-hydroxy-3(2H)-furanone	14.099	0.19
81	1,2-Ethanediol, 1-(2-furanyl)	19.096	0.03
82	5-Hydroxymethylfurfural	19.445	0.36
83	3-Deoxy-d-mannoic lactone	28.924	0.52
Nitrogen-containing compounds			
84	*N*,*N*-Dimethylaminoethanol	5.216	0.12
85	1,3,5-Triazine-2,4,6-triamine	14.778	0.68
86	Acetic acid, 2-(*N*-methyl-*N*-phosphonatomethyl)amino-	15.617	0.11
87	1-Heptadecanamine	18.667	0.07
88	Nonanamide	23.034	0.02
89	Dodecanamide (Lauryl amide)	33.331	0.04
90	Tetradecanamide (Myristic amide)	37.717	0.44
91	Hexadecanamide (Palmitic amide)	41.718	1.26
92	Docosenamide	44.987	6.04
93	Nonadecanamide	45.352	0.32
Sulfur-containing compounds			
94	Sulfurous acid, cyclohexylmethyl hexadecyl ester	23.173	0.67
Hydrocarbons			
95	1-Butene, 4,4-diethoxy-2-methyl-	9.425	0.07
96	1-Methyl-2-octylcyclopropane	12.171	0.07
97	2-Trifluoroacetoxytridecane	13.923	0.03
98	trans-2,3-Epoxynonane	23.642	0.03
99	2-Heptafluorobutyroxypentadecane	23.887	0.04
100	1,2-Epoxyundecane	24.016	0.02
101	Heptacosane	24.357	0.03
102	1-Heptadecene	29.262	0.33
103	Octadecane, 1,1′-[(1-methyl-1,2-ethanediyl)bis(oxy)]bis-	29.426	0.01
104	1-Nonadecene	33.847	0.22
Pyrans			
105	Tetrahydro-4H-pyran-4-ol	17.074	0.03
106	4H-Pyran-4-one, 2,3-dihydro-3,5-dihydroxy-6-methyl-	17.198	0.02
Others			
107	5,6-Dihydroxypiperazine-2,3-dione dioxime	8.320	0.02
108	Tetraethyl silicate	11.807	0.04
109	Silanediol, dimethyl-, diacetate	17.300	0.07
110	D-Allose	26.609	0.19
111	Phenol, 2,4-bis(1,1-dimethylethyl)-	27.430	0.51
112	Oxirane, hexadecyl-	34.898	0.02
113	Ethyl iso-allocholate	36.936	0.06
114	Oleic anhydride	43.700	3.96

RT: Retention time in minutes.

2.3. In vitro *Cytotoxic Activity of MOS*

The cell viability of the MOS extract-treated HCT-116 cells was evaluated using an MTT assay after 48 h. The percentage of cell viability of the MOS extract-treated HEK-293 and HCT-116 cells was determined. The MTT assay examined the percentage of cell viability. The number of viable cells present in the control group was compared with the MOS-treated cells. In Figure 3, we show that cancer cells (control group, without MOS treatment) showed 100% cell viability, whereas cancer cells treated with MOS extract showed a significant decrease, which suggests that MOS extract could induce a significant drop in the viability of cancerous cells compared to control ones (without treatment using the MOS extract).

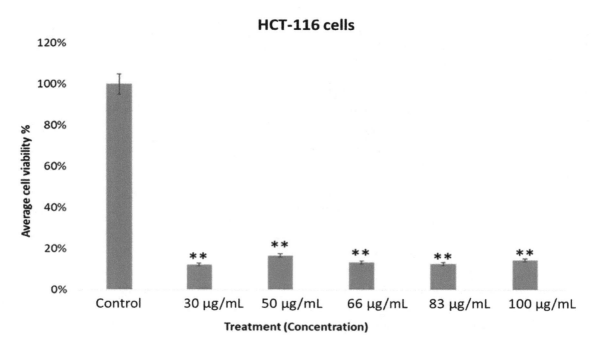

Figure 3. Effect of MOS extract on colon cancer cells (HCT-116) after treatment for 48 h with different concentrations. The average cell viability was calculated by MTT assay (** $p < 0.01$).

The average viability of the MOS extract-treated cancer cells at various concentrations showed quite encouraging outcomes, with $p < 0.01$. The specificity of the MOS extract in the concentration range of 30 to 100 µg/mL on normal cells was inspected using MTT assays after treatment for 48 h (Figure 4). When MOS extract was tested on normal cells (HEK-293), we found no inhibitory action.

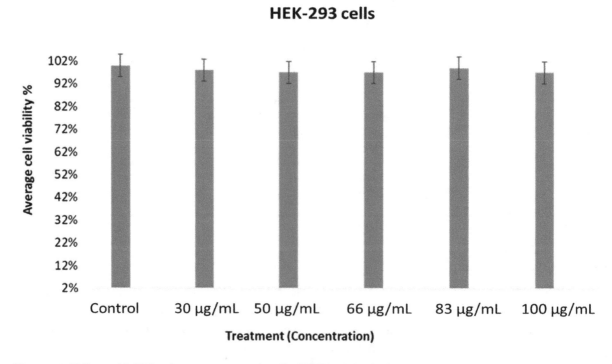

Figure 4. Effect of MOS extract on normal cells (HEK-293) after treatment for 48 h treated different concentrations. The average cell viability was calculated by MTT assay.

The MOS extract showed content-dependent specificity when the data were taken from three replications. A Student's *t*-test was used to understand the difference between the two treated groups and the results are presented as the mean ± standard deviation (SD).

2.4. Nuclear Breakdown of MOS Extract-Treated Cancerous Cells

Figure 5 illustrates the MOS extract-treated and untreated cell morphology that was imaged using confocal scanning microscopy (CSM). The MOS extract-treated cancer cells exhibited stronger inhibitory action (Figure 5A) than the control sample (Figure 5B). The CMS images of the nuclear cell morphology of both control (untreated) and MOS extract-treated (66 µg/mL) samples after stained by DAPI showed a substantial loss (nuclear disintegration) because of the treatments.

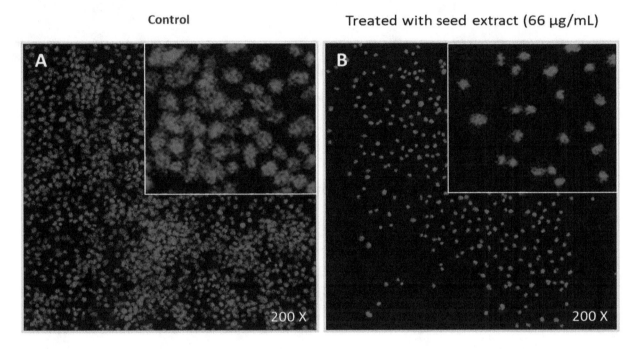

Figure 5. Confocal staining by DAPI. (**A**) The HCT-116 cells (non-treated) and (**B**) HCT-116 cells treated with MOS (66 µg/mL), 200× magnifications.

It was deduced that the MOS extract has strong anti-cancerous activities in colon cancer cells (as supported by the GC-MS analysis).

2.5. Antibacterial Efficacy of MOS Extract

The antibacterial potency of the MOS extract was assessed on Gram-negative and Gram-positive bacteria using the AWD method, wherein the inhibited areas due to antibacterial action around the inoculated wells were measured. This zone of inhibition was produced by the diffusion of the active chemical constituents present in the MOS extract. These results confirm the impact of the MOS extract on *S. aureus* and *E. coli*. Interestingly, the MOS extract was found to produce better antibacterial action in *S. aureus* bacteria than *E. coli*.

In Figure 6, the MOS extract shows concentration-dependent inhibition of *S. aureus* bacteria, with inhibition zones ranging from 18 to 24 mm. On the other hand, the inhibition zones of *E. coli* were found to range from 6 to 20 mm. The maximum and minimum inhibition zone diameters were acquired with the corresponding extract contents of 250 and 50 µg/mL (Figures 6 and 7). No inhibition was observed in *E.coli* with 50 µg/mL, whereas a higher concentration showed inhibition of the bacteria.

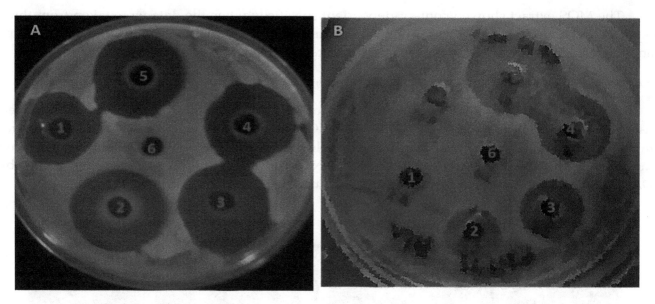

Figure 6. Agar well diffusion (AWD) plates showing the inhibition zones. (**A**) *S. aureus* and (**B**) *E. coli*.
1: 50 μg/mL, **2**: 100 μg/mL, **3**: 150 μg/mL, **4**: 200 μg/mL, **5**: 250 μg/mL of MOS, **6**: Control (DH$_2$O).

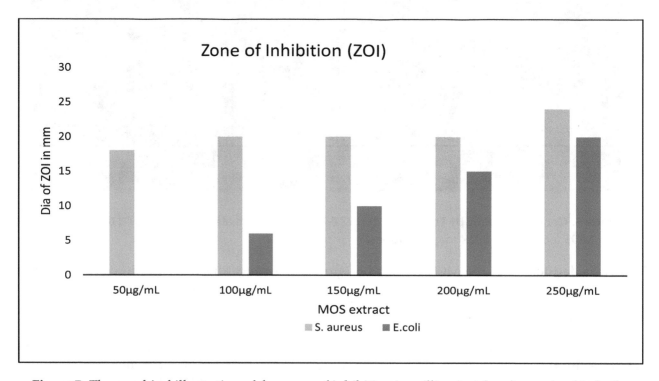

Figure 7. The graphical illustration of the zones of inhibition in millimeters (mm) examined in both *S. aureus* and *E. coli* after treatment using different concentrations of MOS extract. Data are the means ± SD of three different experiments.

The morphological changes in bacteria treated with MOS were studied using SEM. The untreated cells of *E. coli* were seen as regular rod-shaped cells with smooth cell surfaces (Figure 8a). The *E. coli* subjected to treatment with MOS appeared as damaged cells (Figure 8b) and the cell number also showed a reduction with a significant alteration of the cell wall and membrane. Similarly, the treatment of *S. aureus* with MOS extract also showed significant morphological changes in the structure and number of cells (Figure 8d), whereas the control *S. aureus* cells appeared as regular cocci with intact cell surfaces (Figure 8c). The damaged cells lost their cellular integrity, which led to the death of bacterial cells.

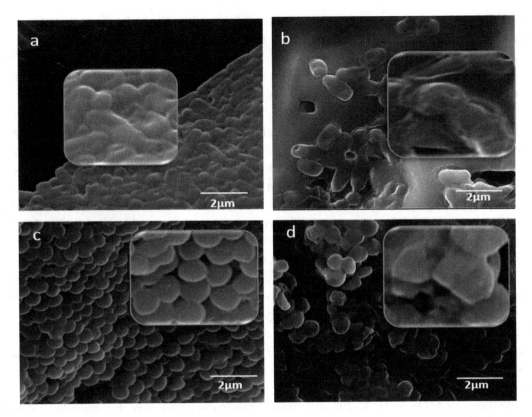

Figure 8. SEM micrographs for the study of morphogenesis by MOS extract. (**a**) *E. coli* cells (non-treated) and (**b**) treated *E. coli* cells, (**c**) *S. aureus* cells (non-treated) and (**d**) treated *S. aureus* cells.

3. Discussion

The LIBS and GC-MS techniques were utilized for the identification and quantitation of the elements existing in the MOS extract. For the first time, the anticancer and antibacterial activities of the MOS extract were assessed. Our results show the presence of diverse elements in MOSs, as confirmed by different methods. The GC-MS results of the MOS extract verified the existence of diverse anticancer and antimicrobial compounds. The spectra from different points on the surface of MOS pellets were examined by the LIBS method. The outcomes proved that MOSs are rich in different minerals that are useful to humans as food and medicine. Besides, the seeds have an influential role in antibacterial activity because of the availability of the following elements: K, Fe, P, Ca, Mg, S, Mn, Na, Se and Zn. It is clear that the amounts of Ca, K and Mg present in the MOSs were greater than the other elements. These results give evidence that MOSs are rich in different minerals, which are highly useful to humans as food supplements and medicine, indicating their remarkable impact in regulating the level of blood pressure, blood lipids, regulating the stomach function, protecting the liver, strengthening the bones, generating protein and enhancing the immunity of the human body [23–25]. Furthermore, the existence of Se in MOSs plays a vital role by protecting from fatal diseases like cancer, cardiovascular disease, cognitive decline, and thyroid disease. Moreover, these seeds exhibit a powerful antibacterial activity due to the presence of the detected elements, which is evidenced clearly by the antimicrobial studies conducted in this work.

The analysis of GC-MS of the MOSs showed the presence of 114 volatile complexes with diverse chemical groups: fatty acids, esters, ketones, alcohols, aldehydes, and hydrocarbons. To form esters, fatty acids and alcohols in plants may undergo esterification [19]. It has been reported that most of these compounds possess anticancer activities. In addition, palmitic acid shows selective cytotoxicity against human leukemic cells. The fatty acids also possess both antifungal and antibacterial activities. The omega-9 fatty acid was a detected primary complex (oleic acid) in the MOSs, which has numerous human health benefits (preventing ulcerative colitis and reducing blood pressure with remarkable antioxidant efficiency [26,27]). Therefore, GC-MS measurement proved the presence of numerous fatty acids and their related esters (cis-9-hexadecenoic acid (palmitoleic), oleic acid, octadecanoic (stearic) acids, n-hexadecenoic acid) and alcohols. It was reported that most of these compounds have anticancer activity. For example, D-allose inhibits cancer cell growth at G1 phase [17]. Palmitic acid has selective cytotoxicity against leukemic cells in humans. Fatty acids also have antifungal and antibacterial effects [28].

In the present study, the biological activities of MOS were evaluated. The cell viability of the MOS extract-treated (for 48 h) HCT-116 (cancer) cells was assessed via MTT assay. The viability status of the extract-treated HEK-293 (normal) and HCT-116 cells was determined. It was inferred that the MOS extract has strong anticancer activity in colon cancer cells. However, few reports done on MOS extract have shown that the enhanced anticancer activity of the extract correlated with the occurrence of high oleic acid and fatty acid contents [21]. Previously, it has been shown that *Moringa* plants (leaves and fruits) have been used for various applications, such as antioxidant, antimicrobial, anticancer, anti-inflammatory, antiulcer, antihypertensive, anti-urolithic, antidiabetic, anti-asthmatic, anti-aging, analgesic, diuretic, cardiovascular, hepatoprotective, hypoglycemic and immunomodulatory uses [22]. As per our knowledge, there is no information on whether *Moringa* leaf extract or seed extract cause any differential response in cancer cells. Nevertheless, it would be interesting to do a comparative study where the effects of *Moringa* seed and *Moringa* leaf extracts are examined in cancer cells. We have used HEK-293 (human embryonic kidney) cells as normal cells to compare the MOS anticancer activity to human colon cancer cell line HCT-116. The purpose was to check whether MOS extracts produce any cytotoxic effects in normal cells or not. In our studies, we have found that MOS extracts produce inhibitory action in colon cancer cells (HCT-116), whereas no inhibitory action was found using the same concentrations of MOS in HEK-293 cells (non-cancerous cells), which suggests that MOS extracts could be non-cytotoxic to normal cells.

MOS has 114 volatile complexes with diverse chemical groups: fatty acids, esters, ketones, alcohols, aldehydes and hydrocarbons. The hypotensive, antibacterial and anticancer efficacies of the MO leaves and fruits are due to presence of sundry distinctive chemical compounds (benzyl glucosinolate, niazimicin, benzyl iso-thiocyanate complexes and pterygospermin) in their structure [6]. Several methods have been improved to extract the initial contents from MOL plants for the production of food supplements medicines (with natural organic components) and the determination of their other health benefits. While we do not know the molecular mechanism of the anticancer activities of MOS extract in cancer cells, the role of the caspase signaling pathway cannot be ruled out in the process of programmed cell death. It would be interesting to study the different caspases, such as caspase-3 and caspase-9 in MOS extract-induced cell death.

The antimicrobial potency of the MOS extract was assessed in the Gram-negative and Gram-positive bacteria via AWD, wherein the inhibited areas around the inoculated wells were measured. Due to the occurrence of varying cell components, there is a discrepancy in the bactericidal action of the MOS extract for the two different types of test bacteria [29].

The study of morphogenesis using SEM showed that MOS extract affects the cell wall at the initial stage, and later penetrates and accumulates at the surface membrane. This leads to an interruption in the metabolic activities of bacterial cells and initiates cell death [30]. The present study illustrates that the MOS extract causes damage to the microbial cell surface, thereby causing significant antibacterial activity. The penetration of the extract into the bacterial cell alters the membrane integrity by structural alterations, the loss of membrane proteins, etc.

Natural compounds like fatty acids, esters, ketones, alcohols, aldehydes and hydrocarbons have been reported in a variety of plants [31]. The mechanisms of the antibacterial activities of such compounds is linked to their high affinity towards lipids due to their hydrophobic characteristics. Their antibacterial actions are evidently related to this lipophilic nature and to the bacterial membrane structure [32]. This leads the compounds to penetrate the cellular membrane of the microbial cell, which enhances the fluidity and permeability of membrane, alters the topology of membrane proteins and inflicts disruption in the respiration chain [33,34].

The present study indicated the presence of phenolic compounds and these are reported to disrupt the cell membrane, leading to the inhibition of cell metabolism causing the leakage of cellular content [35]. It has been found that phenolics inhibit processes associated with the cell membrane, for example, electron transport, ions, protein translocation, phosphorylation and other enzyme-dependent reactions. Therefore, the disturbed permeability of the cytoplasmic membrane may lead to cell death [36]. The interaction of plant bioactive compounds with bacterial cell membranes results in the inhibition of several Gram-positive and Gram-negative bacteria [37]. It has also been indicated that Gram-positive bacteria are more susceptible to the antibacterial action of natural compounds like fatty acids, esters, ketones, alcohols, aldehydes and hydrocarbons, compared to Gram-negative bacteria [38]. This is also concordant with the current study, owing to the fact that Gram-negative bacteria have an outer layer surrounding their cell wall, limiting the access of hydrophobic compounds.

Therefore, MOSs can serve as an antibacterial component that can be further studied and recommended as a potential antimicrobial and anticancer therapy. This natural source can be further evaluated and upgraded for pharmaceutical application.

4. Materials and Procedures

4.1. Seed Assembly and Extract Preparation

All the extracts used in this study were prepared from good quality MOSs procured from a place where they are naturalized, Dammam in Saudi Arabia (originally imported from India). The seeds, without a shell, were crushed to obtain fine powder, followed by compression to get pellets. Figure 9a–c shows different steps of sample production for detailed analysis with the LIBS technique. Diversified ratios of the MOS powder between 5–25 g was mingled with 220 mL of ethanol and were stirred for 5 h, then the MOS solutions were filtered and put into a rotary evaporator to get a dry powder. The samples (MOSs) were subjected to GC-MS and anticancer activity and antibacterial activity tests.

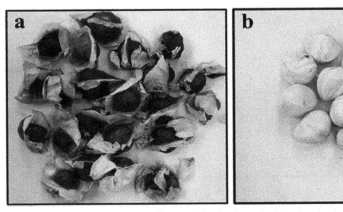
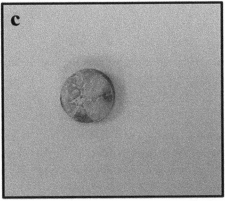

Figure 9. Pictorial view of the pelletization of *Moringa oleifera* seed samples, showing: (**a**) as-purchased *Moringa oleifera* seeds, (**b**) *Moringa oleifera* seeds without coat, (**c**) pelletized seed sample.

4.2. LIBS Setup

Figure 10 depicts the modified LIBS setup that was employed to determine the chemical constituents (elemental compositions) present in the MOS specimens. A quadrupled Q-switched Nd:YAG pulse laser (QUV-266-5) with an energy of 30 mJ, a pulse width of 8 ns, a 266 nm wavelength and a 20 Hz repetition rate was used with a UV convex lens of focal length 30 mm to focus the pulses onto the MOS pellets (which acted as the target) to ablate them. A plasma plume was generated when the target was ablated by the laser source. The emitted plasma was detected/collected using a fiber optic system positioned at 45° and the other end (500 mm) was connected to a spectrometer (Andor SR 500i-A) via grating with approximately 1200 lines per mm. An automated sample holder able to move across the plane was used to mount the pellet to avoid the formation of crusts on the surface of the target as a result of several laser pulses on the sample. The spectrum was recorded by an Intensified charge-coupled device (ICCD) camera (Model iStar 320T, 690 × 255 pixels with delay time setting at 300 ns) and data were transferred to an interfaced online computer (PC).

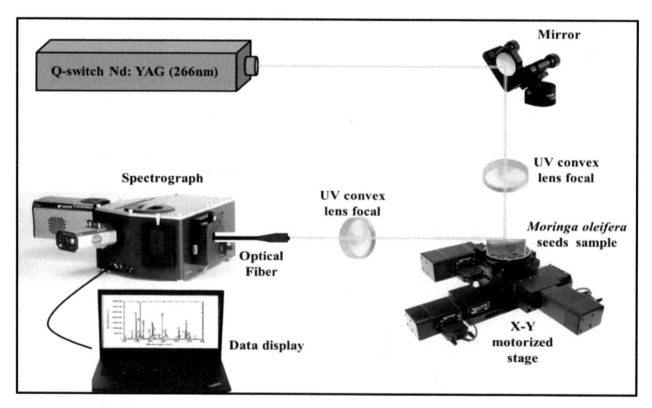

Figure 10. Schematic illustration of the LIBSsetup employed for the detection of vital elements present in MOS.

4.3. GC-MS Measurements

GC-MS (Shimadzu GC-2010 Plus) was applied for the analysis of ethanol MOS extracts that were provided by a split/splitless auto-injector (AOC-20i series) and coupled to a QP2010 Ultra single quadrupole instrument. The secession with GC was accomplished by using an Rxi-5MS fused silica capillary column (Restek, USA) with 30 m long, 0.25 mm wide and 100 μm thick films. The temperature was raised at a constant rate (5 °C/min) from the initial 60 °C (retained for 0.5 min) up to a final 280 °C (kept for 5 min). The temperature of the inlet was 270 °C (in the splitless mode) and helium (used as carrier gas of purity 99.99%) was blown through the MS transfer line (280 °C) at a 1 mL/min rate. The electron impact modes were used to operate the ion source (70 eV of energy at 250°C) and the mass spectrum (full scan) was recorded in the range of 33–550 m/z. The spectrum values were gained by regulating the GC-MS and via a GC-MS solution. The compounds of emanated volatiles were disclosed by means of the NIST-11 and WILEY-9 libraries and by calculating the relative area of each compound.

4.4. Anticancer Activity of MOS Extract

4.4.1. In Vitro Cell Viability and Cell Culture Assay

As already mentioned, the anticancer activities of the MOS extract were evaluated by treating HCT-116 and normal (HEK-293) human cell lines. The cells were obtained from Dr. Khaldoon M. Alsamman, College of Applied Medical Science, Imam Abdulrahman Bin Faisal University, Dammam, Saudi Arabia. First, cells were cultured in 96 well-plates according to the earlier specified method. Dulbecco's modified Eagle's medium (DMEM), supplemented with other reagents (selenium chloride, fetal bovine serum, L-glutamine and antibiotics), was added to the plates for cell growth [29,30].

The cells were treated with varying concentrations of MOS extracts (30–100 µg/mL) for 48 h, whereas in the control, no MOS extract was added. Equal concentrations of a solvent, dimethyl sulfoxide (DMSO) were used in both the control and MOS-treated samples. After 48 h, an MTT assay was performed for 4 h (Molecules, Wellington, New Zealand). Afterward, the growth medium was removed from the plates and (DMSO) was added to every well so the MTT formed formazan crystal. Then, the wells containing the cell cultures were checked at a wavelength of 570 nm via a micro-plate reader (Bio-Rad Labs., Boston, MA, USA). Finally, the recorded readings were analyzed through inbuilt software (Version 5.0, GraphPad Prism) and the statistical significance was studied via ANOVA tests.

4.4.2. Nuclear Staining via DAPI

The cells were treated with MOS extract (at 0.066 µg/mL) for 48 h and, in the control group, no MOS extract was added. The effects of MOS extract on cell nuclei were estimated with DAPI staining. Cold paraformaldehyde (4%) was used to pretreat the cells, which were then washed with 0.1% of Triton X-100 made from phosphate-buffered saline (PBS). At the same time, both the control and MOS- treated cells were stained using PBS with DAPI of 1.0 µg/mL concentration followed by rinsing with X-100 (0.1%). Cell morphologies of both cells (control and the treated) were analyzed *via* (CSM) (CSM-Zeiss, Frankfurt, Germany).

4.5. Antimicrobial Activity Assessment of MOS Extract

The effect of MOS extract on antibacterial efficacy at 50, 100, 150, 200 and 250 µg/mL against the *E. coli* ATCC35218 and *S. aureus* ATCC29213 strains was assessed using the AWD method. The inoculum was made from fresh bacteria grown overnight at 37 °C using nutrient broth (NB). This was followed by the preparation of inoculum to 0.5 McFarland standard and 100 µL of inoculum were disseminated over the surface of Mueller–Hinton agar (MHA) plates and dried in an aseptic environment. Next, the inoculated plates (6 mm) were punched using a sterile cork-borer. From the prepared extract, around 50 µL were added to the wells and further kept at 37 °C for an overnight incubation. Thereafter, the bacterial inhibition zone diameter over the entire well was recorded to evaluate the inhibition by the MOS extracts [29].

4.6. Antimicrobial Activity Assessment of MOS Extract Using SEM

The effect of MOS extract was additionally studied to investigate the structural damage caused to the selected bacteria by using SEM. The adjusted bacterial cell density, as described above, was treated with 250 µg/mL MOS for overnight incubation. The assay was carried out as per the protocol described by Rehman et.al [29].

4.7. Statistical Analysis

In the present study, cell viability data are presented as mean (±) standard deviation (SD), which were obtained from three independent experimental repeats. One-way ANOVA followed by

Dunnett's post hoc test with GraphPad Prism software version 5.0 (GraphPad Software, Inc., La Jolla, CA, USA) was done for the statistical analysis. $p < 0.05$ was considered to indicate a statistically significant difference.

5. Conclusions

The LIBS and GC-MS techniques were used to identify and quantify the elemental compositions of MOS extract. The antibacterial and antiproliferative effectiveness of the MOS extracts was evaluated. The LIBS spectra revealed the presence of various nutritional elements in the MOSs that are important for health. The GC-MS analysis reconfirmed the presence of several bioactive compounds in the MOS extract. The MTT assay and DAPI staining showed a significant impact of the MOS extract on the inhibition of the growth of the HCT-116 cells and the insignificant inhibitory action of the extract on the HEK-293 cells, indicating the excellent specificity of the extracts towards the cancer cells. The MOS extracts showed strong antibacterial activity in terms of the growth inhibition and morphogenic changes against *S. aureus* compared to *E. coli,* owing to their cell wall differences. Therefore, it is established that MOS extract can be a prospective antibacterial and anticancer agent for functional pharmaceutical formulations.

Author Contributions: M.A.G. conceptualized and designed the study; R.K.A., M.A.A., S.R. and F.A.K. carried out the experiments and prepared all the figures; M.A.A., S.R., A.M. and F.A.K. wrote the manuscript; S.R., M.A.A., M.A.G., F.A.K. and A.B. revised and finalized the manuscript. All authors have read and agreed to the published version of the manuscript.

References

1.   Shale, T.L.; Stirk, W.A.; van Staden, J. Screening of medicinal plants used in Lesotho for anti-bacterial and anti-inflammatory activity. *J. Ethnopharmacol.* **1999**. [CrossRef]

2.   Macéé, S.R.H.; Truelstrup, H.L. Anti-bacterial activity of phenolic compounds against Streptococcus pyogenes. *Medicines* **2017**, *4*, 25. [CrossRef]

3.   Nakhjavan, M.; Palethorpe, H.M.; Tomita, Y.; Smith, E.; Price, T.G.; Yool, A.J.; Pei, V.J.; Townsend, A.R.; Hardingham, G.H. Stereoselective anti-cancer activities of ginsenoside rg3 on triple negative breast cancer cell models. *Pharmaceuticals* **2019**, *12*, 117. [CrossRef]

4.   Khor, K.Z.; Lim, V.; Moses, E.J.; Samad, N.A. The in Vitro and in Vivo Anticancer Properties of Moringa oleifera. *Evid.-based Complement. Altern. Med.* **2018**, *2018*, 14. [CrossRef]

5.   Oduro, I.; Ellis, W.O.; Owusu, D. Nutritional potential of two leafy vegetables: Moringa oleifera and Ipomoea batatas leaves. *Sci. Res. Essays* **2008**, *3*, 57–60. [CrossRef]

6.   Vergara-Jimenez, M.; Almatrafi, M.M.; Fernandez, M.L. Bioactive components in Moringa oleifera leaves protect against chronic disease. *Antioxidants* **2017**, *6*, 91. [CrossRef]

7.   Natarajan, S.; Joshi, J.A. Characterisation of moringa (Moringa oleifera Lam.) genotypes for growth, pod and seed characters and seed oil using morphological and molecular markers. *Vegetos* **2015**, *28*, 64–71. [CrossRef]

8.   Stohs, S.J.; Hartman, M.J. Review of the safety and efficacy of Moringa oleifera. *Phytother. Res.* **2015**, *29*, 796–804. [CrossRef]

9.   Retta, N.; Awoke, T.; Mekonnen, Y. Comparison of total phenolic content, free radical scavenging potential and anti-hyperglycemic condition from leaves extract of Moringa stenopetala and Moringa oliefera. *Ethiop. J. Public Heal. Nutr.* **2019**, *1*, 20–27.

10.   El-Hack, M.E.A.; Alagawany, M.; Elrys, A.S.; Desoky, E.-S.M.; Tolba, H.M.N.; Elnahal, A.S.M.; Elnesr, S.S.; Swelum, A.A. Effect of forage moringa oleifera l. (moringa) on animal health and nutrition and its beneficial applications in soil, plants and water purification. *Agriculture (Switzerland)* **2018**, *8*, 145. [CrossRef]

11.   Ferreira, P.M.P.; Farias, D.F.; Oliveira, J.T.D.A.; Carvalho, A.D.F.U. Moringa oleifera: Bioactive compounds and nutritional potential. *Revista de Nutricao* **2008**, *21*. [CrossRef]

12.   Anwar, F.; Zafar, S.N.; Rashid, U. Characterization of Moringa oleifera seed oil from drought and irrigated regions of Punjab, Pakistan. *Grasasy Aceites* **2006**. [CrossRef]

13.   Silva, M.O.; Camacho, F.P.; Ferreira-Pinto, L.; Giufrida, W.M.; Vieira, A.M.S.; Visentaine, J.V.; Vedoy, D.R.L. Cardozo-Filho, L. Extraction and phase behaviour of Moringa oleifera seed oil using compressed propane. *Can. J. Chem. Eng.* **2016**, *94*, 2195–2201. [CrossRef]

14. Gondal, M.A.; Hussain, T.; Yamani, Z.H.; Baig, M.A. Detection of heavy metals in Arabian crude oil residue using laser induced breakdown spectroscopy. *Talanta* **2006**, *69*, 1072–1078. [CrossRef] [PubMed]

15. Sabsabi, M.; Cielo, P. Quantitative analysis of aluminum alloys by Laser-induced breakdown spectroscopy and plasma characterization. *Appl. Spectrosc.* **1995**, *49*. [CrossRef]

16. Zhao, S.; Zhang, D. An experimental investigation into the solubility of Moringa oleifera oil in supercritical carbon dioxide. *J. Food Eng.* **2014**. [CrossRef]

17. Yamaguchi, F.; Takata, M.; Kamitori, K.; Ninaka, M.; Dong, Y.; Tokuda, M. Rare sugar D-allose induces specific up-regulation of TXNIP and subsequent G1 cell cycle arrest in hepatocellular carcinoma cells by stabilization of p27kip1. *Int. J. Oncol.* **2008**, *32*, 377–385. [CrossRef]

18. Sharma, S.; Shukla, N.; Bharti, A.S.; Uttam, K.N. Simultaneous Multielemental Analysis of the Leaf of Moringa oleifera by Direct Current Arc Optical Emission Spectroscopy. *Natl. Acad. Sci. Lett.* **2018**, *41*, 65–68. [CrossRef]

19. Osuntokun, O.T.; Yusuf-Babatunde, M.A.; Fasila, O.O. Components and Bioactivity of Ipomoea batatas (L.) (Sweet Potato) Ethanolic Leaf Extract. *Asian J. Adv. Res. Rep.* **2020**, *10*, 10–26. [CrossRef]

20. Welch, R.; Tietje, A. Investigation of Moringa oleifera leaf extract and its cancer-selective antiproliferative properties. *J. South. Carolina Acad. Sci.* **2017**, *15*, 4.

21. Menendez, J.; Lupu, R. Mediterranean Dietary Traditions for the Molecular Treatment of Human Cancer: Anti-Oncogenic Actions of the Main Olive Oils Monounsaturated Fatty Acid Oleic Acid (18:1n-9). *Curr. Pharm. Biotechnol.* **2006**. [CrossRef]

22. Fahey, J. Moringa oleifera: A Review of the Medical Evidence for Its Nutritional, Therapeutic, and Prophylactic Properties. Part 1. *Trees Life J.* **2005**, *10*, 602–608. [CrossRef]

23. Zhong, J.; Wang, Y.; Yang, R.; Liu, X.; Yang, Q.; Qin, X. The application of ultrasound and microwave to increase oil extraction from *Moringa oleifera* seeds. *Ind. Crops Prod.* **2018**, *120*, 1–10. [CrossRef]

24. Rai, A.; Mohanty, B.; Bhargava, R. Experimental modeling and simulation of supercritical fluid extraction of *Moringa oleifera* seed oil by carbon dioxide. *Chem. Eng. Commun.* **2017**, *204*, 957–964. [CrossRef]

25. Belo, Y.N.; Al-Hamimi, S.; Chimuka, L.; Turner, C. Ultrahigh-pressure supercritical fluid extraction and chromatography of *Moringa oleifera* and *Moringa peregrina* seed lipids. *Anal Bioanal Chem.* **2019**, *411*, 3685–3693. [CrossRef]

26. Almessiere, M.A.; Altuwiriqi, R.; Gondal, M.A.; AlDakheel, R.K.; Alotaibi, H.F. Qualitative and quantitative analysis of human nails to find correlation between nutrients and vitamin D deficiency using LIBS and ICP-AES. *Talanta* **2018**, *185*, 61–70. [CrossRef]

27. Mehta, S.; Rai, P.K.; Rai, N.K.; Rai, A.K.; Bicanic, D.; Watal, G. Role of Spectral Studies in Detection of Antibacterial Phytoelements and Phytochemicals of Moringa oleifera. *Food Biophys.* **2011**. [CrossRef]

28. Pasquini, C.; Cortez, J.; Silva, L.M.C.; Gonzaga, F.B. Laser induced breakdown spectroscopy. *J. Braz. Chem. Soc.* **2007**, *18*, 463–512. [CrossRef]

29. Rehman, S.; Asiri, S.M.; Khan, F.A.; Jermy, B.R.; Ravinayagam, V.; Alsalem, Z.; Jindan, R.A.; Qurashi, A. Biocompatible Tin Oxide Nanoparticles: Synthesis, Antibacterial, Anticandidal and Cytotoxic Activities. *ChemistrySelect* **2019**, *4*, 4013–4017. [CrossRef]

30. Rehman, S.; Asiri, S.M.; Khan, F.A.; Jermy, B.R.; Ravinayagam, V.; Alsalem, Z.; Jindan, R.A.; Qurashi, A. Anticandidal and In Vitro Anti-Proliferative Activity of Sonochemically synthesized Indium Tin Oxide Nanoparticles. *Sci. Rep.* **2020**. [CrossRef]

31. Chávez-González, M.L.; Rodríguez-Herrera, R.; Aguilar, C.N. Essential Oils: A Natural Alternative to Combat Antibiotics Resistance. A Natural Alternative to Combat Antibiotics Resistance. *Antibiot. Resist. Mech. New Antimicrob. Approaches* **2016**, *11*, 227–235.

32. Paduch, R.; Kandefer-Szerszeń, M.; Trytek, M.; Fiedurek, J. Terpenes: Substances useful in human healthcare. *Arch. Immunol. et Ther. Exp.* **2007**, *55*, 27–315. [CrossRef]

33. Bajpai, V.K.; Baek, K.H.; Kang, S.C. Control of Salmonella in foods by using essential oils: A review. *Food Res. Int.* **2012**, *45*, 722–734. [CrossRef]

34. Friedly, E.C.; Crandall, P.G.; Ricke, S.C.; Roman, M.; O'Bryan, C.; Chalova, V.I. In vitro antilisterial effects of citrus oil fractions in combination with organic acids. *J. Food Sci.* **2009**, *74*, M67–M72. [CrossRef]

35. Trombetta, D.; Castelli, F.; Sarpietro, M.G.; Venuti, V.; Cristani, M.; Daniele, C.; Saija, A.; Mazzanti, G.; Bisignano, G. Mechanisms of antibacterial action of three monoterpenes. *Antimicrob. Agents Chemother.* **2005**. [CrossRef]

36. Nithyanand, P.; Shafreen, R.M.B.; Muthamil, S.; Murugan, R.; Pandian, S.K. Essential oils from commercial and wild Patchouli modulate Group A Streptococcal biofilms. *Ind. Crops Prod.* **2015**, *69*, 1–492. [CrossRef]
37. Tajkarimi, M.M.; Ibrahim, S.A.; Cliver, D.O. Antimicrobial herb and spice compounds in food. *Food Control* **2010**, *21*, 1199–1218. [CrossRef]
38. Calo, J.R.; Crandall, P.G.; O'Bryan, C.A.; Ricke, S.C. Essential oils as antimicrobials in food systems—A review. *Food Control* **2015**, *54*, 111–119. [CrossRef]

12

Thymus mastichina: Composition and Biological Properties with a Focus on Antimicrobial Activity

Márcio Rodrigues [1,2,3,*], Ana Clara Lopes [1], Filipa Vaz [1], Melanie Filipe [1], Gilberto Alves [3], Maximiano P. Ribeiro [1,2,3], Paula Coutinho [1,2,3,*] and André R. T. S. Araujo [1,2,4,*]

[1] School of Health Sciences, Polytechnic Institute of Guarda, Rua da Cadeia, 6300-035 Guarda, Portugal; claralopes28@gmail.com (A.C.L.); filipa.a.c.vaz@hotmail.com (F.V.); melaniemfilipe@gmail.com (M.F.); mribeiro@ipg.pt (M.P.R.)

[2] Research Unit for Inland Development (UDI), Polytechnic Institute of Guarda, Av. Dr. Francisco Sá Carneiro, 50, 6300-559 Guarda, Portugal

[3] CICS-UBI—Health Sciences Research Centre, University of Beira Interior, Av. Infante D. Henrique, 6200-506 Covilhã, Portugal; gilberto@fcsaude.ubi.pt

[4] LAQV/REQUIMTE, Department of Chemical Sciences, Faculty of Pharmacy, University of Porto, Rua Jorge Viterbo Ferreira, 228, 4050-313 Porto, Portugal

* Correspondence: marciorodrigues@ipg.pt (M.R.); coutinho@ipg.pt (P.C.); andrearaujo@ipg.pt (A.R.T.S.A.)

Abstract: *Thymus mastichina* has the appearance of a semishrub and can be found in jungles and rocky lands of the Iberian Peninsula. This work aimed to review and gather available scientific information on the composition and biological properties of *T. mastichina*. The main constituents of *T. mastichina* essential oil are 1,8-cineole (or eucalyptol) and linalool, while the extracts are characterized by the presence of flavonoids, phenolic acids, and terpenes. The essential oil and extracts of *T. mastichina* have demonstrated a wide diversity of biological activities. They showed antibacterial activity against several bacteria such as *Escherichia coli*, *Proteus mirabilis*, *Salmonella* subsp., methicillin-resistant and methicillin-sensitive *Staphylococcus aureus*, *Listeria monocytogenes EGD*, *Bacillus cereus*, and *Pseudomonas*, among others, and antifungal activity against *Candida* spp. and *Fusarium* spp. Additionally, it has antioxidant activity, which has been evaluated through different methods. Furthermore, other activities have also been studied, such as anticancer, antiviral, insecticidal, repellent, anti-Alzheimer, and anti-inflammatory activity. In conclusion, considering the biological activities reported for the essential oil and extracts of *T. mastichina*, its potential as a preservative agent could be explored to be used in the food, cosmetic, or pharmaceutical industries.

Keywords: antimicrobial; biological activities; essential oil; extract; *Thymus mastichina*

1. Introduction

Thymus mastichina L. (Figure 1) is an endemic species of the Iberian Peninsula, commonly known as "Bela-Luz", "Sal-Puro", "Tomilho-alvadio-do-Algarve", "Mastic thyme", and "Spanish marjoram" and belongs to the Lamiaceae family [1–4]. *T. mastichina* species can be classified into two subspecies: *T. mastichina* subsp. *donyanae* and *T. mastichina* subsp. *mastichina*; the first of which is present in Algarve (Portugal) and Huelva and Seville (Spain) and the latter extends throughout the Iberian Peninsula [5,6]. This aromatic plant is a semiwoody shrub that grows up to 50 cm tall and is characterized by simple and opposite leaves and bilabiate flower groups in a flower head or capitula, which blossom from April to June [2,7,8]. *T. mastichina* can be found in jungles, uncultivated, ruderal, and rupicolous lands and in dry stony open places, except in calcareous regions [1,8], being very resistant to frost, diseases, and pests. *T. mastichina* is known for its strong eucalyptus odor and it has been used for various health conditions due to its antiseptic, digestive, antirheumatic, and antitussive effects [2,6,9,10].

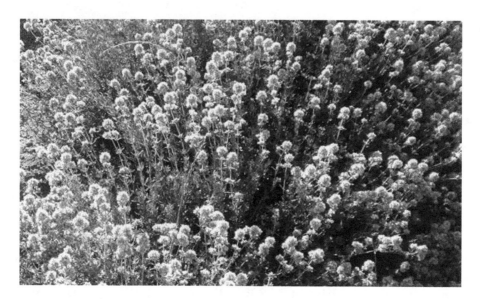

Figure 1. *Thymus mastichina* plant (source Planalto Dourado™ Essential Oils Enterprise, from Freixedas, Guarda, Portugal).

T. mastichina can be used in fresh or dry form and its leaves are traditionally used as a condiment/spices flavoring, in seasoning traditional dishes and salads, to preserve olives, to aromatize olive oil, and as a substitute for salt [10,11]. This medicinal and aromatic plant is also used as a source of essential oil in the cosmetic and perfume industries [10,12]. Infusions with dry parts of the plant have been used to relieve colds, cough, throat irritations, and abdominal pain, while infusions with fresh parts of the plant have been used for indigestion and stomach pain [13]. Thus, there are different products based on *T. mastichina* that are commercially available in Portugal and Spain (e.g., "Bela-Luz" essential oil, "Marjoram Spanish" essential oil, "Tomilho Bela Luz" herbs). In this work, we compiled the available information regarding the chemical composition of the essential oil and extracts of *T. mastichina* to review published studies in which its biological activities have been evaluated.

2. Search Strategy

The search was performed on the following databases: PubMed and Web of Science. Various combinations of the following terms were queried: *T. mastichina*, thyme, antibacterial, antifungal, antimicrobial, anti-inflammatory, anti-Alzheimer, antioxidant, anticancer, antiviral, insecticidal, repellent, essential oil, plant extract, biological activity, and composition. In addition, references cited in related publications were followed up. The selection of articles was performed by its relevance to the purpose of this review. It should be noted that no date or language criteria were defined as filters in the search strategy implemented.

3. Chemical Composition of *T. mastichina* Essential Oils and Extracts

The essential oil of *T. mastichina* is usually obtained mainly by hydrodistillation for 2–4 h, with low yields (from 0.4% to 6.90% (v/w)) (Table 1). Other extraction methods were also used, such as microdistillation, that showed higher amounts of 1,8-cineole plus limonene in comparison with hydrodistillation. However, in general, few differences were found between the different methodologies. The yield may vary depending on several factors, namely the part of the plant used, place of harvest, period of the year, storage time, extraction time, and type of fertilization, among others [14].

Table 1. Obtention features and characterization of the *Thymus mastichina* essential oil and its main constituents (equal or higher than 5%).

Plant Material (Growth Phase)	Period of Year	Source	Yield	Major Constituents	Reference
Flowering branches	May–July	Trás-os-Montes; Beira Alta; Beira Baixa; Estremadura; Ribatejo; Alto Alentejo; Algarve (Portugal)	2.2% (v/w)	1,8-cineole (53.3%); linalool (5.5%)	[15]
Leaves	December; May	Nave do Barão, Algarve (Portugal)	-	1,8-cineole (46.29%); camphor (10.77%); camphene (6.31%); α-pinene (5.23%)	[16]
Leaves	-	Vadofresno, Córdoba (Spain)	-	1,8-cineole (24.81%) 1,8-cineole (18.87%)	[17]
Leaves and flowers	December; May	Algarve (Portugal)	-	1,8-cineole (46.3–50.4%); camphor (9.6–10.8%); camphene (5.0–6.3%); α-pinene (4.0–5.3%);	[18]
Leaves		S. Brás de Alportel, Algarve (Portugal)	0.4–0.9% (v/w)	1,8-cineole (50.2–61.0%); camphor (7.6–10.1%); δ-terpineol (6.5–9.7%); camphene (4.4–6.1%)	[19]
Flowers	-		1.6–2.2% (v/w)	1,8-cineole (46.7–50.2%); δ-terpineol (5.9–8.2%)	
Aerial parts	December; May; June; Octcber January; May, June; October (2 years)	S. Brás de Alportel, Algarve (Portugal)	-	1,8-cineole (42.1–50.43%); camphor (7.4–11.5%); camphene (3.1–6.3%); α-terpineol (3.4–5.7%); *trans*-sabinene hydrate (0.2–5.6%); α-pinene (3.1–5.3%)	[20]

Table 1. *Cont.*

Plant Material (Growth Phase)	Period of Year	Source	Yield	Major Constituents	Reference
Flowers (full flowering phase)		S. Brás de Alportel, Algarve, Sotavento (Portugal)	-	1,8-cineole (46.9%); camphor (6.7%); α-terpineol (5.2%)	[21]
Leaves (full flowering phase)				1,8-cineole (42.4%); camphor (7.7%); borneol (6.8%); α-terpineol (6.1%)	
Aerial parts (beginning of flowering phase)	May	Sesimbra, Estremadura (Portugal)	-	Chemotype A (aerial parts): linalool (44.4%); 1,8-cineole (37.4%) Chemotype B (aerial parts): linalool (61.4%); camphor (5.3%)	
Aerial parts (flowering phase)	-	Algarve (Portugal) Estremadura (Portugal)	-	1,8-cineole (45.3%); camphor (8.5%); camphene (6.6%); α-pinene (5.4%); limonene (5.2%); borneol (5.0%) linalool (52.3%); 1,8-cineole (9.6%); limonene (6.4%); p-cymene (6.2%)	[22]
Aerial parts	October; January; April; June	Nave do Barão, Algarve (Portugal)	0.7–3.6% (v/w)	1,8-cineole (45.1–58.6%); camphor (5.5–8.9%); α-pinene (4.6-6.8%); camphene (4.3–6.0%)	[23]
Aerial parts (vegetative phase and flowering phase)	October; May	Sesimbra (Portugal)	0.7–2.7% (v/w)	linalool (58.7–69%); 1,8-cineole (1.1–10.8%); elemol (0.9–6.6%); camphor (2.4–5.3%)	[24]

Table 1. *Cont.*

Plant Material (Growth Phase)	Period of Year	Source	Yield	Major Constituents	Reference
Aerial parts	January	Direção Regional de Agricultura de Trás-os-Montes (Portugal)	1.3% (v/w)	1,8-cineole (57.8%); limonene (10.8%)	[25]
Aerial parts	-	Direção Regional de Agricultura de Trás-os-Montes, Mirandela (Portugal)	-	1,8-cineole (67.4%)	[26]
Leaves	June	Sesimbra (Portugal)	2.2%	linalool (68.5%); 1,8-cineole (9.4%)	[8]
Flowers			2.6%	linalool (73.5%);	
Leaves		Arrábida (Portugal)	1.7%	1,8-cineole (10.2%) 1,8-cineole (69.2%); linalool (6.3%)	
Flowers			3.5%	1,8-cineole (54.6%); linalool (13.7%)	
Leaves		Mértola (Portugal)	2.0%	1,8-cineole (44.2%)	
Flowers			3.0%	1,8-cineole (39.4%); linalool (8.1%)	
Leaves		S. Brás de Alportel (Portugal)	1.4%	1,8-cineole (49.7%)	
Flowers			2.0%	1,8-cineole (48.5%)	
Aerial parts (flowering phase)		Mirandela (Portugal)	2.4% (v/w)	1,8-cineole (64.1%); α-terpineol (5.6%)	[27]
Aerial parts (vegetative phase)	January	Algarve (Portugal)	2.3% (v/w)	1,8-cineole (49.4%); limonene (9.3%)	[28]
Aerial parts	-	Córdoba (Spain)	-	1,8-cineole (45.67%); linalool (27.88%)	[29]
Aerial parts	-	Mértola (Portugal) Vila Real de Santo António (Portugal) Sesimbra (Portugal)	1.0–1.3% (v/w)	1,8-cineole (61.0%) 1,8-cineole (49.4%) linalool (39.7%); 1,8-cineole (9.6%)	[30]

Table 1. *Cont.*

Plant Material (Growth Phase)	Period of Year	Source	Yield	Major Constituents	Reference
Plants (flowering phase)	-	Direção Regional de Agricultura e Pescas do Algarve (Portugal)	-	1,8-cineole (41.0%); β-pinene + trans-sabinene (7.0%); camphor (6.9%); borneol (6.5%); α-pinene (6.0%); camphene (5.5%)	[31]
Aerial parts (flowering phase)	June	Direção Regional de Agricultura e Pescas do Algarve (Portugal)	4% (w/w)	1,8-cineole (44%); camphor (10%); borneol (7%); camphene (7%); α-pinene (6%); α-terpineol (5%)	[32]
Plant (flowering phase)	Summer	Tordesillas, Valladolid; Truchas, Peradoones, Carrocera, Boñar, León; Almazán, Soria; Riaza, Villacastín, Segovia; Serranilos, Avila; Saldaña, Palencia (Spain)	3.40–6.90%	-	[33]
Aerial parts	-	Direção Regional de Agricultura e Pescas do Algarve (Portugal)	6.3% (w/w)	1,8-cineole (49.4%); α-pinene (7.0%); camphene (6.9%); camphor (5.8%); β-pinene (5.3%)	[14]
Whole plants	-	Barcelona (Spain)	-	1,8-cineole (52.57%); linalool (12.78%)	[34]
Commercial samples: leaves, stem, and flowers	-	Esencias Martinez Lozano, Murcia (Spain)	-	1,8-cineole (51.94%); linalool (19.90%)	[35]
Aerial parts (vegetative phase)	-	Coimbra (Portugal)	1.17% (v/w)	1,8-cineole (46%); limonene (23%)	[36]

Table 1. *Cont.*

Plant Material (Growth Phase)	Period of Year	Source	Yield	Major Constituents	Reference
Aerial parts (flowering phase)	June–July	Béjar, Valdemierque, Mozarbez, Golpejas, Salamanca; Carrocera, Boñar, Truchas, Peranzanes, León; Salas de los Infante, Lerma, Oña, Burgos; Villacastín, Riaza, Coca, Prádena, Segovia; Vinuesa, Aldealpozo, Almazán, Langa de Duero, Soria (Spain)	2.27–6.48% (v/w)	1,8-cineole (56.80–69.60%); linalool (0.62–15.7%); α-terpineol (2.07–5.99%); β-pinene (1.72–5.63%); limonene (1.07–5.10%)	[37]
Aerial parts	-	Vila Chã (Portugal)	-	1,8-cineole (47.4%); thymol (13.7%); p-cymene (9.7%); γ-terpinene (7.3%)	[38]
Flowers and leaves	June	Carrocera, Léon (Spain)	-	1,8-cineole + limonene (61.6%); linalool (6%); β-pinene (5.7%) 1,8-cineole + limonene (69.3%) 1,8-cineole + limonene (64%)	[39]
Plants (flowering phase)	-	Algarve (Portugal)	1.2% (v/w)	1,8-cineole (52.8%); α-pinene (7.2%); camphene (7.2%); camphor (7.2%)	[40]
Plants grown in vitro (all parts except roots)	-	Urbino (Italy)	0.56% (v/w)	1,8-cineole (55.6%); linalool (24.5%); β-pinene (5.9%)	[41]
Commercial samples	-	Planalto Dourado™, Freixedas (Portugal)	-	1.8-cineole (49.94%); linalool (5.66%); α-terpineol (5.59%); β-pinene (5.54%)	[42]

Table 1. *Cont.*

Plant Material (Growth Phase)	Period of Year	Source	Yield	Major Constituents	Reference
Aerial parts	-	Évora, Alentejo (Portugal)	1.1% (v/w)	1,8-cineole (72.0%); α-terpineol (9.0%)	[43]
Flowers		Badajoz (Spain)	-	limonene + 1,8-cineole (71.82%); β-myrcene (9.81%); α-terpineol (5.32%); camphene (5.15%)	[44]
Fruits				limonene + 1,8-cineole (78.37%); β-myrcene (5.69%); α-terpineol (5.05%)	
Leaves	Summer	Alentejo (Portugal)	-	1,8-cineole (74.2%); α-terpenyl acetate (7.9%)	[45]
Leaves	-	UNIQ F&F Co., Ltd. (Seoul, Korea)	-	β-pinene (5.81%); 1,8-cineole (64.61%); linalool (15.28%)	[46]
Aerial parts	July	Murcia (Spain)	1.8–3.6% (v/w)	1,8-cineole (38.8–74.0%); linalool (13.3–42.7%)	[4]
Leaves and stem	-	Ciudad Real (Spain)	-	1,8-cineole (43.26%); linalool (36.72%); linalyl acetate (5.58%)	[47]
Commercial samples	-	Ervitas Catitas (Portugal)		1,8-cineole (55.9%); β-pinene (10.8%)	[48]
Aerial parts	-	Évora, Alentejo (Portugal)	1.06% (v/w)	1,8-cineole (71.2%); α-terpineol (9.7%)	[2]

As shown in Figure 2 and Table 1, the composition of the essential oil of *T. mastichina* is quite diverse, being constituted by hydrocarbon and oxygenated monoterpenes and sesquiterpenes, presenting main constituents of 1,8-cineole (also known as eucalyptol) and linalool. The major constituents of the essential oil of *T. mastichina* have been determined by gas chromatography [2,4,8,14–20,23–32,34–45,47,48]. Table 1 summarizes the major constituents present and it can be seen that their composition varies according to origin. In fact, there are three main subtypes of essential oils, depending on the main compounds present: 1,8-cineole, linalool, and 1,8-cineole/linalool. In Portugal, the chemotypes of linalool and 1,8-cineole/linalool are only found in Estremadura, mainly at Arrábida and Sesimbra, while the 1,8-cineole chemotype is distributed throughout the country [8,21]. As expected, there are differences in the phytochemical composition among different species of Thymus; for instance, the main compound presented in *Thymus vulgaris* is thymol, which is present in low percentages in *T. mastichina* [49].

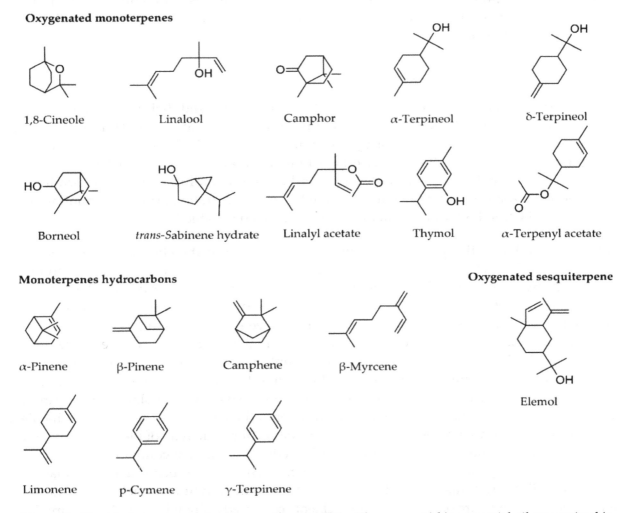

Figure 2. Chemical structures of main constituents of the *Thymus mastichina* essential oil categorized in oxygenated and hydrocarbons monoterpenes and hydrocarbon sesquiterpene.

As presented in Table S1, in addition to *T. mastichina* essential oil, in some cases after hydrodistillation, the decoction water (the remaining hydrodistillation aqueous phase) was also collected [12,14,32,43,50]. Conversely, in some studies, extraction from the aerial parts of the plant was performed using different solvents (hexane, dichloromethane, ethanol, diethyl ether, ethyl acetate, *n*-butanol, and water) [10,13,32,37,43,50,51]. Furthermore, in some cases, the extracts were obtained by ultrasound [9,51]. The extracts obtained from the aerial parts of the plant were characterized by the presence of different polyphenol classes, in particular, flavonoids (apigenin, kaempferol, luteolin, naringenin, quercetin, sakuranetin, sterubin), phenolic acids (caffeic acid, chlorogenic acid, 2-methoxysalicylic acid, 3-methoxysalicylic acid, rosmarinic acid, salvianolic acids I and K and derivatives), phenolic terpene (carnosol) and hexoside and glycoside derivatives; other compounds identified were steroid (β-sitosterol), triterpenoids (oleanolic acid, ursolic acid), and xanthophyll lutein [9,10,12,37,51,52]. In Figure S1 the chemical structures of several compounds present in the extract are presented. In opposition to *T. mastichina* essential oil, in which the composition is extensively characterized, the extract phenolic profile has been less investigated and diverse chromatographic peaks detected during the phytochemical characterization remain unidentified.

4. Biological Properties

The diverse bioactivities of *T. mastichina* essential oil and extracts are related to the chemical composition. Essential oil and extracts from the aerial parts of *T. mastichina* have been mainly described for their antibacterial and antifungal activities, but also for antioxidant, anticancer, antiviral, insecticidal, insect repellent, and anti-enzymatic activities (anti-Alzheimer, anti-inflammatory, α-amylase, and α-glucosidase).

4.1. Antibacterial and Antifungal Activities

The antibacterial and antifungal activities of the essential oils and their main compounds were evaluated by several researchers. The effect of antibacterial activity of essential oils may inhibit the growth of bacteria (bacteriostatic) or destroy bacterial cells (bactericidal). Nevertheless, it is difficult to distinguish these actions, as the antibacterial activity evaluation if frequently based on the most known and basic methods such as disk-diffusion and broth microdilution for the determination of the diameter of the zone of inhibition, minimum inhibitory concentration (MIC), and minimum lethal concentration (MLC), and mixtures of methods, as can be seen in Table 2.

The antimicrobial activity of *T. mastichina* essential oil from the chemotype of Algarve and two chemotypes of Sesimbra (Estremadura) in Portugal, measured by disc agar diffusion method, was confirmed by Faleiro et al. [21]. The tested microorganisms (*Escherichia coli, Proteus mirabilis, Salmonella* subsp., *Staphylococcus aureus, Listeria monocytogenes EGD*) presented different sensitivities. In particular, *T. mastichina* essential oil (3 μL) from Algarve showed the highest activity against *S. aureus* showing a diameter of the zone of inhibition of 13.7 and 15.7 mm for the flower and leaf, respectively, while *T. mastichina* essential oil from Sesimbra (Estremadura) had the highest activity for *S. aureus* showing a diameter of the zone of inhibition of 13.3 mm for chemotype A. Additionally, the antimicrobial activity observed with *T. mastichina* essential oil was explored to determine if it was due to the main constituents present in the different oil chemotypes (linalool, 1,8-cineole and linalool/1,8-cineole (1:1) mixture); for this purpose, the antimicrobial activity of these constituents alone was tested. It was concluded a higher antimicrobial activity of linalool compared with 1,8-cineole. Moreover, possible antagonist and synergistic effects of the various constituents of the essential oil were registered, once *E. coli* was susceptible to linalool but not to the mixture of linalool plus 1,8-cineole, and for *C. albicans* the mixture of linalool plus 1,8-cineole produced a slight increase in the antimicrobial activity whereas was not susceptible to 1,8-cineole. In a previous work of the same authors, and using the same method, the results suggested that the higher antimicrobial activity of the *T. mastichina* essential oil against *Salmonella* was associated to higher amounts of camphor present in *T. mastichina* essential oil comparatively to the essential oils of other plants [16].

Table 2. Antibacterial and antifungal activity of *Thymus mastichina* essential oils and extracts.

Origin	Micro-Organisms	Species	Measured Response and Results Obtained		References
			Diameter of the zone of inhibition (mm), including the diameter of the disc (6 mm)		
			Flower	Leaf	
S. Brás de Alportel, Algarve, Sotavento (Portugal)	Gram-negative bacteria	*Escherichia coli*	8.0	14.0	[21]
		Proteus mirabilis	7.0	7.3	
		Salmonella subsp.	8.0	8.7	
	Gram-positive bacteria	*Staphylococcus aureus*	13.7	15.7	
		Listeria monocytogenes EGD	9.7	12.3	
	Fungus	*Candida albicans*	10.0	11.0	
			Chemotype A	Chemotype B	
Sesimbra, Estremadura (Portugal)	Gram-negative bacteria	*Escherichia coli*	7.5	10.6	
		Proteus mirabilis	7.5	10.0	
		Salmonella subsp.	6.3	7.0	
	Gram-positive bacteria	*Staphylococcus aureus*	13.3	9.6	
		Listeria monocytogenes EGD	ND	11.0	
	Fungus	*Candida albicans*	10.6	13.6	
			MIC (µL/mL)	MLC (µL/mL)	
Direção Regional de Agricultura de Trás-os-Montes, Mirandela (Portugal)	Fungi	*Candida albicans*	2.5	2.5	[26]
		Candida albicans	1.25–2.5	2.5	
		Candida albicans	2.5	5.0	
		Candida tropicalis	2.5–5.0	5.0	
		Candida tropicalis	5.0–10.0	5.0	
		Candida glabrata	1.25–2.5	5.0	
		Candida glabrata	2.5	5.0	
		Candida krusei	1.25–2.5	2.5	
		Candida guilhermondii	1.25	1.25	
		Candida parapsilosis	2.5–5.0	5.0	
			MIC (%, v/v)		
Córdoba (Spain)	Gram-negative bacteria	*Escherichia coli*—origin in poultry	4		[29]
		Salmonella enteritidis—origin in poultry	4		
		Salmonella essen—origin in poultry	4		
		Escherichia coli (ETEC)—origin in pig	4		
		Salmonela choleraesuis—origin in pig	4		
		Salmonella typhimurium—origin in pig	4		

Table 2. *Cont.*

Barcelona (Spain) — Area of the inhibition zone (mm²) excluding the film area

Origin	Micro-Organisms	Species	6%	7%	8%	9%	References
Barcelona (Spain)	Gram-positive bacteria	*Listeria innocua*	NA[a]	0.79[a]	0.79[a]	NF[a]	[34]
		Methicillin-resistant *Staphylococcus aureus*	NA[a]	NA[a]	NA[a]	NF[a]	
	Gram-negative bacteria	*Salmonella enteritidis*	NA[a]	NA[a]	NA[a]	NF[a]	
		Pseudomona fragi	NA[a]	NA[a]	NA[a]	NF[a]	

Monteloeder, SL (Elche, Spain)

Origin	Micro-Organisms	Species	MIC microdilution technique (μg/mL) After 24 h	After 48 h	MIC dilution technique (μg/mL) After 24 h	After 48 h	MBC broth dilution techniques (μg/mL) Microdilution	Tube dilution	References
Monteloeder, SL (Elche, Spain)	Gram-negative bacteria	*Escherichia coli*	12,800[b]	25,600[b]	12,800[b]	25,600[b]	51,200[b]	51,200[b]	[53]
		Salmonella enterica	6400[b]	12,800[b]	12,800[b]	25,600[b]	25,600[b]	51,200[b]	
		Enterobacter aerogenes	12,800[b]	51,200[b]	51,200[b]	102,400[b]	51,200[b]	102,400[b]	
	Gram-positive bacteria	*Bacillus cereus*	1600[b]	3200[b]	3200[b]	3200[b]	6400[b]	6400[b]	
		Methicillin-resistant *Staphylococcus aureus*	400[b]	800[b]	800[b]	1600[b]	1600[b]	3200[b]	

Esencias Martinez Lozano (Murcia, Spain)

Origin	Micro-Organisms	Species	Diameter of the inhibition zone (mm) including disc diameter (9 mm)	MIC (μL/mL)	References
Esencias Martinez Lozano (Murcia, Spain)	Gram-positive bacteria	*Listeria innocua*	26.83	3.75	[35]
	Gram-negative bacteria	*Serratia marcescens*	12.36	7.5	
		Pseudomonas fragi	11.68	3.75	
		Pseudomonas fluorescens	9.0	3.75	
		Aeromonas hydrophila	11.29	3.75	
		Shewanella putrefaciens	9.0	3.75	
		Achromobacter denitrificans	10.69	3.75	
		Enterobacter amnigenus	12.51	7.5	
		Enterobacter gergoviae	12.14	7.5	
		Alcaligenes faecalis	23.50	3.75	

Esencias Martinez Lozano (Murcia, Spain) — Diameter of the inhibition zone (mm) including disc diameter (10 mm)

Origin	Micro-Organisms	Species	1%	2%	References
Esencias Martinez Lozano (Murcia, Spain)	Gram-positive bacteria	*Listeria innocua*	17.92[c]	25.51[c]	[54]
	Gram-negative bacteria	*Serratia marcescens*	21.15[c]	32.36[c]	
		Enterobacter amnigenus	NA[c]	NA[c]	
		Alcaligenes faecalis	18.42[c]	28.29[c]	

Table 2. *Cont.*

Origin	Micro-Organisms	Species	Measured Response and Results Obtained			References
			Diameter of the inhibition zone (mm) including disc diameter (9 mm)			
			Minced beef	Cooked ham	Dry-cured sausage	
Esencias Martinez Lozano (Murcia, Spain)	Gram-positive bacteria	Listeria innocua	34.98	15.23	19.45	[55]
	Gram-negative bacteria	Achromobacter denitrificans	11.29	13.29	15.87	
		Alcaligenes faecalis	16.91	15.34	16.03	
		Aeromonas hydrophila	14.7	12.13	24.94	
		Enterobacter amnigenus	10.97	10.69	17.31	
		Enterobacter gergoviae	10.82	13.81	9	
		Pseudomonas fluorescens	12.07	12.86	16.7	
		Pseudomonas fragi	11.61	11.78	14.19	
		Serratia marcescens	11.84	12.69	11.49	
		Shewanella putrefaciens	13.09	14.34	15.82	
			MIC (µg/mL)	MFC (mg/mL)		
Urbino (Italy)	Fungi	Fusarium culmorum	1500	2		[41]
		Fusarium graminearum	1500	2		
		Fusarium poae	1500	2		
		Fusarium avenaceum	1500	2		
		Fusarium equiseti	2100	2.4		
		Fusarium semitectum	2000	2.4		
		Fusarium sporotrichoides	2000	2.4		
		Fusarium nivale	2000	2.4		
			MIC (mg/mL)	MBC (mg/mL)		
Alentejo (Portugal)	Gram-positive bacteria	Methicillin-sensitive Staphylococcus aureus	20	40		[45]
		Bacillus subtilis	15	30		
	Gram-negative bacteria	Escherichia coli	15	30		
		Pseudomonas aeruginosa	20	70		
			ED_{50}			
Ciudad Real (Spain)	Fungi	Botrytis cinerea	-			[47]
		Sclerotinia sclerotiorum	14.87			
		Fusarium oxysporum	58.0			
		Phytophthora parasitica	22.0			
		Alternaria brassicae	>100			
		Cladobotryum mycophilum	14.1			
		Trichoderma agressivum	-			

Table 2. *Cont.*

Origin	Micro-Organisms	Species	Measured Response and Results Obtained		References
			MIC (mg/mL)	MBC (mg/mL)	
Murcia (Spain)	Gram-negative bacteria	*Escherichia coli*	2.3–9.4	2.3–9.4	[4]
	Gram-positive bacteria	Methicillin-sensitive *Staphylococcus aureus*	2.3–4.7	4.6–4.7	
	Fungus	*Candida albicans*	2.3–4.7	2.3–4.7	
			Inhibition growth zone (mm)	MIC (µg/mL)	
Ervitas Catitas (Portugal)	Gram-positive bacteria	Methicillin-sensitive *Staphylococcus aureus* (isolates)	9.0–11.8	500–4000 (or higher)	[48]
		Staphylococcus epidermidis (isolates)	ND; 9.0–13.8	4000–4000 (or higher)	
			Inhibition growth zone (mm)	MIC (µL/mL)	
Évora, Alentejo (Portugal)	Gram-positive bacteria	Methicillin-sensitive *Staphylococcus aureus*	19	>2	[2]
		Staphylococcus epidermidis	21	>2	
		Enterococcus faecalis	21	>2	
		Escherichia coli	11	>2	
		Morganella morganii	17	1.1	
	Gram-negative bacteria	*Proteus mirabilis*	9	0.5	
		Salmonella enteritidis	11	0.1	
		Salmonella typhimurium	8	>2	
		Pseudomonas aeruginosa	17	1.1	

ED$_{50}$ (effective dose 50), concentration that inhibits mycelial growth by 50%; MBC, minimum bactericidal concentration; MFC, minimal fungicidal concentration; MIC, minimum inhibitory concentration; MLC, minimum lethal concentration; NA, not active; ND, not determined; NF, no film formed. [a] Whey protein isolate films incorporated with *T. mastichina* essential oil [b] Mixture of *Rosmarinus officinalis*, *Salvia lavandulifolia*, and *T. mastichina* and chitosan [c] Chitosan edible film disks incorporated with *T. mastichina* essential oil.

T. mastichina essential oils with origin in different bioclimatic zones from Murcia (Spain) showed activity (growth inhibition) against Gram-positive (methicillin-sensitive *S. aureus*), Gram-negative (*E. coli*), and fungi (*C. albicans*). However, some differences were identified among them, probably due to the influence of the clime in the composition of the essential oil. In particular, *T. mastichina* essential oil from the Supra-Mediterranean bioclimatic zone (Moratalla, Spain) produced higher inhibition against *C. albicans* than the *T. mastichina* essential oils from other bioclimatic zones (Caravaca de la Cruz and Lorca, Spain) due to the high concentration of linalool [4]. However, other studies reported lower antibacterial activities of *T. mastichina* essential oil than those found in this study [29,45]. Recently Arantes et al. [2] described the *T. mastichina* essential oil broad spectrum of antibacterial activity against several strains. It was observed higher susceptibility (lower MICs) observed in Gram-negative bacteria (*E. coli, Morganella morganii, P. mirabilis, Salmonella enteritidis, Salmonella typhimurium*, and *Pseudomonas aeruginosa*) than in Gram-positive ones (methicillin-sensitive *S. aureus, Staphylococcus epidermidis*, and *Enterococcus faecalis*) for both agar disc diffusion assay and MICs determination by broth microdilution assay. The higher antibacterial activity against Gram-negative is suggested to be correlated with the presence of monoterpene and phenolic compounds capable of disintegrating the outer membrane of Gram-negative strains. In fact, essential oils are characterized by unique antibacterial potential due to the high number of chemical compounds present in their composition, which act simultaneously, preventing resistance mechanisms in bacteria. Furthermore, synergistic interactions between compounds of essential oils can potentiate their natural antimicrobial effect. Thus, antimicrobial potential cannot be associated with only one component or mechanism of action. Nevertheless, due to the lipophilic character of essential oils, the mechanism of action could be related to the alteration of cell membrane properties.

The antifungal activity of *T. mastichina* essential oils from Sesimbra (Estremadura, Portugal) was observed against *C. albicans* [21]. The antifungal capacity of the *T. mastichina* essential oil against *Candida* spp. have also been evaluated through the macrodilution method that enables the determination of MIC and MLC [26]. Flow cytometry was also used as a complementary method for the study of the mechanisms responsible for antifungal activity. *T. mastichina* essential oil showed higher inhibition compared to the other *Thymus* species tested, with a lower MIC concentration obtained for *T. mastichina* against *Candida* spp. varied from 1.25 to 10.00 µL/mL, depending on the species of *Candida*, while the MLC remained at 5 µL/mL for almost all species. This study described the potent antifungal activity of *T. mastichina* essential oil against *Candida* spp., warranting future therapeutic trials on mucocutaneous candidosis. Compared with other studies, similar MIC values for *Candida* were found using *T. mastichina* essential oil from Portugal [4]. A remarkable increase in antifungal activity of the mixture of extracts of *Rosmarinus officinalis, Salvia lavandulifolia, T. mastichina*, and chitosan against different yeasts (*C. albicans, Pichia anomala, Pichia membranaefaciens*, and *Saccharomyces cerevisiae*) and filamentous fungi (*Aspergillus niger* and *Penicillium digitatum* strains belonging to the collection of fungi isolated from citrus) was observed [53]. However, the results obtained did not enable the determination of MICs or minimum fungicidal concentrations (MFCs) because the values were higher than the maximum concentrations tested. Additionally, the fungicide activity of *T. mastichina* extracts (at 20–25 mg/mL) from plants micropropagated in vitro against *Aspergillus fumigatus* was demonstrated for the first time [56]. In another study, the antifungal capacity of *T. mastichina* essential oil was determined against *Fusarium* spp. using the agar dilution method. *T. mastichina* essential oil showed antifungal activity against pathogenic fungi strains of the genus *Fusarium* with MICs and MFCs ranging from 1500 to 2100 µg/mL and from 2.0 to 2.4 mg/mL, respectively. In this study, the antifungal activity of the two main constituents, 1,8-cineole and linalool, was also evaluated and considering the obtained MICs and MFCs, the antifungal activity of the essential oil seemed to be due to the presence of major constituents [41].

On the other hand, the potential use of *T. mastichina* essential oil as an active and functional ingredient in food products, and the antimicrobial activity against zoonotic and food spoilers and foodborne microorganisms was evaluated in several studies.

The effect of *T. mastichina* essential oil was evaluated on several bacteria of the Enterobacteriaceae family (*E. coli, Salmonella* spp.) with an origin in poultry and pigs species, was registered with MIC values with 4% (*v/v*) [29], as well as in other studies against methicillin-sensitive *S. aureus* and *S. epidermidis* isolates from ovine mastitic milk [48].

Gram-negative bacteria (*E. coli, Salmonella enterica*, and *Enterobacter aerogenes*) and Gram-positive bacteria (*Bacillus cereus* and methicillin-resistant *S. aureus*) were used for determination of MIC, through dilution and microdilution techniques, of a mixture of extracts of *Rosmarinus officinalis, Salvia lavandulifolia, T. mastichina*, and chitosan [53]. All tested extracts demonstrated noticeable antimicrobial activities against spoilage and foodborne pathogens such as *B. cereus*, methicillin-resistant *S. aureus, E. coli, E. aerogenes, S. enterica*, and yeast-like fungi, without interference in sensory properties. Vieira et al. [45] also observed *T. mastichina* essential oil activity, with MIC values of 15 mg/mL (*Bacillus subtilis* and *E. coli*) and 20 mg/mL (methicillin-sensitive *S. aureus* and *P. aeruginosa*); and the same pattern for MLC, with a value of 40 mg/mL for *S. aureus*, 30 mg/mL for *B. subtilis* and *E. coli*, and 70 mg/mL for *P. aeruginosa*, and suggesting this aromatic plant to be used in control pathogenic microorganisms in deteriorating foods. In another study, the antibacterial activity of *T. mastichina* essential oil was assayed in vitro by a microdilution method against both Gram-positive (*Listeria innocua*, methicillin-resistant *S. aureus*, and *B. cereus*) and Gram-negative bacteria (*S. enterica* and *E. coli*). In this study, the inhibition percentage increased with the *T. mastichina* essential oil concentration and higher inhibition was observed for *L. innocua* [44]. Furthermore, the antimicrobial activity of whey protein isolate-based edible films incorporated with *T. mastichina* essential oil were tested against Gram-positive bacteria (*L. innocua* and methicillin-resistant *S. aureus*) and Gram-negative bacteria (*S. enteritidis* and *Pseudomonas fragi*) to be useful as a coating in the food industry. In this context, it should be highlighted that the antimicrobial activity was only observed against *L. innocua* and using the whey protein films containing 7% and 8% of *T. mastichina* essential oil [34]. This work suggests the possibility of using films incorporating essential oils on food systems.

The active antimicrobial activity of *T. mastichina* essential oil (30 μL) applied through the disk-diffusion method was confirmed by Ballester-Costa et al. [35] against *L. innocua* and *Alcaligenes faecalis, Serratia marcescens, Enterobacter amnigenus*, and *Enterobacter gergoviae*, but not active against *P. fragi, Pseudomonas fluorescens, Aeromonas hydrophila, Shewanella putrefaciens, Achromobacter denitrificans*, and *E. gergoviae*. Additionally, MIC of *T. matichina* essential oil determined by microdilution assay was between 3.75 and 7.5 μL/mL for all strains. The differences obtained in both methods are related to the lower dispersion of the essential oils on a solid medium and consequently reduced ability to access to the microorganism in the disk diffusion method, confirming the unreliability of this method for essential oil evaluation. Posteriorly, the same authors tested the effect of chitosan edible film disks incorporated with the essential oil of *T. mastichina* at concentrations of 1% and 2% against *L. innocua, S. marcescens, E. amnigenus*, and *A. faecalis*. At both concentrations, antibacterial activity was observed for *S. marcescens, L. innocua*, and *A. faecalis*, with activity against *S. marcescens* being higher. However, antibacterial activity against *E. amnigenus* was not registered [54]. Besides, in the following year, they evaluated the activity of *T. mastichina* essential oil (30 μL), applied through the disk-diffusion method, against the bacteria *A. denitrificans, A. faecalis, A. hydrophila, E. amnigenus, E. gergoviae, L. innocua, P. fluorescens, P. fragi, S. marcescens*, and *S. putrefaciens* using, as culture medium, extracts from meat homogenates (minced beef, cooked Ham, or dry-cured sausage). *T. mastichina* essential oils were extremely active against *L. innocua* in minced beef and active for *A. hydrophila* in dry-cured sausage, while for the remaining bacteria only moderate activity or absence of activity was found [55]. In this way, it was suggested the use of *T. mastichina* essential oil as a "green" preservative agent in the food industry, per se or incorporated in edible films. In addition, it should be highlighted that its efficacy as an antibacterial agent has been demonstrated in model systems that closely simulate food composition.

Due to the serious damage caused by fungal pathogens of agricultural interest, the possible future application of the essential oils as alternative antifungal agents was evaluated by [47]. In this study, *T. mastichina* essential oil showed either partial or complete antifungal activity against plant and mushroom pathogenic fungi (*Sclerotinia sclerotiorum, Fusarium oxysporum, Phytophthora parasitica, Alternaria brassicae*, and *Cladobotryum mycophilum*) by the disk-diffusion assay; the inhibitory effect of essential oils was dose-dependent on the eight tested fungi enabling the determination of ED_{50} values for most of them.

Rapid antibacterial screening of essential oils using the agar diffusion technique is usually conducted. However, the lack of standardized methods makes direct comparison of results between studies difficult [57]. The problems related to oils dispersion and lipophilic constituents in aqueous media, and varying methods for determining numbers of viable bacteria remaining after the addition of the oil were the main causes of unreliability and inconsistent results obtained from disc diffusion, well diffusion, and agar dilution methods. Nevertheless, the broth dilution method, using emulsifier, seems to be the most accurate method for testing the antimicrobial activity of the hydrophobic and viscous essential oils.

4.2. Antioxidant Activity

The use of antioxidants is useful in the food industry to avoid rancidity and/or deterioration of foods [58] and also to prevent reactive oxygen species (ROS) formation, such as superoxide anion, hydrogen peroxide, and hydroxyl radicals. The ROS are capable of inducing lipid peroxidation, which may result in damage of membranes, lipids, lipoproteins, and induce DNA mutations that are linked to several diseases such as rheumatoid arthritis, atherosclerosis, ischemia, carcinogenesis, and aging [31]. The antioxidant properties of different *T. mastichina* plant extracts, essential oils, and pure compounds have been evaluated using a quite diverse number of in vitro assays, namely, those that evaluate lipid peroxidation, free radical scavenging ability, and chelating metal ions. In a study conducted by Miguel et al. [22], *T. mastichina* essential oil, as well as its main constituents (1,8-cineole and linalool), evaluated through the peroxide values expressed as percentage of inhibition, showed antioxidant activity higher than that shown by the synthetic antioxidant butylated hydroxytoluene (BHT). Nevertheless, the results cannot be explained only by some of its constituents because there may be synergistic or antagonistic effects among them. Due to the demonstrated antioxidant activity, essential oils of this species seem to be a good alternative to some synthetic antioxidants. Miguel et al. [25] conducted another study, in which *T. mastichina* essential oil was tested by a modified thiobarbituric acid-reactive substances (TBARS) assay in which the antioxidant capacity was evaluated measuring the ability to inhibit lipid peroxidation. In this modified TBARS assay egg yolk was used (as a lipid-rich medium) in the presence or absence of the radical inducer of lipid peroxidation, 2,2′-azobis (2 amidinopropane) dihydrochloride (ABAP). At concentrations of 62.5–500 mg/L of essential oil, the antioxidant capacity in the absence of the peroxyl radical inducer ABAP, presented values between 9.6% and 38.9% and in the presence of the peroxyl radical inducer, ABAP lower values were achieved (−19.5–16.0%). In 2007, the same research group compared the antioxidant activity of *T. mastichina* essential oils, over a concentration range (160–1000 mg/L), isolated from different populations. The highest differences in the antioxidant activities of these essential oils were observed at the lowest concentration tested (160 mg/L), in which the *T. mastichina* essential oil from Mértola showed the lowest activity (20%), whereas *T. mastichina* essential oil from Sesimbra exhibited the highest activity (42%). Similarly, for the highest concentration tested (1000 mg/L), *T. mastichina* essential oil from Mértola showed an antioxidant index of 59% and *T. mastichina* essential oil from Sesimbra presented an inhibition percentage of 79%. At a concentration of 1000 mg/L, the *T. mastichina* essential oils from Vila Real de Santo António and Sesimbra showed a higher ability to inhibit lipid oxidation than α-tocopherol and were within the same range of activity of BHA. In comparison with assays without ABAP, the presence of the radical inducer reduced the ability of *T. mastichina* essential oils to prevent oxidation, particularly at concentrations of 160, 800, and 1000 mg/L [30].

In a study conducted by Galego et al. [31], the antioxidant activity of *T. mastichina* essential oil was determined using different methods, such as TBARS, measuring the scavenging effect of the substances on the 2,2-diphenyl-1-picrylhydrazyl (DPPH) radicals, determining the ferric reducing antioxidant power (FRAP) based on the principle that substances, which have reduction potential, react with potassium ferricyanide (Fe^{3+}) to form potassium ferrocyanide (Fe^{2+}), which then reacts with ferric chloride to form ferric–ferrous complex, and also monitoring the chelating effect on ferrous ions (Fe^{2+}). The results showed that even at higher concentrations of *T. mastichina* essential oil (1000 mg/L), the antioxidant index was around 50% as observed with the TBARS method, while for the synthetic antioxidants, BHA and BHT, the antioxidant index was approximately 100%. In other methods, the difference between the activity of the essential oil and synthetic antioxidants BHA and BHT was more accentuated showing lesser antioxidant activity.

According to Bentes et al. [32], the antioxidant activities of *T. mastichina* essential oil were screened by five different methods: DPPH free radical scavenging, modified TBARS (using egg yolk as a lipid-rich medium) for measuring the inhibition of lipid peroxidation, FRAP assay based on the reduction of ferric iron (Fe^{3+}) to ferrous iron (Fe^{2+}) by antioxidants present in the samples, chelating activity on ferrous ions (Fe^{2+}), and superoxide anion radical scavenging. With the DPPH free radical scavenging assay, *T. mastichina* essential oil was almost totally ineffective as an antioxidant, in contrast to the remaining water-soluble hydrodistillation-aqueous phase extract that showed similar activity to that of α-tocopherol, particularly at higher concentrations (75 and 100 mg/L). This result suggests that a considerable portion of the antioxidant compounds were retained in the remaining hydrodistillation-aqueous water. In this study, the FRAP assay of *T. mastichina* essential oil was also compared. However, the correlation between DPPH and the FRAP assay activities was not as clear in the evaluation of different extracts. Whereas the hydrodistillation-aqueous phase extracts were the best antioxidants when evaluated by DPPH, the *T. mastichina* methanolic extract had a greater capacity for reducing Fe^{3+} than the hydrodistillation-aqueous phase extract. In addition, in the superoxide anion assay, only the hydrodistillation-aqueous phase and methanolic extracts were able to scavenge superoxide radicals, but the first ones were the most effective. The superoxide radical scavenging capacity of these extracts was even higher than that of the positive control (ascorbic acid, particularly at 500 mg/L). *T. mastichina* methanol extracts were powerful superoxide radical scavengers with 40–60% activity.

To determine the antioxidant activity in plant extracts, four different methods were used: the DPPH radical scavenging assay, the TBARS assay in brain homogenates, the FRAP assay of ferric iron (Fe^{3+}) to ferrous iron (Fe^{2+}), and the system β-carotene/linoleic acid based on the inhibition of β-carotene bleaching in the presence of linoleic acid radicals. The IC_{50} in the β-carotene/linoleic acid assay was achieved at a value of 0.90 mg/mL, in the DPPH radical scavenging assay, the value obtained was 0.69 mg/mL, the TBARS assay yielded a value of 0.43 mg/mL, and in the FRAP assay, the lowest value was obtained at 0.23 mg/mL [13].

As Asensio-S.-Manzanera et al. [33] reported, the DPPH and FRAP assays were used to evaluate the antioxidant activity on dry plant extracts of *T. mastichina* and dry residues after hydrodistillation. In the dry plant extracts, a scavenging effect was observed through the assays of DPPH (EC_{50} 0.59–1.78 mg/mL) and FRAP (EC_{50} 0.77–2.05 mg/mL). While for the hydrodistilled residue, the EC_{50} values were higher, showing less antioxidant activity. These results could be related to the higher phenol content in the dry extracts compared with the hydrodistilled residue, indicating that a considerable amount of antioxidants were retained in the remaining hydrodistilled water and *T. mastichina* essential oil.

Albano et al. [14], evaluated the antioxidant activity of *T. mastichina* essential oil and decoction water extract. The DPPH method was used with the essential oil and decoction water extract, while the scavenging activity of the superoxide anion radical was only used successfully with decoction water extract. For the DPPH method, the IC_{50} of the essential oil was much higher (6706.8 µg/mL) than that of the extract (4.2 µg/mL). The evaluation of the antioxidant activity by the superoxide anion scavenging activity method in the extract revealed that the IC_{50} of *T. mastichina* was 14.8 µg/mL. In this study, no correlation was detected between total phenols and removal of superoxide anion radicals.

The antioxidant activity of *T. mastichina* ethanolic extracts, obtained by the *Soxhlet* system or ultrasound method, was also evaluated through the β-carotene/linoleate model system, FRAP, DPPH radical scavenging, and iron and copper ion chelation. In general, good antioxidant activities were obtained; in particular, for the *T. mastichina* extract obtained by Soxhlet extraction, which was even comparable to the antioxidant standard red grape pomace [51].

In a study conducted by Delgado et al. [37], the DPPH and FRAP assays of the methanolic extracts and essential oils from 20 different populations were examined. All methanolic extracts and essential oils presented a similar concentration-dependent pattern, increasing the scavenging activity against DPPH with the increase in concentration. However, much higher DPPH radical scavenging abilities were obtained with the methanolic extracts than with the essential oils. The results of the inhibition of DPPH radicals ranged between 86.6% and 93.9% when the highest methanolic extract concentration was used. In contrast, the essential oils of *T. mastichina* presented a much lower DPPH radical scavenging activity, varying between 30.8% and 57.7%, even when the highest concentration was used. Relative to the reductive power assay, it was only determined for the methanolic extracts because it was not possible to perform the assay correctly with the essential oils. Interestingly, in this study, the authors tried to relate the antioxidant activity to their chemical composition. In fact, *T. mastichina* methanolic extracts were rich in rosmarinic acid, which is a polyphenol carboxylic acid, known for possessing antioxidant activity, whereas the essential oils had low contents of thymol, among others, that could explain the low antioxidant activity.

The antioxidant activity of 14 populations of *T. mastichina* methanolic extracts grown in an experimental plot was analyzed by DPPH and FRAP assays to determine antioxidant activity. Population means for DPPH activity ranges were 44–98 mg TE/g dry weight (DW), while FRAP antioxidant capacity was 52–115 mg of Trolox equivalents (TE)/g DW. In general, populations with high DPPH free radical scavenging assay also showed high FRAP antioxidant activity and vice-versa. In this study, the rosmarinic acid contributed mainly to the FRAP antioxidant capacity and total phenolic content, while the unknown compound (peak 3) contributed mainly to the DPPH assay. This study showed high intrapopulation variability and, above all, high interpopulation variability [9].

Chitosan edible films incorporated with *T. mastichina* essential oil (concentrations of 1% and 2%) were tested by DPPH and FRAP methods. The DPPH method demonstrated lower values (0.29 and 0.44 mg/g, respectively) compared to the FRAP method (2.21 and 3.99 mg/g, respectively) [54]. These investigators also evaluated the antioxidant activity but under different conditions. The concentrations used ranged from 0.23 to 30 mg/mL of *T. mastichina* essential oil for DPPH methods, 2,2'-azino-bis(3-ethylbenzothiazoline-6-sulfonic acid) (ABTS) radical cation scavenging activity assay, and FRAP assay, while the concentrations used ranged from 0.15 to 20 mg/mL of *T. mastichina* essential oil for the ferrous ion-chelating ability assay. The DPPH method showed the lowest IC_{50} values (3.11 mg/mL), followed by the ABTS radical scavenging method (3.73 mg/mL), followed by the ferrous ion-chelating activity (9.61 mg/mL). Relative to the FRAP assay, the results were 19.26 mg TE/mL. *T. mastichina* essential oil can be used in general by the food and pharmaceutical industry as a potential natural additive, replacing or reducing the use of chemical substances, since it has antioxidant properties [55].

In the study conducted by Delgado-Adámez et al. [44], the antioxidant activity of *T. mastichina* essential oil showed an antioxidant activity lower than 4 g Trolox/L determined by the ABTS radical method.

In another study, the antioxidant activities of *T. mastichina* essential oil and aqueous extract were evaluated. The essential oil in the β-carotene/linoleic acid method presented an IC_{50} of 0.622 mg/mL, while the aqueous extract presented values of 0.017 mg/mL activity. In the radical DPPH method, the IC_{50} values were 9.052 and 0.104 mg/mL for the essential oil and aqueous extract, respectively. Finally, for the FRAP test, the IC_{50} values presented the same pattern (18.687 and 0.109 mg/mL for the essential oil and aqueous extract, respectively). Thus, it was clear that the extract showed higher antioxidant activity than the essential oil due to the high content of phenolic compounds in extracts [43]. These results are in accordance with the study of Albano et al. [14], in which the extracts also showed higher scavenging ability. In a recent study from the same investigators, the antioxidant activity of *T. mastichina* essential oil was corroborated through the DPPH radical method, FRAP assay, and β-carotene/linoleic acid system. This activity could be related to the high content of oxygenated monoterpenes (85.9%), which act as radical scavengers and ferric reducers with high activity to protect the lipid substrate [2].

The antioxidant activities of *T. mastichina* essential oils have been evaluated using several complementary methods: oxygen radical absorbance capacity (ORAC) that measures the antioxidant capacity against peroxyl radicals, ABTS, DPPH, TBARS, and chelating power. The results obtained in the different methods were the following: ORAC method (163.5–735.1 mgTE/g), ABTS method (0.8–4.3 mg TE/g), DPPH assay (53.5–76.1 mg TE/kg), TBARS method (0.9–1.2 mg BHT equivalents (BHTE)/g), and chelating power (0.6–1.6 mg ethylenediaminetetraacetic acid equivalents (EDTAE)/g). In general, the different antioxidant activities were related to the individual constituents that were also tested in these assays [4].

Taghouti et al. [10] showed that the *T. mastichina* hydroethanolic extract presented a significantly higher scavenging activity of the ABTS radical cation ($\approx$1.48 mmol TE/g extract) than the aqueous decoction extract ($\approx$0.96 mmol TE/g extract). For the hydroxyl radical and nitric oxide radical scavenging assays, both extracts showed a similar capacity for scavenging. These screening assays showed that *T. mastichina* extracts may be a potential source of phenolic compounds with relevant antioxidant activities, inclusively using the decoction that is the traditional method of consumption.

4.3. Anticancer Activity

Dichloromethane and ethanol extracts from the aerial parts of *T. mastichina* were evaluated regarding anticancer activity on the colon cancer cell line HCT, presenting IC_{50} values of 2.8 and 12 μg/mL, respectively. Additionally, one constituent of the extract, ursolic acid, was found to have an IC_{50} value of 6.8 μg/mL, while the other compounds in the extract were inactive with an $IC_{50} >$ 20 μg/mL. A mixture of oleanolic and ursolic acid showed higher cytotoxicity than pure ursolic acid (IC_{50} of 2.8 μg/mL). The presence of these constituents identified by colon cancer cytotoxicity-guided activity indicates that *T. mastichina* extracts may have a protective effect against colon cancer [52].

The cytotoxic effects of *T. mastichina* essential oil were evaluated on human epithelioid cervix carcinoma (HeLa) and human histiocytic leukemia (U937) cell lines. A dose-dependent decrease in the survival of both tumor cell lines was observed after treatment with *T. mastichina* essential oil; this decrease was statistically significant at a concentration of 0.1% (*v/v*) *T. mastichina* essential oil [44].

The antiproliferative effect of *T. mastichina* essential oil against human breast carcinoma cell line MDA-MB-231 was also evaluated, showing an IC_{50} value of 108.5 μg/mL. From the literature, studies reported that antiproliferative activity could be related to 1,8-cineole content and are dependent on the monoterpenes content and their ability to affect oxidative stress [2]. It has been appointed that the preventive effect of essential oils on cancer disorders could be related to the promotion of cell cycle arrest, stimulating cell apoptosis and DNA repair mechanisms, inhibiting cancer cell proliferation, metastasis formation, and multidrug resistance, which makes them potential candidates for adjuvant anticancer therapeutic agents.

In a recent study, a *T. mastichina* aqueous decoction and hydroethanolic extract presented a dose and time-dependent inhibitory effect on the cell viability of a human colon adenocarcinoma (Caco-2) cell line and human hepatocellular carcinoma (HepG2) cell line. The hydroethanolic extract presented higher antiproliferative activity/cytotoxicity on Caco-2 cells (IC_{50}: 71.18 and 51.30 μg/mL after 24 and 48 h of incubation, respectively) than the aqueous decoction extracts (IC_{50}: 220.68 and 95.65 μg/mL after 24 and 48 h of incubation, respectively), which was correlated with its higher phenolic content. In addition, it should be noted that the Caco-2 cells were more sensitive than HepG2 cells, as it presented lower IC_{50} values for both extracts [10].

4.4. Antiviral Activity

T. mastichina essential oil was evaluated for its ability to reduce or eliminate the most emergent foodborne viruses in the food industry, evaluating its potential to inactivate two model nonenveloped viruses, a human norovirus surrogate, murine norovirus (MNV-1) with RNA genome, and a human adenovirus serotype 2 (HAdV-2) with DNA genome. However, no significant reduction of virus titers was observed when *T. mastichina* essential oil was used at different temperatures and times [59].

The influenza virus is associated with respiratory tract complications. Thus, in a study conducted by Choi [46], *T. mastichina* essential oil demonstrated interesting anti-influenza activity of reducing visible cytopathic effects of the A/WS/33 virus. This anti-influenza A/WS/33 activity of *T. mastichina* essential oil appeared to be associated with the constituent linalool.

4.5. Insecticidal and Insect Repellent Activity

In recent years, plants have been identified for their insecticidal or larvicidal properties and used to control insect vectors offering an economically viable and ecofriendly approach. One of the studies was based on exposing *Spodoptera littoralis* larvae to *T. mastichina* essential oil and verifying larval mortality. The essential oil was highly toxic with a lethal concentration at 50% (LC_{50}) of 19.3 mL/m^3 when applied by fumigation. After topical application, *T. mastichina* essential oil was also highly toxic with a LC_{50} of 0.034 µL/larvae [60]. The same investigator also evaluated the topical and fumigant activity of essentials oils on the adult house fly (*Musca domestica* L.) and determined a topical LD_{50} of 33 µg/fly and fumigant LD_{50} of 7.3 $µg/cm^3$ [61].

4.6. Anti-Alzheimer Activity

Alzheimer's disease is characterized by the loss of cholinergic neurons, leading to the progressive reduction of acetylcholine in the brain and cognitive impairment. Inhibition of acetylcholinesterase (AChE) and butyrylcholinesterase (BChE) has great potential in the treatment of Alzheimer's disease and special focus has been directed to these targets.

Albano et al. [14] reported the AChE inhibition activity of *T. mastichina* essential oil for the first time, with IC_{50} values of 45.8 µg/mL related to the 1,8-cineole constituent. However, the assessment of decoction water extracts was not possible for AChE inhibition capacity. Aazza et al. [40] also reported AChE inhibition activity of *T. mastichina* essential oil but poor activity was observed (IC_{50} of 0.1 mg/mL), despite the fact that the main constituent was also 1,8-cineole.

In another study, *T. mastichina* essential oil revealed a high ability to inhibit cholinesterase activity with an IC_{50} of 78.8 and 217.1 µg/mL for AChE and BChE, respectively. The aqueous extract also showed AChE activity, with IC_{50} values of 1003.6 and 779.1 µg/mL for AChE and BChE, respectively. These results suggest that the essential oils and extracts of this aromatic plant could be useful in the treatment of Alzheimer's disease [43].

Finally, *T. mastichina* essential oil was also reported to have AChE inhibition activity with an IC_{50} of 57.5–117.2 µg/mL. These results support the possible use of *T. mastichina* essential oils as an aid in the treatment of Alzheimer's disease or in its prevention for people with family precedents [4].

4.7. Anti-Inflammatory Activity

The 5-lipoxygenase (5-LOX) activity is an assay used to evaluate both anti-inflammatory and antioxidant activities.

Albano and Miguel [50] evaluated the 5-LOX activity of deodorized (divided into three fractions: the first one suspended in methanol; the second fractionated with water and chloroform; the third with chloroform), organic (diethyl ether, ethyl ether, and *n*-butanol), and aqueous extracts of *T. mastichina*. This study reported that lower IC_{50} values (12.2 µg/mL) were obtained for the water-insoluble deodorized chloroformic fraction of deodorized extract. In contrast, a higher IC_{50} was obtained using diethyl ether, with an IC_{50} of 62.5 µg/mL. Finally, for the deodorized fraction suspended in methanol and the aqueous extract, it was not possible to determine the IC_{50}. For most of these extracts in the 5-LOX assay, there was a correlation between phenol content and IC_{50} values, meaning that a higher phenolic content in the extract resulted in a lower 5-LOX activity.

The *T. mastichina* essential oil revealed anti-inflammatory activity, being able to inhibit 5-LOX, with an IC_{50} of 1084.5 µg/mL, whereas the extracts showed an IC_{50} of 66.7 µg/mL. The constituents of the *T. mastichina* essential oil have also been shown to be as effective as 5-LOX inhibitors, such as 1,8-cineole [14]. In another study, a similar IC_{50} of 0.73 mg/mL for the *T. mastichina* essential oil was also reported [40].

T. mastichina essential oil was reported to present 5-LOX inhibition activity that was expressed as the degree of inhibition (DI (%)). *T. mastichina* essential oil, at a concentration of 150 µg/mL, showed a DI between 40.8% and 56.7% [4].

4.8. α-Amylase and α-Glucosidase Activity

Inhibition of α-amylase and α-glucosidase activity was also studied for *T. mastichina* essential oil, with reported IC_{50} values of 4.6 and 0.1 mg/mL, respectively [40]. The inhibition of these enzymes could result in the slow and prolonged release of glucose into circulation and, consequently, the retardation of sudden hyperglycemia after the consumption of a meal.

5. Conclusions

T. mastichina essential oil was obtained mainly by hydrodistillation, consisting mainly of 1,8-cineole (eucalyptol), linalool, limonene, camphor, borneol, and α-terpineol, as well as other volatile compounds. Conversely, despite being lesser studied, *T. mastichina* extracts using different solvents were also characterized, being composed of 2-methoxysalicylic acid, 3-methoxysalicylic acid apigenin, caffeic acid, chlorogenic acid, kaempferol, luteolin, quercetin, rosmarinic acid, sakuranetin, sterubin, salvianolic acid derivatives, and hexoside and glycoside derivatives, among other constituents.

T. mastichina has been traditionally used as a flavoring for food and in the treatment of health conditions due to its antiseptic, digestive, antirheumatic, and antitussive effects. Regarding the biological activities reported in different studies, *T. mastichina* essential oil and/or extracts also have antibacterial, antifungal, antioxidant, insecticide, repellent, antiviral, anti-Alzheimer, and anti-inflammatory activities. The antibacterial and antifungal activities of *T. mastichina* are an important characteristic for the use of these plants for production as natural antimicrobial agents that could be used as preservatives against diverse Gram-positive and negative bacteria and fungi. In addition, the antioxidant activity of *T. mastichina* was also largely explored through different assays, representing an interesting alternative to synthetic antioxidants. Although little attention has been paid to other activities, such as insecticide, repellent, antiviral, anti-Alzheimer, and anti-inflammatory activities, *T. mastichina* also showed interesting potential for these activities. In some studies, these effects were related to the composition and were tested to understand if some compounds were primarily responsible for the observed activity.

In conclusion, attending to its traditional use and reported biological activities, *T. mastichina* essential oil and/or extracts could present a noteworthy role as preservatives and salt substitutes in food industries, as perfumes in cosmetic industry, and as sources of bioactive compounds for pharmaceutical industries.

Author Contributions: Conceptualization, M.R., A.R.T.S.A.; writing—original draft preparation, M.R., A.C.L., F.V., M.F.; writing—review and editing, G.A., M.P.R., P.C., A.R.T.S.A.; funding acquisition, M.R., M.P.R., P.C., A.R.T.S.A. All authors have read and agreed to the published version of the manuscript.

Acknowledgments: The authors would like to thank to Conceição Matos from Planalto Dourado™ Essential Oils Enterprise for kindly providing the photos of *Thymus mastichina* from Freixedas, Guarda, Portugal.

References

1. Utad, J.B. Ficha da Espécie *Thymus mastichina*. Available online: https://jb.utad.pt/especie/Thymus_mastichina (accessed on 23 July 2020).
2. Arantes, S.M.; Piçarra, A.; Guerreiro, M.; Salvador, C.; Candeias, F.; Caldeira, A.T.; Martins, M.R. Toxicological and pharmacological properties of essential oils of *Calamintha nepeta*, *Origanum virens* and *Thymus mastichina* of Alentejo (Portugal). *Food Chem. Toxicol.* **2019**, *133*, 110747. [CrossRef] [PubMed]
3. Póvoa, O.; Delgado, F. Tipos e Espécies de PAM. Guia Para a Produção de Plantas Aromáticas e Medicinais em Portugal. 2015. Available online: http://epam.pt/guia/tipos-e-especies-de-pam/ (accessed on 18 September 2020).
4. Cutillas, A.-B.B.; Carrasco, A.; Martinez-Gutierrez, R.; Tomas, V.; Tudela, J. *Thymus mastichina* L. essential oils from Murcia (Spain): Composition and antioxidant, antienzymatic and antimicrobial bioactivities. *PLoS ONE* **2018**, *13*, e0190790. [CrossRef] [PubMed]
5. Girón, V.; Garnatje, T.; Vallès, J.; Pérez-Collazos, E.; Catalán, P.; Valdés, B. Geographical distribution of diploid and tetraploid cytotypes of *Thymus* sect. *mastichina* (Lamiaceae) in the Iberian Peninsula, genome size and evolutionary implications. *Folia Geobot.* **2012**, *47*, 441–460.
6. Méndez-Tovar, I.; Martín, H.; Santiago, Y.; Ibeas, A.; Herrero, B.; Asensio-S-Manzanera, M.C. Variation in morphological traits among *Thymus mastichina* (L.) L. populations. *Genet. Resour. Crop Evol.* **2015**, *62*, 1257–1267. [CrossRef]
7. Miguel, G.; Guerrero, C.; Rodrigues, H.; Brito, J.; Venâncio, F.; Tavares, R.; Duarte, F. Effect of substrate on the essential oils composition of *Thymus mastichina* (L.) L. subsp. *mastichina* collected in Sesimbra region (Portugal). In *Natural Products in the New Millennium: Prospects and Industrial Application*; Springer: Dordrecht, The Netherlands, 2002; pp. 143–148.
8. Miguel, M.G.; Duarte, F.L.; Venâncio, F.; Tavares, R. Comparison of the main components of the essential oils from flowers and leaves of *Thymus mastichina* (L.) L. ssp. *mastichina* collected at different regions of portugal. *J. Essent. Oil Res.* **2004**, *16*, 323–327.
9. Méndez-Tovar, I.; Sponza, S.; Asensio-S-Manzanera, M.C.; Novak, J. Contribution of the main polyphenols of *Thymus mastichina* subsp: *Mastichina* to its antioxidant properties. *Ind. Crops Prod.* **2015**, *66*, 291–298. [CrossRef]
10. Taghouti, M.; Martins-Gomes, C.; Schäfer, J.; Santos, J.A.; Bunzel, M.; Nunes, F.M.; Silva, A.M. Chemical characterization and bioactivity of extracts from *Thymus mastichina*: A *Thymus* with a distinct salvianolic acid composition. *Antioxidants* **2019**, *9*, 34. [CrossRef]
11. Barros, L.; Carvalho, A.M.; Ferreira, I.C.F.R. From famine plants to tasty and fragrant spices: Three Lamiaceae of general dietary relevance in traditional cuisine of Trás-os-Montes (Portugal). *LWT Food Sci. Technol.* **2011**, *44*, 543–548. [CrossRef]
12. Asensio-S-Manzanera, M.C.; Mendez, I.; Santiago, Y.; Martin, H.; Herrero, B. Phenolic compounds variability in hydrodistilled residue of Thymus mastichina. In *VII Congreso Iberico de Agroingeniería y Ciencias Hortícolas: Innovar y Producir Para el Futuro*; UPM: Madrid, Spain, 2014; pp. 2086–2091.
13. Barros, L.; Heleno, S.A.; Carvalho, A.M.; Ferreira, I.C.F.R. Lamiaceae often used in Portuguese folk medicine as a source of powerful antioxidants: Vitamins and phenolics. *LWT Food Sci. Technol.* **2010**, *43*, 544–550. [CrossRef]
14. Albano, S.M.; Sofia Lima, A.; Graça Miguel, M.; Pedro, L.G.; Barroso, J.G.; Figueiredo, A.C. Antioxidant, anti-5-lipoxygenase and antiacetylcholinesterase activities of essential oils and decoction waters of some aromatic plants. *Rec. Nat. Prod.* **2012**, *6*, 35–48.
15. Salgueiro, L.R.; Vila, R.; Tomàs, X.; Cañigueral, S.; Da Cunha, A.P.; Adzet, T. Composition and variability of the essential oils of *Thymus* species from section *mastichina* from Portugal. *Biochem. Syst. Ecol.* **1997**, *25*, 659–672. [CrossRef]
16. Faleiro, L.; Miguel, G.M.; Guerrero, C.A.C.; Brito, J.M.C. Antimicrobial activity of essential oils of *Rosmarinus officinalis* L., *Thymus mastichina* (L) L. ssp *Mastichina* and *Thymus albicans* Hofmanns & link. *Acta Hortic.* **1999**, *501*, 45–48.

17. Jiménez-Carmona, M.M.; Ubera, J.L.; Luque De Castro, M.D. Comparison of continuous subcritical water extraction and hydrodistillation of marjoram essential oil. *J. Chromatogr. A* **1999**, *855*, 625–632. [CrossRef]

18. Miguel, M.G.; Guerrero, C.A.C.; Brito, J.M.C.; Venâncio, F.; Tavares, R.; Martins, A.; Duarte, F. Essential oils from *Thymus mastichina* (L.) L. ssp. *mastichina* and *Thymus albicans* Hoffmanns & link. *Acta Hortic.* **1999**, *500*, 59–63.

19. Miguel, M.G.; Duarte, F.; Venâncio, F.; Tavares, R. Chemical composition of the essential oils from *Thymus mastichina* over a day period. *Acta Hortic.* **2002**, *597*, 87–90. [CrossRef]

20. Miguel, M.G.; Duarte, F.; Venâncio, F.; Tavares, R.; Guerrero, C.; Martins, H.; Carrasco, J. Changes of the chemical composition of the essential oil of portuguese *Thymus mastichina* in the course of two vegetation cycles. *Acta Hortic.* **2002**, *576*, 83–86. [CrossRef]

21. Faleiro, M.L.; Miguel, M.G.; Ladeiro, F.; Venâncio, F.; Tavares, R.; Brito, J.C.; Figueiredo, A.C.; Barroso, J.G.; Pedro, L.G. Antimicrobial activity of essential oils isolated from Portuguese endemic species of *Thymus*. *Lett. Appl. Microbiol.* **2003**, *36*, 35–40. [CrossRef]

22. Miguel, M.G.; Figueiredo, A.C.; Costa, M.M.; Martins, D.; Duarte, J.; Barroso, J.G.; Pedro, L.G. Effect of the volatile constituents isolated from *Thymus albicans*, *Th. mastichina*, *Th. carnosus* and *Thymbra capitata* in sunflower oil. *Nahr. Food* **2003**, *47*, 397–402. [CrossRef]

23. Miguel, M.G.; Guerrero, C.; Rodrigues, H.; Brito, J.; Duarte, F.; Venâncio, F.; Tavares, R. Essential oils of Portuguese *Thymus mastichina* (L.) L. subsp. *mastichina* grown on different substrates and harvested on different dates. *J. Hortic. Sci. Biotechnol.* **2003**, *78*, 355–358.

24. Miguel, M.G.; Guerrero, C.; Rodrigues, H.; Brito, J.C.; Duarte, F.; Venâncio, F.; Tavares, R. Main components of the essential oils from wild portuguese *Thymus mastichina* (L.) L. ssp. *mastichina* in different developmental stages or under culture conditions. *J. Essent. Oil Res.* **2004**, *16*, 111–114. [CrossRef]

25. Miguel, G.; Simões, M.; Figueiredo, A.C.; Barroso, J.G.; Pedro, L.G.; Carvalho, L. Composition and antioxidant activities of the essential oils of *Thymus caespititius*, *Thymus camphoratus* and *Thymus mastichina*. *Food Chem.* **2004**, *86*, 183–188. [CrossRef]

26. Pina-Vaz, C.; Rodrigues, A.G.; Pinto, E.; Costa-de-Oliveira, S.; Tavares, C.; Salgueiro, L.; Cavaleiro, C.; Gonçalves, M.J.; Martinez-de-Oliveira, J. Antifungal activity of *Thymus* oils and their major compounds. *J. Eur. Acad. Dermatol. Venereol.* **2004**, *18*, 73–78. [CrossRef] [PubMed]

27. Moldão-Martins, M.; Beirão-da-Costa, S.; Neves, C.; Cavaleiro, C.; Salgueiro, L.; Luísa Beirão-da-Costa, M. Olive oil flavoured by the essential oils of *Mentha × piperita* and *Thymus mastichina* L. *Food Qual. Prefer.* **2004**, *15*, 447–452. [CrossRef]

28. Miguel, M.G.; Falcato-Simões, M.; Figueiredo, A.C.; Barroso, J.M.G.; Pedro, L.G.; Carvalho, L.M. Evaluation of the antioxidant activity of *Thymbra capitata*, *Thymus mastichina* and *Thymus camphoratus* essential oils. *J. Food Lipids* **2005**, *12*, 181–197.

29. Peñalver, P.; Huerta, B.; Borge, C.; Astorga, R.; Romero, R.; Perea, A. Antimicrobial activity of five essential oils against origin strains of the Enterobacteriaceae family. *APMIS* **2005**, *113*, 1–6. [CrossRef]

30. Miguel, M.G.; Costa, L.A.; Figueiredo, A.C.; Barroso, J.G.; Pedro, L.G. Assessment of the antioxidant ability of *Thymus albicans*, *Th. mastichina*, *Th. camphoratus* and *Th. carnosus* essential oils by TBARS and Micellar Model systems. *Nat. Prod. Commun.* **2007**, *2*, 399–406.

31. Galego, L.; Almeida, V.; Gonçalves, V.; Costa, M.; Monteiro, I.; Matos, F.; Miguel, G. Antioxidant activity of the essential oils of *Thymbra capitata*, *Origanum vulgare*, *Thymus mastichina*, and *Calamintha baetica*. *Acta Hortic.* **2008**, *765*, 325–334. [CrossRef]

32. Bentes, J.; Miguel, M.G.; Monteiro, I.; Costa, M.; Figueiredo, A.C.; Barroso, J.G.; Pedro, L.G. Antioxidant activities of essential oils and extracts of Portuguese *Thymbra capitata* and *Thymus mastichina*. *Ital. J. Food Sci.* **2009**, *XVIII*, 1–125.

33. Asensio-S-Manzanera, M.C.; Martín, H.; Sanz, M.A.; Herrero, B. Antioxidant activity of *Lavandula latifolia*, *Salvia lavandulifolia* and *Thymus mastichina* collected in Spain. *Acta Hortic.* **2011**, *925*, 281–290. [CrossRef]

34. Fernández-Pan, I.; Royo, M.; Ignacio Maté, J. Antimicrobial activity of whey protein isolate edible films with essential oils against food spoilers and foodborne pathogens. *J. Food Sci.* **2012**, *77*, M383–M390.

35. Ballester-Costa, C.; Sendra, E.; Fernández-López, J.; Pérez-Álvarez, J.A.; Viuda-Martos, M. Chemical composition and in vitro antibacterial properties of essential oils of four *Thymus* species from organic growth. *Ind. Crops Prod.* **2013**, *50*, 304–311. [CrossRef]

36. Faria, J.M.S.; Barbosa, P.; Bennett, R.N.; Mota, M.; Figueiredo, A.C. Bioactivity against *Bursaphelenchus*

xylophilus: Nematotoxics from essential oils, essential oils fractions and decoction waters. *Phytochemistry* **2013**, *94*, 220–228. [CrossRef] [PubMed]

37. Delgado, T.; Marinero, P.; Asensio-S-Manzanera, M.C.; Asensio, C.; Herrero, B.; Pereira, J.A.; Ramalhosa, E. Antioxidant activity of twenty wild Spanish *Thymus mastichina* L. populations and its relation with their chemical composition. *LWT Food Sci. Technol.* **2014**, *57*, 412–418. [CrossRef]

38. Miguel, M.G.; Gago, C.; Antunes, M.D.; Megías, C.; Cortés-Giraldo, I.; Vioque, J.; Lima, A.S.; Figueiredo, A.C. Antioxidant and antiproliferative activities of the essential oils from *Thymbra capitata* and *Thymus* species grown in Portugal. *Evid. Based Complement. Altern. Med.* **2015**, *2015*, 1–8.

39. Méndez-Tovar, I.; Sponza, S.; Asensio-S-Manzanera, C.; Schmiderer, C.; Novak, J. Volatile fraction differences for Lamiaceae species using different extraction methodologies. *J. Essent. Oil Res.* **2015**, *27*, 497–505. [CrossRef]

40. Aazza, S.; El-Guendouz, S.; Miguel, M.G.; Dulce Antunes, M.; Leonor Faleiro, M.; Isabel Correia, A.; Cristina Figueiredo, A. Antioxidant, anti-inflammatory and anti-hyperglycaemic activities of essential oils from *Thymbra capitata, Thymus albicans, Thymus caespititius, Thymus carnosus, Thymus lotocephalus* and *Thymus mastichina* from Portugal. *Nat. Prod. Commun.* **2016**, *11*, 1029–1038.

41. Fraternale, D.; Giamperi, L.; Ricci, D. Chemical Composition and antifungal activity of essential oil obtained from in vitro plants of *Thymus mastichina* L. *J. Essent. Oil Res.* **2003**, *15*, 278–281.

42. Ibáñez, M.D.; Blázquez, M.A. Herbicidal value of essential oils from oregano-like flavour species. *Food Agric. Immunol.* **2017**, *28*, 1168–1180. [CrossRef]

43. Arantes, S.; Piçarra, A.; Candeias, F.; Caldeira, A.T.; Martins, M.R.; Teixeira, D. Antioxidant activity and cholinesterase inhibition studies of four flavouring herbs from Alentejo. *Nat. Prod. Res.* **2017**, *31*, 2183–2187. [CrossRef]

44. Delgado-Adámez, J.; Garrido, M.; Bote, M.E.; Fuentes-Pérez, M.C.; Espino, J.; Martín-Vertedor, D. Chemical composition and bioactivity of essential oils from flower and fruit of *Thymbra capitata* and *Thymus* species. *J. Food Sci. Technol.* **2017**, *54*, 1857–1865.

45. Vieira, M.; Bessa, L.J.; Martins, M.R.; Arantes, S.; Teixeira, A.P.S.; Mendes, Â.; Martins da Costa, P.; Belo, A.D.F. Chemical composition, antibacterial, antibiofilm and synergistic properties of essential oils from *Eucalyptus globulus* Labill. and seven mediterranean aromatic plants. *Chem. Biodivers.* **2017**, *14*, e1700006. [CrossRef] [PubMed]

46. Choi, H.-J. Chemical constituents of essential oils possessing anti-influenza A/WS/33 virus activity. *Osong Public Health Res. Perspect.* **2018**, *9*, 348–353. [CrossRef] [PubMed]

47. Diánez, F.; Santos, M.; Parra, C.; Navarro, M.J.; Blanco, R.; Gea, F.J. Screening of antifungal activity of 12 essential oils against eight pathogenic fungi of vegetables and mushroom. *Lett. Appl. Microbiol.* **2018**, *67*, 400–410. [CrossRef] [PubMed]

48. Queiroga, M.C.; Pinto Coelho, M.; Arantes, S.M.; Potes, M.E.; Martins, M.R. Antimicrobial activity of essential oils of Lamiaceae aromatic spices towards sheep mastitis-causing *Staphylococcus aureus* and *Staphylococcus epidermidis*. *J. Essent. Oil Bear. Plants* **2018**, *21*, 1155–1165. [CrossRef]

49. Salehi, B.; Mishra, A.P.; Shukla, I.; Sharifi-Rad, M.; del Mar Contreras, M.; Segura-Carretero, A.; Fathi, H.; Nasrabadi, N.N.; Kobarfard, F.; Sharifi-Rad, J. Thymol, thyme, and other plant sources: Health and potential uses. *Phyther. Res.* **2018**, *32*, 1688–1706. [CrossRef]

50. Albano, S.M.; Miguel, M.G. Biological activities of extracts of plants grown in Portugal. *Ind. Crops Prod.* **2011**, *33*, 338–343. [CrossRef]

51. Sánchez-Vioque, R.; Polissiou, M.; Astraka, K.; de los Mozos-Pascual, M.; Tarantilis, P.; Herraiz-Peñalver, D.; Santana-Méridas, O. Polyphenol composition and antioxidant and metal chelating activities of the solid residues from the essential oil industry. *Ind. Crops Prod.* **2013**, *49*, 150–159. [CrossRef]

52. Gordo, J.; Máximo, P.; Cabrita, E.; Lourenço, A.; Oliva, A.; Almeida, J.; Filipe, M.; Cruz, P.; Barcia, R.; Santos, M.; et al. *Thymus mastichina*: Chemical constituents and their anti-cancer activity. *Nat. Prod. Commun.* **2012**, *7*, 1491–1494.

53. Giner, M.J.; Vegara, S.; Funes, L.; Martí, N.; Saura, D.; Micol, V.; Valero, M. Antimicrobial activity of food-compatible plant extracts and chitosan against naturally occurring micro-organisms in tomato juice. *J. Sci. Food Agric.* **2012**, *92*, 1917–1923. [CrossRef]

54. Ballester-Costa, C.; Sendra, E.; Fernández-López, J.; Viuda-Martos, M. Evaluation of the antibacterial and antioxidant activities of chitosan edible films incorporated with organic essential oils obtained from four

Thymus species. *J. Food Sci. Technol.* **2016**, *53*, 3374–3379. [CrossRef]

55. Ballester-Costa, C.; Sendra, E.; Viuda-Martos, M. Assessment of antioxidant and antibacterial properties on meat homogenates of essential oils obtained from four *Thymus* species achieved from organic growth. *Foods* **2017**, *6*, 59. [CrossRef] [PubMed]

56. Leal, F.; Coelho, A.C.; Soriano, T.; Alves, C.; Matos, M. Fungicide activity of *Thymus mastichina* and *Mentha rotundifolia* in plants in vitro. *J. Med. Food* **2013**, *16*, 273. [CrossRef]

57. Hood, J.R.; Wilkinson, J.M.; Cavanagh, H.M.A. Evaluation of common antibacterial screening methods utilized in essential oil research. *J. Essent. Oil Res.* **2003**, *15*, 428–433. [CrossRef]

58. Figueiredo, A.; Barroso, J.G.; Pedro, L.G.; Salgueiro, L.; Miguel, M.G.; Faleiro, M.L. Portuguese *Thymbra* and *Thymus* species volatiles: Chemical composition and biological activities. *Curr. Pharm. Des.* **2008**, *14*, 3120–3140. [CrossRef]

59. Kovač, K.; Diez-Valcarce, M.; Raspor, P.; Hernández, M.; Rodríguez-Lázaro, D. Natural plant essential oils do not inactivate non-enveloped enteric viruses. *Food Environ. Virol.* **2012**, *4*, 209–212.

60. Pavela, R. Insecticidal activity of some essential oils against larvae of *Spodoptera littoralis*. *Fitoterapia* **2005**, *76*, 691–696. [CrossRef] [PubMed]

61. Pavela, R. Insecticidal properties of several essential oils on the house fly (*Musca domestica* L.). *Phyther. Res.* **2008**, *22*, 274–278. [CrossRef] [PubMed]

13

Screening of Bacterial Quorum Sensing Inhibitors in a *Vibrio fischeri* LuxR-Based Synthetic Fluorescent *E. coli* Biosensor

Xiaofei Qin [1,2], Celina Vila-Sanjurjo [2,3], Ratna Singh [4], Bodo Philipp [5] and Francisco M. Goycoolea [2,6,*] ⓘ

[1] Department of Bioengineering, Zhuhai Campus of Zunyi Medical University, Zhuhai 519041, China; iamxfqin@njtech.edu.cn

[2] Laboratory of Nanobiotechnology, Institute of Plant Biology and Biotechnology, University of Münster, Schlossplatz 8, D-48143 Münster, Germany; celina.vila@usc.es

[3] Department of Pharmacology, Pharmacy and Pharmaceutical Technology, University of Santiago de Compostela, Campus Vida, s/n, 15782 Santiago de Compostela, Spain

[4] Laboratory of Molecular Phytopathology and Renewable Resources, Institute of Plant Biology and Biotechnology, University of Münster, Schlossplatz 8, D-48143 Münster, Germany; singhr@uni-muenster.de

[5] Institute of Molecular Microbiology and Biotechnology, University of Münster, Corrensstraße 3, D-48149 Münster, Germany; bodo.philipp@uni-muenster.de

[6] School of Food Science and Nutrition, University of Leeds, Leeds LS2 9JT, UK

[*] Correspondence: F.M.Goycoolea@leeds.ac.uk

Abstract: A library of 23 pure compounds of varying structural and chemical characteristics was screened for their quorum sensing (QS) inhibition activity using a synthetic fluorescent *Escherichia coli* biosensor that incorporates a modified version of lux regulon of *Vibrio fischeri*. Four such compounds exhibited QS inhibition activity without compromising bacterial growth, namely, phenazine carboxylic acid (PCA), 2-heptyl-3-hydroxy-4-quinolone (PQS), 1H-2-methyl-4-quinolone (MOQ) and genipin. When applied at 50 μM, these compounds reduced the QS response of the biosensor to 33.7% ± 2.6%, 43.1% ± 2.7%, 62.2% ± 6.3% and 43.3% ± 1.2%, respectively. A series of compounds only showed activity when tested at higher concentrations. This was the case of caffeine, which, when applied at 1 mM, reduced the QS to 47% ± 4.2%. In turn, capsaicin, caffeic acid phenethyl ester (CAPE), furanone and polygodial exhibited antibacterial activity when applied at 1mM, and reduced the bacterial growth by 12.8% ± 10.1%, 24.4% ± 7.0%, 91.4% ± 7.4% and 97.5% ± 3.8%, respectively. Similarly, we confirmed that *trans*-cinnamaldehyde and vanillin, when tested at 1 mM, reduced the QS response to 68.3% ± 4.9% and 27.1% ± 7.4%, respectively, though at the expense of concomitantly reducing cell growth by 18.6% ± 2.5% and 16% ± 2.2%, respectively. Two QS natural compounds of *Pseudomonas aeruginosa*, namely PQS and PCA, and the related, synthetic compounds MOQ, 1H-3-hydroxyl-4-quinolone (HOQ) and 1H-2-methyl-3-hydroxyl-4-quinolone (MHOQ) were used in molecular docking studies with the binding domain of the QS receptor TraR as a target. We offer here a general interpretation of structure-function relationships in this class of compounds that underpins their potential application as alternatives to antibiotics in controlling bacterial virulence.

Keywords: compounds screening; quorum sensing inhibition; antibacterial; molecular docking

1. Introduction

Bacteria communicate with secreted chemical signalling molecules that act as autoinducers in a phenomenon known as quorum sensing (QS) which allows them to fulfil a variety of functions, including bioluminescence, virulence and biofilm formation, among others [1]. In the case of Gram-negative bacteria, the autoinducer molecules belong mostly to the family of the acyl homoserine lactones (AHLs), which accumulate to particular threshold concentrations once the population of cells grow to sufficient [2,3].

AHL synthesis relies on the synthase LuxI family, while AHL reception depends on LuxR-type transcriptional regulators, which include the nominal LuxR protein from *Vibrio fischeri*, but also the related TraR and LasR from *Agrobacterium tumefaciens* and *P. aeruginosa*, among others. These act as transcriptional activators or repressors of the target QS genes [4–7]. The canonical LuxR protein from *V. fischeri* comprises two domains. The N-terminal domain is responsible of AHL binding and also can mediate protein dimerisation [8]. In contrast, the C-terminal domain contains a helix-turn-helix (HTH) motif, which is thought to make sequence-specific binding to DNA and to drive RNA polymerase binding to target promoters [9]. Much research has been conducted in recent years on mutant- LuxR-type proteins [10–16]. Among these, the TraR protein from *Agrobacterium tumefaciens* has been thoroughly studied, and its crystal structure has been solved, revealing the presence of the above mentioned two functional domains. In TraR, the N-terminal domain binds to N-3-oxooctanoyl-L-homoserine lactone (OOHL), and the C-terminal domain interacts with the DNA binding domain of the tra box [7,17]. TraR is a dimer in the presence of OOHL, and the TraR-OOHL-*tra* DNA ternary complex can be used as a prototype for the large family of AHL-induced transcription activators. The LasR protein of *Pseudomonas aeruginosa* shares 70% homology with TraR of *A. tumefaciens*, and the 3D model of the TraR active site closely resembles the X-ray structure of the LasR active site [18]. The signal binding sites in both apo-proteins are highly accessible, so TraR constitutes a useful model receptor which allows predicting the ability of putative QS inhibitors (QSIs) to block QS-based mechanisms in the human pathogen *P. aeruginosa* [19,20].

The development of strategies aimed to block or disrupt QS is gaining momentum. These efforts are directed to inhibit the production of virulence factors at the site of infection by dismantling the collective power of bacterial pathogens, an approach known as quorum quenching (QQ) or QS inhibition [21,22]. In the last years, QSIs have attracted significant attention from the scientific community and are considered as potential weapons and new generation antimicrobials in the therapeutic arsenal against infections caused by drug-resistant bacteria [23–25].

There are three major approaches to target bacterial QS using QSIs: (i) destruction of the signalling molecule, (ii) inhibition of signal production, and (iii) inhibition of the receptor [26]. To the date, most of the literature on QQ is centred in the investigation of AHL-degrading enzymes [27] and more abundantly, in QSIs that targeted to specific QS regulators of diverse species [26]. These QSIs may structurally resemble the natural ligand or may on the contrary, have an entirely different molecular structure [28,29]. QSIs include compounds of diverse sources, both natural and synthetic, and include fungal metabolites, plant substances, antibiotics, and synthetic derivatives of QS autoinducers or natural antagonists, to name a few [26–29]. Identification of QSIs is commonly performed through the screening of compound libraries and biosensor-based analysis of the QS response alone or combined with computer modelling analysis. These methods have allowed expanding the catalogue of available QSIs, which includes a variety of AHL analogues, brominated furanones, polyphenolic compounds and polypeptides [23,26,30–32].

Regarding computer modelling, docking-based screening of candidate QSIs is normally carried out by using a genetic algorithm on a library of 2344 compounds and calculates their binding free energy, hence identifying those candidates able to interact with target conserved residues in the binding site of a LuxR-type model receptor [33]. In-silico screening of ligand databases has thus become an important strategy towards the discovery of novel QSIs. GRID molecular interaction fields (GRID-MIFs) is accepted as an efficient method in virtual screening of candidate molecules which target protein binding sites. It is a computational procedure for detecting energetically favourable binding regions in proteins and small molecule drugs of known 3D structure. The energies are calculated using the electrostatic, hydrogen-bond, Lennard Jones, and entropic interactions of chemically selective probes with the chosen biological target. The program works by defining a three-dimensional grid of points that contains the chosen substrate binding site. The above mentioned calculations are repeated for each node in the three-dimensional grid and for each probe being considered. The results of these calculations are a collection of three-dimensional matrices, one for each probe-target interaction. A detailed description of the GRID program, the force field parameters, and details of calculations can be found elsewhere [34,35]. Briefly, a grid is projected inside the protein regions and cavities of interest. The probes are functional groups that can move stepwise from grid point to grid point. The calculated interaction energies of the probes are computed to create the MIFs, which represents the potential interaction of the protein with a particular chemical group. GRID-MIFs is considered as a high-throughput screening method to virtually analyse protein-ligand interactions [36,37].

In this study, we have screened 23 potential QS inhibition compounds, representing five groups according to their chemical structures. We found that seven of them were potent, dose-dependent inhibitors of the *V. fisheri* LuxR-based system expressed on recombinant *E. coli* biosensor cells, including two unprecedented ones. Another five compounds have shown antibacterial activity, while the remaining eleven compounds were inert at the tested doses. Moreover, we performed in silico GRID-MIFs-based computational molecular docking on the 3D crystal structure of TraR that allowed us to propose a hypothesis on the disparate effects observed experimentally for compounds of chemically related structure. We propose that our biosensor- and docking-based approaches have a high potential for drug designing purposes.

2. Results

2.1. Screening a Panel of Potential Quorum Sensing Inhibitors

We selected a panel of 23 pure compounds with the potential to act as inhibitors of LuxR-AHL-mediated QS. These comprised the following groups, namely: Group (1) lactone analogues, Group (2) aromatic ring structures, Group (3) heterocyclic compounds, Group (4) *Pseudomonas spp-* relevant compounds, and Group (5) structurally unrelated compounds. Figure 1 shows the chemical structures of the cognate AHL molecules of LuxR and TraR regulators, namely *N*-3-oxohexanoyl-L-homoserine lactone (3OC$_6$HSL) and OOHL, respectively.

All 23 compounds were tested using the *E. coli* Top10 pSB1A3-BBaT9002 biosensor, which expresses a synthetic version of the *lux* regulon of *V. fischeri* and produces a fluorescent as a response to external (3OC6HSL) [38]. The rate of the density-normalised fluorescence of the *E. coli* biosensor as a function of the 3OC6HSL concentration displays a Hill behaviour, with a k_{Hill} of $7.48 \times 10^{-10} \pm 9.03 \times 10^{-11}$ M. At 3OC6HSL concentrations higher than 1×10^{-9} M, the fluorescence response is saturated, while the fluorescence levels are undetectable at a 3OC6HSL concentration of 1×10^{-10} M [38]. We evaluated the QS inhibitory effect of our panel of compounds by their ability to reduce the fluorescence response of this *E. coli* biosensor without compromising cell growth.

214

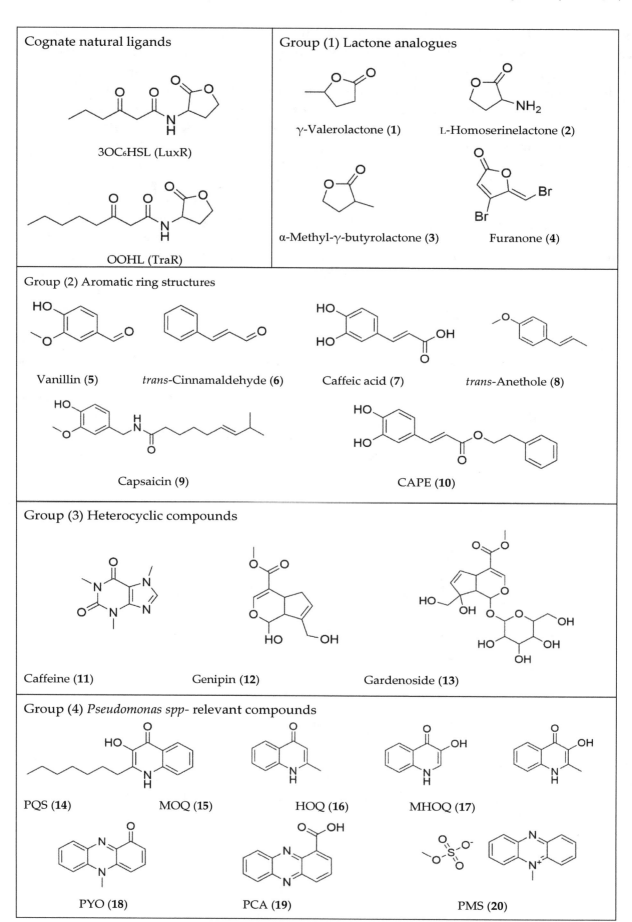

Figure 1. *Cont.*

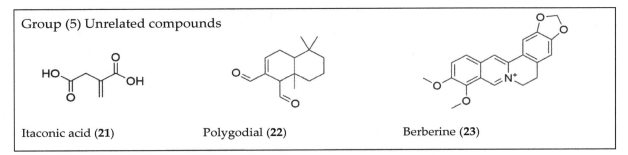

Figure 1. Chemical structures of studied compounds. Group (1) lactone analogues, Group (2) aromatic ring structures, Group (3) heterocyclic compounds, Group (4) *Pseudomonas* spp.-relevant compounds, and Group (5) structurally unrelated compounds. In the Figure are also shown the structure of natural LuxR and TraR ligands, namely 3OC6HSL and OOHL. Other details of the series of compounds are given in Materials and Methods section.

Screening of the 23 compounds revealed that they could be classified into three main categories based on their QS inhibition activity, relative to their effects on bacterial growth. The first category refers to compounds that have not shown QS inhibition nor antibacterial activities (i.e., no apparent effect on the fluorescent response and growth of the *E. coli* biosensor). The second includes compounds with the ability to reduce the QS response of the biosensor without compromising cell growth. While the third one comprises compounds with the ability to reduce the QS response at the expense of hampering cell growth. Figure 2 shows representative dose-response curves of compounds belonging to the classes 1, 2, 3, namely gardenoside (13) (Figure 2a,d,g), caffeine (11) (Figure 2b,e,h) and furanone (4) (Figure 2c,f,i) on the fluorescence (Figure 2a–c), growth (Figure 2d–f) and density-normalized fluorescence (Figure 2g–i) of the *E. coli* biosensor. A selection of dose-response effects of other compounds is available as Supporting Information, as discussed below.

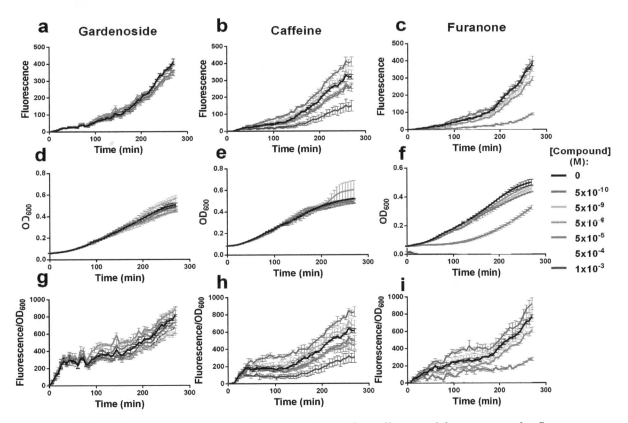

Figure 2. Effect of increasing concentrations of gardenoside, caffeine and furanone on the fluorescence (**a–c**), growth (**d–f**) and density-normalised fluorescence (**g–i**) of the *E. coli* biosensor over time.

The three compounds are chosen as representatives of the following categories: no inhibition (gardenoside; **a,d,g**), QS inhibition in the absence of growth reduction (caffeine; **b,e,h**) and QS and growth inhibition (furanone; **c,f,i**). Results from additional experiments on other compounds are available in Supporting Information. Data shows the mean and standard deviation of a representative experiment with triplicated treatments.

Next, we calculated the end-point effect of the 23 candidate compounds on the QS-based response and growth of the biosensor, relative to those of untreated cells. Figure 3 shows end-point, relative reduction of density-normalised fluorescence and cell density of compounds tested at fixed concentrations of 5×10^{-5} M (Figure 3a,b) and 1×10^{-3} M (Figure 3c,d). The rationale behind the chosen concentrations was based on the maximum water solubility of the compounds. Relative values close to 1.0 indicate none or negligible effect of a given compound on the density-normalised response and/or growth of the biosensor. In turn, we considered that relative fluorescence values significantly lower than 1.0 as were a diagnose of inhibition of the QS-based response, proven that the relative OD_{600} values stayed close to 1.0. This condition applied to vanillin (**5**), caffeine (**11**) and *trans*-cinnamaldehyde (**6**) applied at 1×10^{-3} M (Figure 3a,b); and to phenazine carboxylic acid (PCA, **19**), 2-heptyl-3-hydroxy-4-quinolone (PQS, **14**), genipin (**12**) and 1*H*-2-methyl-4-quinolone (MOQ, **15**) applied at 5×10^{-5} M. In all cases, the relative QS and OD_{600} data were compared statistically against itaconic acid, due to its negligible effect on both parameters.

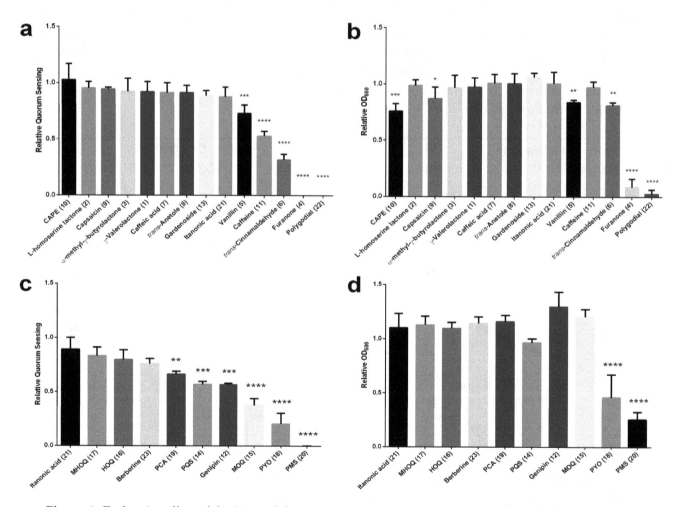

Figure 3. End-point effect of the 23 candidate compounds on the QS-based response and growth of the *E. coli* biosensor. (**a**) Effect of compounds **10, 2, 9, 3, 1, 7, 8, 13, 21, 5, 11, 6, 4, 22**; applied at 1×10^{-3} M on the density-normalised fluorescence of treated cells relative to control cells.

Relative fluorescence was calculated as follows: the mean of the last ten values of density-normalised fluorescence over time, corresponding to 246–300 min of incubation (see Figure 2) was divided by the corresponding values of untreated cells. (b) Effect of compounds **10, 2, 9, 3, 1, 7, 8, 13, 21, 5, 11, 6, 4, 22;** applied at 1×10^{-3} M on cell density of treated cells relative to control cells. Relative OD_{600} was calculated as follows: the mean of the last 10 OD_{600} values over time, corresponding to 246–300 min of incubation (see Figure 2) was divided by the corresponding values of untreated cells. (c). Effect of compounds **21, 17, 16, 23, 19, 14, 12, 15, 18, 20;** applied at 5×10^{-5} M on the density-normalised fluorescence of treated cells relative to control cells. Relative fluorescence was calculated as in (a,d) Effect of compounds **21, 17, 16, 23, 19, 14, 12, 15, 18, 20;** applied at 5×10^{-5} M on cell density of treated cells relative to control cells. Relative OD_{600} was calculated as in (b) *t*-Student statistical comparisons were made using itaconic acid as a reference treatment (* $p < 0.05$, ** $p < 0.01$, *** $p < 0.001$ and **** $p < 0.0001$). Data show the mean and standard deviation of three independent experiments with triplicated treatments.

Figure 3a shows that the compounds *trans*-cinnamaldehyde (**6**) ($p < 0.0001$), caffeine (**10**) ($p < 0.0001$), and, to a less extent, vanillin (**5**) ($p < 0.001$) can significantly reduce the QS-based fluorescence of the biosensor when applied at 1×10^{-3} M. Importantly, the QS inhibitory effect of caffeine (**10**) was not accompanied by any compromise of cell growth (Figure 3b). As for vanillin (**5**) ($p < 0.01$) and *trans*-cinnamaldehyde (**6**) ($p < 0.01$), they slightly reduced cell growth by 16.0% and 18.6%, respectively (Figure 3b). Furanone (**4**) ($p < 0.0001$), and polygodial (**21**) ($p < 0.0001$), which abolished the QS-based fluorescence of the biosensor at the tested concentration, they concomitantly exerted a dramatic antibacterial effect (cf. Figure 3a,b). Figure 3c shows that compounds PCA (**19**) ($p < 0.01$), PQS (**14**) ($p < 0.001$), genipin (**12**) ($p < 0.001$) and MOQ (**15**) ($p < 0.0001$) significantly reduced the density-normalized fluorescence of the biosensor when tested at 5×10^{-5} M (Figure 3a) and, importantly, they did not exert a significant effect on bacterial growth (Figure 3b). By contrast, compounds PYO (**18**) ($p < 0.0001$) and PMS (**20**) ($p < 0.0001$), showed a strong deleterious effect both on the QS response of the biosensor and its growth (cf. Figure 3c,d). We carried out a series of experiments to confirm that inhibition of the density-normalised fluorescence observed with PYO (**18**) and genipin (**12**) at sub-lethal doses was in fact due to interference with the QS response of the biosensor and not due to GFP fluorescence quenching. To this end, we used a control *E. coli* strain Top10 pBCA9445-jtk28282::sfGFP, which constitutively expresses a super folded version of GFP (sfGFP). We compared the effects of both compounds in the *E. coli* biosensor and control strains (Figures S2–S8). In our hands, neither of them at concentrations in the range 1×10^{-8} M to 1×10^{-4} M (Figures S3–S5) acted as quenchers of sfGFP fluorescence in the control strain *E. coli* Top10 pBCA9445-jtk28282::sfGFP. We observed a high degree of experimental variability and not apparent dose-response effects of PYO at sub-lethal concentrations ranging from 1×10^{-8} to 1×10^{-4} M (Figure S5). The implications of these disparate observations are further considered in the Discussion section.

2.2. Computation of GRID-MIFs

The three-dimensional molecular crystal structure of TraR receptor was obtained from the protein data bank (PDB No. 1L3L). Information about the binding region where the natural ligand OOHL interacts with TraR was described elsewhere [17]. Favorable interaction points at the binding site of the receptor was studied with GRID-MIFs. To define the GRID maps at TraR binding site, the Autogrid utility inbuilt in AutoDockTools 1.5.6 software was applied. Three different chemical probes (HD, HA, DRY) were used, representing the potentially significant functional group at the binding site. In Figure 4a the GRID-MIFs generated at TarR binding site is shown. Here, the green patch generated by DRY probe accounts for the favourable hydrophobic interaction ligand and receptor; blue contours were generated by HD (donor) probe responsible for favourable hydrogen bonds between receptor and ligand, and red contours were generated by HA (acceptor) probe, which informs about favourable hydrogen bonds between ligand and receptor amino acid residues. Comparing with the natural substrate OOHL (Figure 4b) the dry probe matches with the ring and all carbons in the substrate, the HD (blue) probe matches the NH group of substrate and HA (red) matches the O functional group present in the substrate.

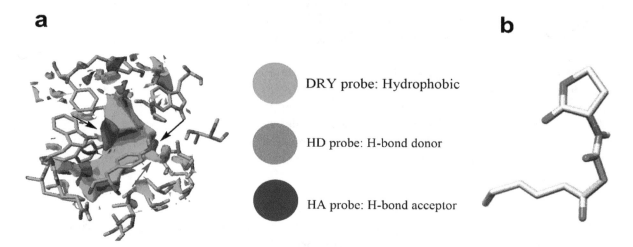

Figure 4. (**a**) GRID-MIFs for TraR protein with DRY probe (green) showing favorable hydrophobic interaction sites. GRID-MIFs for TraR protein with HD (blue) and HA (red) probes showing favorable hydrogen bond (blue for hydrogen bond donor and red for hydrogen bond acceptor) binding sites. (**b**) Natural substrate OOHL.

2.3. Docking and Interaction of Selected Compounds

We docked six selected compounds, based on their generated GRID-MIFs, over the binding domain of TraR. We included the cognate OOHL ligand as a reference. This enabled to gain Information on dock score, hydrogen bond and hydrophobic interactions. We selected ligand conformations using that of the natural ligand OOHL into the binding site as a reference (Figure 5a). Thus, we fixed docked ligand binding poses to that of the natural ligand. In other words, superimposition of the docked ligand on OOHL conformation in TraR's crystal structure implied that the aromatic ring of the ligand coincided with the lactone ring of the natural substrate. Table 1 lists the estimated binding energy values for the docked compounds. Strikingly, PCA (19) and PQS (14) showed a more negative docking score (i.e., predicted free energy of binding) than that estimated for the cognate ligand OOHL, which would in principle indicate a stronger affinity of these two compounds towards the binding site of TraR (Table 1). Figure 5b shows the docking-predicted binding pose of PCA into TraR's binding pocket. Two ligand conformations were identified for PQS (14), namely PQS-conf A (Figure 5c) and PQS-conf B (Figure 5d and Table 1). Both conformations were similar to OOHL binding pose, only differing in ring flip, which affects hydrogen bond interactions between ligand and receptor (cf. Figure 5a–c). The estimated docking score for PQS (14)-conf A was more negative than that of OOHL, whereas the predicted value for PQS-conf B was less negative, indicating a potential stronger affinity of conf B vs conf A towards the binding site of TraR (Table 1). Docking scores of smaller ligands, namely MOQ, HOQ and MHOQ were less negative than that of OOHL, predicting poorer affinities for these ligands towards TraR (Table 1).

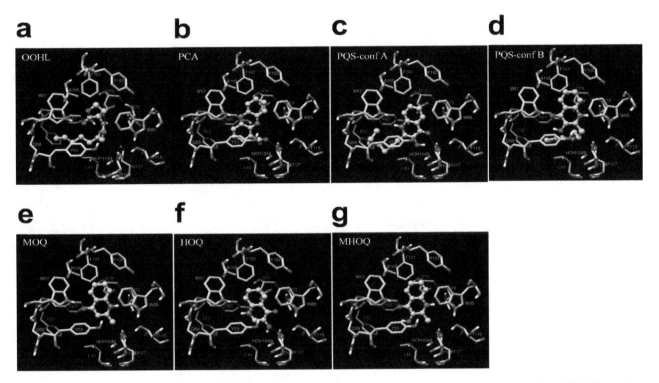

Figure 5. Interaction of TraR receptor with (**a**) OOHL; (**b**) PCA, (**c**) and (**d**) PQS; (**e**) MOQ; (**f**) HOQ and (**g**) MHOQ. (**c**) shows us the PQS conf A and (**d**) shows PQS conf B. Close-up view of all compounds binding site, oxygen carbon and nitrogen are colored in red yellow and blue, respectively, hydrogen bonds are shown as blue line.

Table 1. Cumulative results for the compounds docked against TraR protein.

Compound	Hydrogen Bonding Interactions	Dock Score (Kcal/mol)	Hydrophobic Interactions
OOHL	4 (including Trp 57)	−7.58	Leu 40, Tyr 53, Gln 58, Trp 85, Phe101, Ala 105, Ile 110.
MOQ (**15**)	1 (including Trp 57)	−6.16	Tyr 53, Val 72, Trp 85, Phe 101, Tyr 102, Ala 105, Met 127
HOQ (**16**)	0	−5.72	Trp 57, Tyr 61, Asp 70, Val 72, Trp 85, Phe 101, Met 127
MHOQ (**17**)	1 (including Trp 57)	−5.83	Tyr 53, Asp 70, Val 72, Trp 85, Phe 101, Tyr 102, Ala 105, Met 127, Thr 129
PCA (**19**)	3 (including Trp 57)	−8.01	Leu 40, Tyr 53, Tyr 61, Val 72, Trp 85, Phe101, Tyr 102, Ala 105, Met 127
PQS (**14**) (conf A)	2	−8.04	Leu 40, Tyr 53, Tyr 61, Val 72, Val 73, Trp 85, Phe 101, Tyr 102, Ala 105, Met127, Thr 129
PQS (**14**) (conf B)	1 (including Trp 57)	−6.59	Ala 38, Leu 40, Ala 49, Thr 51, Gln 58, Tyr 61, Phe 62, Val 72, Trp 85, Phe 101, Met127

We studied in detail the docking-predicted poses of selected candidates to elucidate the mechanisms of receptor-ligand possible interactions (Table 1). Figure 5 shows interaction maps of the six selected compounds (Table 1) with TraR's binding pocket. Clear from Figure 5a are the presence of four hydrogen bonds established between the cognate substrate OOHL and specific amino acids at the binding pocket of the receptors The H- bonds are located as follows: (1) between Trp 57 in TraR and keto group present in the lactone ring, (2) between Tyr 53 in TraR and the 1-keto group of the lactone, (3) between Asp 70 in TraR and the imino group in OOHL and (4) between Tyr 61 in TraR and the 3-keto group of OOHL (Figure 5a). Apart from these bonds, the cognate ligand also establishes strong hydrophobic interactions with nearby residues, as shown in Table 1. Altogether, it seems that both hydrophobic and hydrogen bond interactions are important for ligand selectivity. Our docking results confirm previous docking predictions of binding and pose conformations for OOHL in TraR's binding site [18]. Figure 5b shows the docking-predicted map for PCA (19)-TraR interaction (19). Importantly, our predictions show the presence of three hydrogen bonds with TraR's binding pocket, namely: (1) between Trp 57 in TraR and the deprotonated N present in the aromatic group of PCA, (2) and (3) between Thr 129 in TraR, an intermediate water molecule and the carboxylic acid functional group of PCA (Figure 5b). Again, our docking predicted several hydrophobic interactions between specific aminoacids of the binding site of TraR and the aromatic and heterocyclic rings of PCA (19) (Table 1). Figure 5c shows the predicted maps for PQS-confA and the binding site of TraR. In this case, two hydrogen bonds are predicted to form, namely: (1) between Thr129 and the keto group present in the aromatic ring of PQS (14), (2) between a hydroxyl group in PQS and a molecule of water (Figure 5c). In turn the predicted map for PQS-conf B and TraR interaction (Figure 5d shows one hydrogen bond formed between Trp 57 in TraR and the keto group present in the aromatic ring ofPQS (14). Both PQS-conf A and -confB are expected to establish strong hydrophobic interactions with the binding pocket of TraR, as listed in Table 1 and the long carbon chain of PQS in both poses cover most of the hydrophobic patch generated by GRID (cf. Figures 4 and 5c,d). Panels e, f and g of Figure 5, illustrate the prediction interaction maps for TraR and MOQ (15), HOQ (16) and MHOQ (17), respectively. Docking-predicted poses in the binding site of the receptor are very similar (cf. Figure 5e–g); hence, the predicted interaction sites for the three of them did not very much. However, in the case of both MOQ (15) and MOQH (17) an hydrogen bond was predicted between Trp 57 in TraR and the keto group in the aromatic ring of the ligands (cf. Figure 5e,g), while this interaction was not observed in HOQ (15) (Figure 5f). Strikingly, a relative inhibition of the QS-based response of the *E. coli* biosensor was found to be significantly higher for MOQ (15) than that of HOQ (16) and MOQH (17) (Figure S9). This, in principle would indicate that the specific position of H-bonding between these kind of molecules and the binding site of TraR would not necessarily explain *per se* towards LuxR-based proteins.

3. Discussion

QSIs are gaining momentum as potent alternatives to the use of classical antibiotics in the context of rising resistance spread and with enormous potential in many fields, from food science to agriculture and medicine [39,40]. QSIs are structurally diverse molecules that can be synthesised or extracted from natural sources. Here, we screened a total of 23 chemically diverse compounds with potential QS inhibition activity to identify their impact on LuxR-regulated QS models. To this end, we used a well-established *E. coli* Top10 biosensor assay and in silico modelling to recreate the structural interactions between the ligand candidates and the LuxR-like receptor.

The candidate compounds were classified into five broad groups according to with their chemical structure (Table 1). Group 1 comprised the alkyl-substituted lactones (Table 1): γ-valerolactone (**1**), L-homoserine lactone (**2**), α-methyl-γ-butyrolactone (**3**), and furanone **4**. In this group, only furanone (4) showed a significant inhibition (≥37.5%) of the fluorescent- QS-based response of the biosensor at concentrations $\geq 5 \times 10^{-6}$ M 37.5% (Figure 3a and Figure S10). At 1×10^{-3} M, furanone completely abolished the QS-based response of the biosensor, albeit a dramatic, deleterious effect on cell growth (Figure 3b and Figure S10).

γ-Butyrolactones were the first class of small signalling molecules identified from Gram-positive species *Streptomyces griseus*. They were found to induce streptomycin production and sporulation [41]. Even though the chemical structure of γ-butyrolactones is rather similar to that of AHLs, except for the carbon side-chain, it is known that the receptors of γ-butyrolactone do not bind to AHL receptors and that AHL do not bind to γ-butyrolactone receptors. Also, both receptors have low structural similarity [41]. The functions of the signalling molecules also differ as AHLs i.a. are known to regulate QS in Gram-negative bacteria, while γ-butyrolactones mainly regulate the production of antibiotics and differentiation.

From our results, we found that neither α-methyl-γ-butyrolactone, γ-valerolactone nor L-homo-serine lactone showed any QS inhibition activity. These results are consistent with the notion that the carbon side chain is important for binding to the LuxR receptor. Also, it is not unexpected that γ-valerolactone did not show activity, as the methyl substituent is in a different position of the lactone ring than that in 3-oxohexanoylhomoserine. As suggested in previous studies, our results support the proposal that the LuxR receptor does not recognise α-methyl-γ-butyrolactone nor other related lactones (e.g., γ-valerolactone).

Halogenated furanones which resemble AHLs structurally were first discovered in the marine red alga *Delisea pulchra* and proved to preventing swarming motility with the opportunistic human pathogen *Proteus mirabilis* and *S. liquefaciens* without affect growth rate [42,43]. These compounds were the first QSIs found to occur in nature. After that, Manefield et al. further obtained proof-of-principle of the QS inhibition activity of the same type of halogenated furanones by specifically interfering with AHL-mediated gene expression at the level of the LuxR protein [44]. Furthermore, Ren et al. found that (5Z)-4-bromo-5-(bromomethylene)-3-butyl-2(5H)-furanone is a non-specific intercellular signal antagonist [45]. Later, Defoirdt et al. proved that this furanone disrupts quorum sensing-regulated gene expression in *Vibrio harveyi* by decreasing the DNA-binding activity of the transcriptional regulator protein LuxR [46]. Besides halogenated furanones with side alkyl chains that have QS inhibition activity, some synthetic halogenated furanones lacking alkyl chain also have anti-biofilm formation activity through interference with QS, and have been found to protect surfaces from being colonised by *S. epidermidis* [47]. Compound (5Z)-4-bromo-5-(bromomethylene)-3-butyl-2(5H)-furanone included in our library, a synthetic derivate of natural furanone has been reported as a potent antagonist of bacterial QS that not only can increase bacterial susceptibility to tobramycin and SDS when it is applied for action with *P. aeruginosa* biofilms but also can inhibit virulence factor expression because of targeting QS systems [48]. Several previous studies have shown that halogenated furanones can interact with the LuxR protein and induce conformational changes due to rapid proteolytic degradation of the furanone-LuxR complex, which in turn destabilises the AHL-dependent transcriptional activator [49]. However, independent studies confirmed that halogenated furanones without alkyl chains were strongly toxic to the planktonic cell. While furanones with long alkyl chains were shown not to reduce the biofilm formation [50,51]. The present study confirmed that furanone without alkyl chains has high toxicity against the *E. coli* Top10 pSB1A3-BBaT9002 strain, as it reduced 50% the bacterial growth when dosed at 5×10^{-5} M. In fact, at 1×10^{-3} M, indeed, furanone can kill all bacteria, diagnostic that the lack of alkyl chain is at play in the induced toxicity. It has been suggested that the increase of water solubility may explain this effect [51]. Interestingly, when dosed at 5×10^{-6} M, the results showed that furanone could reduce the fluorescence production at no detrimental expense of the bacterial growth (Figure 2c). A possible explanation to these phenomena might be that some compounds when applied at sub-lethal concentrations will not kill bacterial but delay the QS activity because bacteria become weaker than at the normal condition. This phenomenon gave us the illusion that those compounds were QSIs, but when we increased the dose, we noticed that they had an antibacterial activity. The observed antimicrobial effect at furanone concentrations $\geq 5 \times 10^{-6}$ M (Figure S10) prompted us to search QSIs with lower associated toxicity. Closer attention should be paid to this phenomenon to discriminate between potential QSIs more carefully.

Group 2 candidates included compounds with at least one aromatic ring. Vanillin (**5**), proposed as a less toxic alternative to brominated furanones, revealed a relative reduction of the biosensor's fluorescent response of 27.1 % when applied at 1×10^{-3} M (Figure 3a and Figure S7), an effect that was accompanied by a discrete, 16.0% reduction of cell growth (Figure 3b and Figure S7). Belonging to the same group, the well-reported QSI, *trans*-cinnamaldehyde (**6**) revealed a potent capacity to reduce the QS-based response of the biosensor to up to 68.3% (Figure 3a and Figure S7) when applied at 1×10^{-3} M, with a slight reduction of cell growth (18.6%; Figure 3b and Figure S7). Surprisingly, related compounds caffeic acid (**7**) and *trans*-anethole (**8**) were apparently innocuous to the *E. coli* biosensor even at concentrations of 1×10^{-3} M (Figure 3a,b) while capsaicin (**9**) and CAPE (**10**) inhibited cell growth by 12.8 and 24.4%, respectively (Figure 3b).

Vanillin (**5**) is a well-known food flavouring agent and is a major constituent of vanilla pods. Its QS inhibition activity has recently been demonstrated in *Aeromonas hydrophila*, *Agrobacterium tumifaciens* NTL-4, *Chromobacterium violaceum* CV026 when applied at 250 µg/mL (1.64 mM), where it showed significant inhibition in short-chain AHLs (C4-HSL (69%) and 3OC8-HSL (59.8%)), followed by C6-HSL(32%), and C8-HSL (28%), but lower inhibition in long-chain AHLs (C14-HSL (13.5%) and C10-HSL (12%)). It also reduces the biofilm formation on the reverse osmosis membrane of *A hydrophila* [52]. Our own experiments confirmed that vanillin at 1×10^{-3} M can inhibit the QS activity with 3OC6HSL 27.1%. It has been speculated that the possible mechanism whereby vanillin inhibits QS activity is that it interferes with the binding of the short-chain AHLs to their cognate receptor [52]. Our study offers experimental evidence that vanillin may also interfere with binding of 3OC6HSL to its cognate LuxR receptor.

trans-Cinnamaldehyde (**6**) is a component of cinnamon and cassia essential oils, and it is commonly present in food as a flavouring agent and fungicide. In a previous study, it was shown that 200 µM cinnamaldehyde can reduce by 70% the fluorescence intensity due to the expression of GFP, induced by 3-oxo-C6-HSL in a bioreporter *E. coli* ATCC 33,456 pJBA89, and also effective at inhibiting AI-2 mediated QS [53]. Furthermore, Brackman et al. proved *trans*-cinnamaldehyde at concentrations < 1 mM shifts the SDS-PAGE mobility of LuxR-DNA. They concluded that *trans*-cinnamaldehyde and cinnamaldehyde derivatives interfere with AI-2 based QS in various *Vibrio* spp. by decreasing the DNA-binding ability of LuxR [54]. Recent molecular docking analysis studies suggested that *trans*-cinnamaldehyde interacts with LasI and EsaI substrate binding sites thus inducing the QS inhibition activity [55]. Our own studies also confirm that *trans*-cinnamaldehyde inhibits the LuxR-mediated GFP production in the *E. coli* Top 10 biosensor by 68.3% at 1×10^{-3} M concentration. This strain does not express the LuxI gene, thus it cannot produce LuxI synthase of 3-oxo-C6-HSLs but can constitutively overexpress LuxR protein. In our related study, we have shown that *trans*-cinnamaldehyde not only inhibits the expression of GFP, but it also retards its kinetics [38]. We suggest that there are maybe two mechanisms at play for QS inhibition involving LuxR. Firstly, the three-carbon aliphatic side chain of *trans*-cinnamaldehyde could interfere with the binding of 3OC6HSL to LuxR receptor; secondly, it can also decrease the DNA-binding ability of LuxR dimers, as previously suggested.

trans-Cinnamaldehyde (**6**)-related compounds, namely caffeic acid (**7**) and *trans*-anethole (**8**), were also tested on their QS inhibition activity. The results showed that neither of them had QS inhibition activity nor antibacterial effect at the tested concentration of 1×10^{-3} M. Caffeic acid is a phenolic acid that has various documented beneficial biological properties. Besides being a powerful antioxidant, it also has anticancer, anti-inflammatory and antiviral activities [56]. *trans*-Anethole, in turn, is also a natural component of anise seeds and fruits and it is used as a flavouring ingredient. Until now, its antibacterial and QS inhibitory activities have not been tested.

Comparing the chemical structures of caffeic acid and *trans*-anethole with that of *trans*-cinnamaldehyde, we can clearly see that neither the catechol phenolic nor the aromatic ester groups of caffeic acid and trans-anethole, respectively, have any effect on increasing the binding affinity with the LuxR protein. These results may reflect the importance of the unsubstituted aromatic ring in *trans*-cinnamaldehyde to make π-π interactions with the receptor residues at the binding site of LuxR. In this regard, the phenolic residues of caffeic acid can act as the H-bond donors, but not acceptors, at the hydrogen bond acceptor binding domain of the binding pocket of LuxR, hence, decreasing its overall binding efficiency. Similarly, in trans-anethole, the presence of the methyl ester substituent at the aromatic ring may be is enough to prevent its efficient binding with the binding site of LuxR. However, vanillin, with one phenolic, one methyl ester and an aldehyde substituent at the aromatic ring, does show QS inhibition activity as discussed above. Therefore, our study is consistent with the idea that the role of the presence of H-bond acceptor groups along with the the π-π interactions of the aromatic ring, is what determines the overall affinity of compounds to bind with LuxR receptor.

Capsaicin (**9**), structurally related to vanillin (**5**), is a natural alkaloid extracted from fruit of Capsicum family and it is responsible for the pungency of chili peppers. Its structure has an aromatic ring and a long hydrophobic aliphatic chain with a polar amide group. Most studies with capsaicin have addressed its pharmacology and clinical applications [57]. Only a few studies have focused on the inhibition activity of the growth of the gastric pathogen *Helicobacter pylori* [58,59]. One such study found that capsaicin did not inhibit the growth of a human fecal commensal *E. coli* strain [58]. So far, the QS inhibitory activity of capsaicin has not been documented. Our results show that even at the concentration of 1×10^{-3} M, capsaicin did not significantly reduce the QS activity of the *E. coli* Top10 pSB1A3-BBaT9002 biosensor, and it decreased the bacterial growth only by 12.8% ($p < 0.05$). If we compare the structures of capsaicin with that of vanillin, we can observe that they share identical substitution positions in their aromatic ring, except that vanillin has not the long aliphatic chain, but only a strong aldehyde H-bond acceptor group. Our results indicate that the increase in the length of the aliphatic chain does not lead to an increase in binding affinity. CAPE (**10**) is the main active component of propolis extract. Its chemical structure is described as the ester of caffeic acid and phenetyl alcohol; hence, it is a catechol ring with an ester chain bearing another aromatic ring. CAPE has known bioactivities such as antimicrobial, anti-inflammatory and cytotoxic activities. About the antimicrobial activity of CAPE, it has been reported that can inhibit the 60% *E. coli* growth when the concentration is over 60.6 µM. This has been explained as the result of the synthesis of reactive oxygen species that damage the outer membrane of the bacteria-induced by CAPE [60,61]. Our experiments contrast with this study, as we found that CAPE only inhibits the growth of the *E. coli* Top10 pSB1A3-BBaT9002 strain by 24.4% when applied at 1×10^{-3} M. As a possible explanation for the observed discrepancies between the results of our study and the previous ones may stem in the distinct protocols of the assays to quantify the bacterial growth rate. Overall, no QS inhibition activity was shown on the surviving bacteria after treatment with CAPE.

Group 3, comprised by heterocyclic compounds, revealed candidates with important QSI capacity, namely caffeine (**11**) and genipin (**12**), which have been shown to reduce the QS-based response of the biosensor by 47% and by 43.3% when applied at 1×10^{-3} M and 5×10^{-5} M, respectively (Figure 3a,c, Figures S7 and S8) and with negligible effects on cell growth (Figure 3b–d, Figures S7 and S8). Belonging to the same group, gardenoside (**13**) did not show any apparent effect on the *E. coli* biosensor at the doses tested (Figure 3a,b).

Caffeine (**11**) is yet another alkaloid which occurs in coffee cherry and tea. Documented uses of caffeine include as a pesticide to kill certain larvae, insects and beetles. Some studies have shown that caffeine, applied at 2.5 mg/mL ($\approx$12.8 mM), can retard the growth of *E. coli*, *Enterobacter aerogenes*, *Proteus vulgaris*, and *P. aeruginosa* within a short time. The first time caffeine was tested as QS inhibition compound against *C. violaceum* CV026 and *P. aeruginosa* PA01 strains, it was found that when applied at 0.3–1.0 mg/mL ($\approx$1.5–5.0 mM), it inhibits violacein production in *C violaceum* CV026, and short chain AHLs production and swarming motility in *P. aeruginosa* PA01 [62]. Our experiments also proved that caffeine, applied at 1×10^{-3} M to the *E. coli* Top10 pSB1A3-BBaT9002 biosensor strain, it can inhibit 47% GFP production without affecting bacterial growth. Our results, along with previous studies [62], suggest that caffeine has a broad spectrum of QS inhibition activities in different bacterial species; interestingly, all share in common to contain the AHL-regulated QS system. As earlier reported by Norizan et al. Caffeine did not degrade C6-HSL [62], so we hypothesise here that it can be a competitor that binds with AHL receptors because the keto groups from the aromatic ring can also form strong hydrogen bonds with type I QS LuxI/LuxR receptors.

Also in Group 3, genipin (**12**) is an iridoid compound isolated from *Gardenia jasminodies* Ellis fruits. It is the aglycone derivative of geniposide. It was initially identified as a protein cross-linking agent but can also inhibit the production of nitric oxide by downregulating the activity of nuclear factor-κB (NF-κB) [63]. It is also a cell-permeable inhibitor with anti-inflammatory and anti-angiogenic activity mediated by the induction of apoptosis in hepatoma and hepatocarcinoma cell lines [64]. A number of studies have also shown that genipin cross-links chitosan nano- and microparticles, thus allowing them to be used for QS inhibition and the delivery of antimicrobial drugs [65,66]. We found, for the first time, that genipin on its own can inhibit GFP production in the *E. coli* Top10 pSB1A3-BBaT9002 biosensor, without exhibiting significant toxicity, more effectively than a diverse spectrum of alternative compounds. Knowing that genipin possesses inherent fluorogenic properties, we wondered whether the observed effect on the fluorescent response of our biosensor could be due to an artefact associated with the direct fluorescence quenching [67]. We performed a series of extra experiments where we tested genipin on the control *E. coli* strain Top10 pBCA9445-jtk28282::sfGFP strain (Supporting Information). We found that genipin concentrations ranging from 9.95×10^{-10} to 1.19×10^{-4} M did not exert significant fluorescence quenching on the control strain (Figures S2 and S3). Nevertheless, the fact that the fluorescence over growth profiles of both bacterial strains widely differ (Figure S1) make these comparisons a difficult task. Moreover, both strains express different GFP species (namely GFPmut3b and sfGFP in the biosensor and control strain, respectively) and their expression vectors widely diverge (see Supporting Information) [68,69]. Future efforts should be focused on validating the effects of genipin by using a control *E. coli* Top10 strain expressing GFPmut3b constitutively from a modified version of the pSB1A3-BbaT9002 plasmid. On our hands, genipin and related compounds are promising candidates for the development of novel therapeutic approaches based on the inhibition of QS in bacteria. Our data showed a significant difference between the QS inhibition activities of genipin and the closely related glycosylated iridoid compound, gardenoside. These two iridoids share similar structures, differing only with respect to the glycosylation in the hydroxyl group of C1, and in the hydroxyl group at position C8 of the heterocyclic structure, in gardenoside. This result may have a biological significance in host-pathogen interactions via inhibition of QS, as glucose oxidase (GOD) is synthesised by many plants, fungi and bacteria. This hypothesis would need further experimental validation.

Quinolone- and phenazine- like compounds belonging to Group 4 (Table 1) are reported to play important roles in QS-regulated phenotypes of *Pseudomonas spp* [70]. These comprise the alkylquinolone PQS (**14**) signal of *P. aeruginosa* and three structurally-related synthetic quinolones, namely MOQ (**15**), HOQ (**16**) and MHOQ (**17**) (Table 1); bearing a bicyclic core structure with different substituents. Among these three structurally-related synthetic compounds, only MOQ demonstrated significant relative QS inhibition activity of 62.2%. The rest of tested compounds, namely HOQ and MHOQ, did not have any detectable activity, neither QS inhibition nor antibacterial (Figure 3c,d and Figure S9). Also, compound PQS comprised not only one six-carbon ring but also a long carbon chain at the six-member heterocyclic ring, which showed an important QSI activity, by inhibiting the QS-based response of the biosensor by 43.1%, with a negligible effect on cell growth (Figure 3c,d and Figure S8). Compounds PYO (**18**), PCA (**19**) and PMS (**20**) are similarly with three rings, but only PYO and PMS have high GFP inhibition and high toxicity, compound PCA also has QQ activity, inhibiting GFP production by 33.7%, but no toxicity (Figure 3c,d).

Group 4, comprised heterocyclic compounds, some of which can be produced naturally, such as the *Pseudomonas* spp. metabolites (PQS, PCA, PYO), while the rest are synthetic [70]. It is well known that phenazines have antimicrobial activity [71]. Moreover, some of these compounds are known to act as signalling molecules that regulate the QS systems in *P. aeruginosa* as discussed in detail below.

Compound PQS has been found as a QS signal that participates in the *P. aeruginosa* QS network and acts as a link between las and rhl quorum sensing, which either directly or indirectly, mediates the expression of 182 genes in *P. aeruginosa* [72,73]. Besides the intraspecific signalling role of PQS in *P. aeruginosa* involving interactions with its cognate LasR-like PqsR receptor and non-cognate-LuxR-like-RhlI, there is no evidence to the date on PQS interference with other LuxR-based QS regulation circuitries. Despite the fact that there is currently no crystal structure available for RhlI, it is known that it shows significant sequence divergence from TraR, our prototype for docking studies. Thus, it is unknown how PQS binds to RhlI in *P. aeruginosa*. A recent paper from Mukherjee et al. explored ligand-receptor binding of PqsR with C4HSL, by generating a homology model based on the *E. coli* SdiA structure, which is a LuxR-like closest homolog of PqsR [74]. In SdiA and other LuxR-type proteins, the highly conserved amino acids Trp68 and Asp81 interact with the amide group-oxygen and the amide group-nitrogen, respectively, of the cognate C4HSL. Other conserved residues, such as Tyr72 and Trp96, are required for hydrophobic and van der Waals interactions with the ligands [74]. These interactions seem to correlate with our docking predictions of OOHL establishing H-bonding with Trp57 and hydrophobic interactions with Tyr53 and Trp85 in the binding site of TraR (Figure 5a and Table 1). A similar scheme of PQS predicted H-bonding and hydrophobic interactions with Trp57 and Tyr61 (Figure 5c,d and Table 1) would in principle serve as a rationale for a strong affinity of PQS to LuxR homologs and the observed quorum quenching effect on the biosensor's LuxR-regulated response (Figure 3c and Figure S8).

Phenazines are a well-known family of pigments that are secreted from *P. aeruginosa*. Among phenazines, PYO is widely known due to its cytotoxic and redox activities [75]. Importantly, PYO is a terminal signalling factor in the QS network of *P. aeruginosa* [76]. PYO is also an intercellular signal that triggers specific responses in enteric *E. coli* and *Salmonella enterica*, via the SoxR regulon. Whether this kind of signal transduction is also involved in our *E. coli* biosensor in the presence of PYO is a question that we cannot elucidate at present [77]. Also, it is well known that PYO interacts with molecular oxygen to form ROS species that change the redox balance of the cells and that GFP fluorescence can be affected by the presence of ROS species [78,79]. To shed some light on extra effects of PYO on fluorescence quenching and/or the metabolism of *E. coli* Top 10 cells, we decided to perform extra experiments applying increasing PYO concentrations on both the *E. coli* Top10 pSB1A3-T9002 (Figure S4) biosensor and the *luxR*-deficient *E. coli* Top10 pBCA9445-jtk28282::sfGFP (Figures S5 and S6). Strikingly, we found a lack of dose-response effect of PYO on the fluorescence of both strains (Figures S4–S6), together with strong variability among experiments (cf. Figures S5 and S6). These disparate results could arise from some of the transductory and/or redox activity of PYO on our *E. coli* Top10 cells and need further investigation.

PCA (**19**) is yet another redox-active phenazine pigment that is produced from *P. aeruginosa* [80]. PCA is known to be a broad-spectrum activity compound that inhibits the growth of several plant pathogenic species (e.g., *Corynebacterium fascians*, *Agrobacterium tumefaciens*, *Erwinia aroideae*, *Diplodia zeae*) [81,82]. Further studies have found that PCA is precursor for more complex phenazine metabolites, such as 1-hydroxyphenazine, phenazine-1-carboxamide and PYO [76]. Yun Wang et al. found that PCA may shift the redox equilibrium between Fe(III) and Fe(II) in *P. aeruginosa* [83]. Even though PCA and PYO, both are redox-active phenazines, in our study, we found that, at 5×10^{-5} M, PYO has strong toxicity to *E. coli* Top 10 pSB1A3-BBaT9002 strain, while PCA only inhibits the fluorescence intensity but has no effect on bacterial growth. The different effect of PYO and PCA can be attributed to the fact that PCA may help the *E. coli* alleviate Fe(III) limitation by reducing it to ferrous iron [Fe(II)], thus promoting the bacterial growth [83], thus allowing to observe the QS inhibition activity. We will discuss further this aspect in the context of the in silico molecular docking results below.

PMS is a simple phenazonium salt and an electron acceptor and carrier in biochemical oxidation/reduction studies [84,85]. It is also a O_2^- generating agent that can increase intracellular H_2O_2 levels and lead to the formation of free radicals that can affect bacterial growth [85]. This explains why in our experiments PMS shows strong toxic effect against *E. coli* Top 10 pSB1A3-BBaT9002 strain. As explained above, this strain is lacking the SoxR regulon to confer resistance against redox stress.

Previous studies have proved that phenazines are antibiotic compounds that can inhibit microbial growth because of the redox-active effect. From our own studies, it can be argued that when phenazines (namely, PCA, PYO, PMS) are applied at the same concentration of 5×10^{-5} M, only PYO and PMS are toxic to the *E. coli* Top10 pSB1A3-BBaT9002 strain, as we mentioned above. Interestingly, PCA, does not inhibit bacterial growth but has QS inhibition activity. Several studies have also noticed this phenomenon. Morales et al. found that lower concentrations of PCA, PYO and PMS inhibited the fungal yeast-to-filament transition and affected the development of *C. albicans* wrinkled colony biofilms but allowed growth. However, those phenazines have anti-candida activity when the concentration is higher than 500 µM, which means that those compounds have different biological effects at different concentrations [86]. Furthermore, Skindersoe et al. used sub-inhibitory concentrations of antibiotics in *P. aeruginosa* and found that lower doses of antibiotics could modulate gene expression, so that they interfere with QS signalling [87]. To the best of our knowledge, this dual concentration-dependent activity of phenazines had not been reported before to operate in a mutant *E. coli* Top10 pSB1A3-BBaT9002 strain. However, recently, it has been hypothesised that it is a general mechanism of action of many compounds [88].

For the identification of functional group and their arrangement in the binding site required for binding ligand, GRID map was generated by using three different chemical probes i.e., H bond donor (HD), H bond acceptor (HA) and DRY probe. Grid-MIFs generated for TraR indicated (Figure 4) that acceptor interaction points and hydrophobic patches are dominant in comparison to donor interactions points at the binding. Comparing the functional group present in ligands with the GRID-MIFs (Figure 4) it is clear that because of big hydrophobic patch in the center of cavity, hydrophobic interaction from carbon either from aromatic ring or long chain carbon make very favorable interaction. Apart this one donor group at one side of aromatic ring makes favorable interaction with the Trp 57. Hydrogen bond interaction with Trp 57 is identified as important interaction in receptor substrate interaction. Apart from HOQ we found this interaction in all other five ligands. Whereas at the other side of ring one donor or one acceptor would also make favorable interaction with the Thr129 or water.

Consequently, we identified that in the same ringside two functional groups e.g. an OH group just next to the O (acceptor group), do not make a favourable interacting group. This can be observed in the docking score results for HOQ and MHOQ both with lower scores than MOQ. This might explain that in vitro HOQ and MHOQ, did not exhibit QS inhibition activity, while MOQ, that lacks the 3-hydroxyl group did exhibit QS inhibition activity experimentally. PQS showed better score, i.e., PQS-conf A (−8.04) and PQS-conf B (−6.59), in comparison to HOQ and MHOQ because of the long alkyl chain and an overall more favourable hydrophobic interaction (Table 1). In the PQS-conf A (−8.04), the H-bond between the Trp 57 and ligand is missing in this conformation, but because of PQS has a longer alkyl chain than OOHL, a H-bond with Thr 129 and putative H-bond with water, PQS-conf A has a better score than the other compounds. Whereas in PQS-conf B (−6.59) the H-bond is present between ligand O and Trp 57, but because of the OH just next to O is not a favourable interaction (according to GRID-MIFs), hence its lower score. This analysis clearly indicates that OH next to O is not a favourable functional group for interaction in ligand PQS, which affects the pose and docking score. Moreover, because of the H-bond interactions and more hydrophobic interactions in comparison to natural ligand OOHL, this compound is better over other ligands. Along with PQS, PCA has also shown a high dock score compared to other ligands. We argue that this is the result of the combined effect of the three aromatic rings making more hydrophobic interaction, the deprotonated N present in the aromatic group involved in H-bond interaction with Trp57, and the carboxylate function group involved in H-bond interaction with Thr129 and also probably with water. These favourable interactions might explain the high QS inhibition activity observed for PQS and PCA.

Finally, Group 5 contained a more diverse collection of organic molecules with complex structures. Experimentally, with the exception of compounds itaconic acid at 1×10^{-3} M and berberine at 5×10^{-5} M, none of these compounds showed QS inhibition activity. However, we found that polygodial exhibited strong bacterial growth inhibition. Polygodial is a bicyclic sesquiterpene dialdehyde, isolated from different traditional medicinal plants such as *Polygonum hydropiper* and *P. punctatum* [89]. Kubo et al. showed that polygodial has the antibacterial activity against various bacteria, not only as a surfactant to form the pyrrole with primary amine groups at the plasma membrane, thereby disturbing the balance of the membranes, but also may react with various intracellular components when it enters into the cells after the membrane damaged [89]. We also proved that polygodial has high antibacterial activity that suppressed almost completely the growth of *E. coli* Top10 pSB1A3-BBaT9002 strain when dosed at 1×10^{-3} M.

Berberine is an isoquinoline-type alkaloid isolated from *Coptidis rhizomaand* ("huang lian" in Chinese), a plant used in traditional Chinese medicine, and from other plants. It has been reported that when the concentration is at 30-45 μg/mL could exhibit an antibacterial effect and inhibit biofilm formation of *Staphylococcus epidermidis*. Whether the biofilm formation inhibition of berberine observed in Gram-positive bacteria is connected with the QS regulation is not confirmed [90]. However, recent studies have shown that berberine inhibits the QS in Gram-negative bacteria including antimicrobial-resistant *E. coli* strains, *P. aeruginosa PA01*, *C. violaceum* and *Salmonella enterica* [91,92]. Sun et al. investigated the QS inhibition activity of berberine in antimicrobial-resistant (AMR) *E. coli* strains and found that berberine inhibited biofilm formation and downregulated QS-related genes *luxS*, *pfS*, *hflX*, *ftsQ*, and *ftsE* of AMR *E. coli* strains at 1/2 (640 μg/mL) or 1/4 (320 μg/mL) minimal inhibitory concentration (MIC) [90]. Thus the tested berberine concentrations of berberine were tested by Sun et al. were $\geq$ 9.5 times higher than ours (cf. $\geq$ 160 μg/mL and 16.8 μg/mL in Sun et al.'s and our study, respectively). Moreover, the AMR *E. coli* QS system is a LuxS/AI-mediated system, unrelated to the LuxR-based circuitry present in our biosensor. Under our setting, we found no QS inhibition at a berberine concentration of 50μM (16.8 μg/mL). The lower concentration tested in our assays may explain the observed lack of QS inhibition activity. We decided to limit berberine concentration to 50 μM due to solubility problems at higher concentrations. Further efforts should be focused on testing the QS inhibition potential of berberine and other related compounds at concentrations comparable to those of Sun et al.'s and exploring whether the strong effect observed on LuxS-based QS systems can be extrapolated to LuxR-regulated circuitries.

4. Materials and Methods

4.1. Library of Tested Chemical Compounds

Compounds were selected according to their chemical structure and were divided into five groups. They were in all cases of high purity ($\geq$90%) and were either commercially available or synthesised. They were shipped in glass vials as powders or in liquid form and were dissolved in water or organic solution (ethanol or methanol) before use. The details for each compound are given in Table 2. Each is assigned a reference number used throughout this manuscript. 3-Oxohexanoyl-homoserine lactone (3OC6HSL) and all other chemicals were of analytical grade and, unless otherwise stated, were purchased from Merck KGaA (Darmstadt, Germany).

Table 2. List of screened compounds.

Number	Compounds	Group [1]	Solvent/Method	Supplier
1	γ-Valerolactone	Group (1) Lactone analogues	Water	Sigma (St. Louis, MO, USA)
2	L-Homoserine lactone		Water	Santa Cruz Biotechnology
3	α-Methyl-γ-butyrolactone		Water	Sigma (St. Louis, MO, USA)
4	Furanone((Z-)-4-Bromo-5-(bromomethy-lene)-2 (5H)-furanone)		First dissolved in ethanol, then diluted with water	Sigma (St. Louis, MO, USA)
5	Vanillin	Group (2) Aromatic ring structures	Water	Sigma (St. Louis, MO, USA)
6	*trans*-Cinnamaldehyde		First dissolved in ethanol, then diluted with water	Sigma (St. Louis, MO, USA)
7	Caffeic acid		First dissolved with ethanol, then diluted with water	Sigma (St. Louis, MO, USA)

Table 2. *Cont.*

Number	Compounds	Group [1]	Solvent/Method	Supplier
8	*trans*-Anethole		Water	Sigma (St. Louis, MO, USA)
9	Capsaicin		First dissolved with ethanol, then diluted with water	Merck KGaA (Darmstadt, Germany)
10	CAPE (caffeic acid phenethyl ester)		First dissolved with ethanol, then diluted with water	Merck KGaA (Darmstadt, Germany)
11	Caffeine	Group (3) Heterocyclic compounds	water	Merck KGaA (Darmstadt, Germany)
12	Genipin		Water	Challenge Bioproducts Co., Ltd.
13	Gardenoside		water	Nanjing Zelang Medical Technology Co.,Ltd
14	PQS (2-heptyl-3-hydroxy-4-quinolone)		First dissolved with methanol, then diluted with water	Merck KGaA (Darmstadt, Germany)
15	MOQ (1*H*-2-methyl-4-quinolone)		First dissolved with methanol, then diluted with water	Prof. Fetzner's [2]
16	HOQ (1*H*-3-hydroxyl-4-quinolone)	Group (4) Quinolone- and phenazine-based compounds relevant to QS systems of *Pseudomonas* spp	First dissolved with methanol, then diluted with water	Prof. Fetzner's [3]
17	MHOQ (1*H*-2-methyl-3-hydroxyl-4-quinolone)		First dissolved with methanol, then diluted with water	Prof. Fetzner's [4]
18	PYO (pyocyanine)		First dissolved with methanol, then diluted with water	Merck KGaA (Darmstadt, Germany)
19	PCA (Phenazine carboxylic acid)		First dissolved with methanol, then diluted with water	Key Organics Ltd. (Camelford, UK)
20	PMS (Phenazine methosulfate)		First dissolved with methanol, then diluted with water	Sigma (St. Louis, MO, USA)
21	Itaconic acid		First dissolved in ethanol, then diluted with water	Sigma (St. Louis, MO, USA)
22	Polygodial	Group (5) Structurally unrelated compounds	Water	Santa Cruz Biotechnology
23	Berberine		First dissolved in ethanol, then diluted with water	Sigma (St. Louis, MO, USA)

[1] The Group column refers to the classification based on chemical structural features (Figure 1), as explained in the text; [2] Synthesised by Prof. Susane Fetzner according to the method of Eiden et al. [93]. HPLC and UV absorption analysis indicated a purity of over 90%; [3] Synthesised by Prof. Susane Fetzner according to the method of Evans and Eastwood [94]. HPLC and UV absorption analysis indicated a purity of over 90%; [4] Synthesised by Prof. Susane Fetzner according to the method of Cornforth and James [95]. HPLC and UV absorption analysis indicated a purity of over 90%.

4.2. Bacterial Strains

The QQ activity of the 23 selected compounds was determined using the *E. coli* Top 10 strains listed below. The BioBrick standard biological sequence BBa_T9002, ligated into vector psb1a3 (http://partsregistry.org/Part:BBa_T9002), was a gift from Prof. Anderson (UC Berkeley, CA, USA). The sequence BBa_T9002 was introduced by chemical transformation into *E. coli* Top 10 (Invitrogen, Life Technologies Co., Leicestershire, UK) and single-colony cultures from the transformed strain were stored as 30% glycerol stocks at −80 °C as described in Section 2.3 below. The sequence BBa_T9002 comprised the transcription factor (LuxR), which is constitutively expressed, but it is active only in the presence of the exogenous autoinducer signalling molecule 3OC6HSL. At an adequate concentration, two molecules of 3OC6HSL bind to two molecules of LuxR and activate the expression of GFP (output), under the control of the lux pR promoter from *Vibrio fischeri*. The fluorescence biosensor was calibrated for different 3OC6HSL concentrations, as described in our previous studies [4]. An *E. coli* strain Top10 (Invitrogen, Life Technologies Co., U.K.) was transformed with plasmid pBCA9445-jtk2828, carrying a superfolder version of the *gfp* gene (*sfgfp*), which was kindly donated by Prof. Anderson Lab (UC Berkeley, Berkeley, CA, USA). The transformed strain expresses sfGFP constitutively and was used as control culture to test possible fluorescence quenching artefacts of genipin and PYO that could account for the effects observed in the fluorescence *E. coli* Top10 pSB1A3-BBaT9002 biosensor (Supporting Information).

4.3. Growth Media and Glycerol Stocks Preparation

Bacterial strains were cultivated using on Luria-Bertani (LB) and M9 minimal medium purchased from BD GmbH (Heidelberg, Germany). We inoculated 10 mL of LB broth supplemented with 200 µg/mL ampicillin with a single colony from a freshly streaked plate of Top10 containing BBa_T9002 and incubated the culture for 18 h at 37 °C, shaking at 100 rpm. Glycerol stocks were prepared as described in our previous studies [38]. Briefly, a 500 µL aliquots of overnight bacterial culture were mixed with 500 µL 30% sterile glycerol in 1.5 mL plastic vials and stored at −80 °C. Prior to each experiment, an aliquot of a glycerol stock from the single culture was diluted 1:1000 into 20 mL M9 minimal medium supplemented with 0.2% casamino acids, 1 mM thiamine hydrochloride and 200 µg/mL ampicillin (AppliChem GmbH, city, Germany). The culture was maintained under the same conditions until the OD600 reached ~0.15 (~5 h).

4.4. E. coli Top10 Fluorescent Biosensor Assay

Each tested compound was dissolved in MilliQ water or 100% organic solution (ethanol or methanol) according to their solubility at a high concentration of 200 mM, then diluted with MilliQ water to produce samples at six concentrations: 2×10^{-2}, 1×10^{-2}, 1×10^{-3}, 1×10^{-4}, 1×10^{-7} and 1×10^{-8} M; however, some compounds can only be prepared at a maximal concentration of 50 µM given by their water solubility. The 3OC6HSL was dissolved in acetonitrile to a stock concentration of 100 mM and stored at –20 °C kept in a sealed glass vial. Prior to each experiment, serial dilutions from the AHL stock solution were prepared in water to produce solutions with a concentration ranging from 100 mM to 10 nM. We then mixed 10 µL 3OC6HSL solution with 10 µL of the diluted compounds at different concentrations in the wells of a flat-bottomed 96-well plate (cat. # M3061, Greiner Bio-One, city, state abbrev if USA, country) and each well was then filled with 180 µL aliquots of the bacterial culture to test for QS inhibition activity. The final inhibitor concentrations, therefore, ranged from 1×10^{-3} M to 5×10^{-10} M. Several controls were also set up. Blank 1 contained 180 µL of M9 medium and 20 µL of MilliQ water to measure the absorbance background. Blank 2 wells contained 180 µL of bacterial culture and 20 µL of MilliQ water to measure the absorbance background-corrected for the cells. Finally, positive control wells contained 10 µL of water plus 10 µL 3OC6HSL solution and 180 µL of the bacterial culture to measure the fluorescence background. The plates were incubated in a Safire Tecan-F129013 Microplate Reader (Tecan, Crailsheim, Germany) at 37 °C and fluorescence measurements were taken automatically using a repeating procedure ($\lambda_{ex} = 480$ nm and $\lambda_{em} = 510$ nm, 40 µs, 10 flashes, gain 100, top fluorescence), absorbance measurements (OD_{600}) ($\lambda = 600$ nm absorbance filter, 10 flashes) and shaking (5 s, orbital shaking, high speed). The interval between measurements was 6 min. For each experiment, the fluorescence intensity (FI) and OD_{600} data were corrected by subtracting the values of absorbance and fluorescence backgrounds and expressed as the average for each treatment. Data were presented as FI/OD_{600} versus incubation time. All measurements were taken in triplicate.

4.5. Protein Structure File, Ligand Database

The X-ray crystal structure of *Agrobacterium tumefaciens* TraR was downloaded from the Protein Data Bank (PDB ID 1L3L) and used for computer docking. All the water molecules were removed except one molecule in the binding pocket, which plays an important role in interaction and forms the hydrogen bond with the autoinducer OOHL of TraR protein. To define the grid box of TraR protein, OOHL was used as a ligand to select spheres and also followed with the Information from the previous study [18]. The 2D structures of six compounds (OOHL, MOQ, HOQ, MHOQ, PCA and PQS) were drawn manually using Marvin sketch v6.1.3 (ChemAxon Ltd., Budapest, Hungary) and saved as MDL mol files. The mol files were merged into a single mol file and likewise converted to 3D structures using Discovery Studio 3.5 client software. PyMol was used for visualisation and molecular modelling.

4.6. Molecular Docking Studies

For the generation of GRID-MIFs (molecular interaction fields) at the TarR binding site where a given chemical group can interact favourably, Autogrid program inbuilt in AutoDockTools 1.5.6. was used. For MIF generation, mainly three probed were applied i.e., DRY probe representing hydrophobic interaction, HA probe to representing H bond acceptor groups, and HD probe to representing H bond donor groups. Docking guided by the grid map was performed using Autodock tool. Fifty conformations were generated for each docked substrate. Binding scores between the ligand and protein was evaluated using the autodock utility autoscorer considering the hydrogen bond forces, electrostatic forces, van der Waals forces, solvation energy and entropy.

4.7. Statistical Analysis

All the experiments were performed in triplicates to validate reproducibility and the P values were calculated statistically by Student's *t*-test. Values were expressed as mean ±SD. A comparison analysis was performed between tests and control.

5. Conclusions

In this study, we have screened the QS inhibition activity of a library of 23 structurally different compounds against an *E. coli* Top10 pSB1A3-BBaT9002 reporter of AHL-regulated QS. This library included a selection of natural and synthetic compounds that occur naturally in plants and in bacteria species such as *P. aeruginosa*. We were able to establish cues of structure-function relationships for compounds with QS inhibitory activity (e.g., *trans*-cinnamaldehyde, vanillin, caffeine, PQS, PCA). We showed, for the first time, that genipin and MOQ have QS inhibition activity. We also conducted molecular simulations using GRID-MIFs on a selection of compounds (e.g., MOQ, HOQ, MHOQ). Our results aid in the future rational design of novel QS inhibition compounds. For example, the introduction of a 3-methyl group in MOQ may increase the binding affinity substantially to the TraR receptor and hence the QS inhibition activity. This hypothesis could be validated experimentally in future studies. The results of this study may pave the way to future works aimed to fully realise the potential of QS inhibition as an alternative strategy to overcome antimicrobial resistance and biofilms in clinical and other settings.

Author Contributions: Conceptualiazation, F.M.G., X.Q., C.V.-S. and R.S.; methodology, X.Q. and C.V.-S.; formal analysis, X.Q. and R.S.; resources, B.P. and C.V.-S.; writing—original draft preparation, X.Q.; writing—review and editing X.Q., B.P., R.S., C.V.-S. and F.M.G.; supervision, F.M.G. and B.P.; project administration, F.M.G.; funding acquisition, F.M.G. All authors have read and agreed to the published version of the manuscript.

Acknowledgments: X.Q. was recipient of a fellowship from China Scholarship Council. CVS was supported by a pre-doctoral fellowship of the Xunta de Galicia and by a FPU fellowship of the "Ministerio de Educación y Ciencia" of Spain, by a research fellowship of the DAAD (Germany), and research fellowship of the Fundación Pedro Barrié de la Maza (Spain). We acknowledge support from D.F.G., Germany (Project GRK 1549 International Research Training Group 'Molecular and Cellular GlycoSciences'); the research leading to these results has also received funding from the European Union's Seventh Framework Programme for research, technological development and demonstration under grant agreement no. 613931. We are also indebted to Antje von Schaewen for generous access to the Safire Tecan-F129013 Microplate Reader.

References

1. Fuqua, W.C.; Winans, S.C.; Greenberg, E.P. Quorum Sensing in Bacteria: The LuxR-LuxI Family of Cell Density-Responsive Transcriptional Regulatorst. *J. Bacteriol.* **1994**, *176*, 269–275. [CrossRef] [PubMed]
2. Rutherford, S.T.; Bassler, B. Bacterial Quorum Sensing: Its Role in Virulence and Possibilities for Its Control. *Cold Spring Harb. Perspect. Med.* **2012**, *2*, a012427. [CrossRef] [PubMed]
3. Bassler, B.; Losick, R. Bacterially Speaking. *Cell* **2006**, *125*, 237–246. [CrossRef] [PubMed]
4. Passador, L.; Cook, J.; Gambello, M.; Rust, L.; Iglewski, B. Expression of Pseudomonas aeruginosa virulence genes requires cell-to-cell communication. *Science* **1993**, *260*, 1127–1130. [CrossRef]
5. Ochsner, U.A.; Reiser, J. Autoinducer-mediated regulation of rhamnolipid biosurfactant synthesis in Pseudomonas aeruginosa. *Proc. Natl. Acad. Sci. USA* **1995**, *92*, 6424–6428. [CrossRef]
6. Singh, P.K.; Schaefer, A.L.; Parsek, M.R.; Moninger, T.O.; Welsh, M.J.; Greenberg, E.P. Quorum-sensing signals indicate that cystic fibrosis lungs are infected with bacterial biofilms. *Nature* **2000**, *407*, 762–764. [CrossRef]
7. Vannini, A.; Volpari, C.; Gargioli, C.; Muraglia, E.; Cortese, R.; De Francesco, R.; Neddermann, P.; Di Marco, S. The crystal structure of the quorum sensing protein TraR bound to its autoinducer and target DNA. *EMBO J.* **2002**, *21*, 4393–4401. [CrossRef]
8. Hanzelka, B.L.; Greenberg, E.P. Evidence that the N-terminal region of the Vibrio fischeri LuxR protein constitutes an autoinducer-binding domain. *J. Bacteriol.* **1995**, *177*, 815–817. [CrossRef]
9. Stevens, A.M.; Dolan, K.M.; Greenberg, E.P. Synergistic binding of the Vibrio fischeri LuxR transcriptional activator domain and RNA polymerase to the lux promoter region. *Proc. Natl. Acad. Sci. USA* **1994**, *91*, 12619–12623. [CrossRef]
10. Chai, Y.; Winans, S.C. Site-directed mutagenesis of a LuxR-type quorum-sensing transcription factor: Alteration of autoinducer specificity. *Mol. Microbiol.* **2004**, *51*, 765–776. [CrossRef]
11. Choi, S.H.; Greenberg, E.P. The C-terminal region of the Vibrio fischeri LuxR protein contains an inducer-independent lux gene activating domain. *Proc. Natl. Acad. Sci. USA* **1991**, *88*, 11115–11119. [CrossRef] [PubMed]
12. Kiratisin, P.; Tucker, K.D.; Passador, L. LasR, a Transcriptional Activator of Pseudomonas aeruginosa Virulence Genes, Functions as a Multimer. *J. Bacteriol.* **2002**, *184*, 4912–4919. [CrossRef] [PubMed]
13. Lamb, J.R.; Patel, H.; Montminy, T.; Wagner, V.E.; Iglewski, B.H. FunctionalDomains of the RhlR Transcriptional Regulator ofPseudomonasaeruginosa. *J. Bacteriol.* **2003**, *185*, 7129–7139. [CrossRef] [PubMed]
14. Luo, Z.-Q.; Smyth, A.J.; Gao, P.; Qin, Y.; Farrand, S.K. Mutational Analysis of TraR. *J. Boil. Chem.* **2003**, *278*, 13173–13182. [CrossRef] [PubMed]
15. Shadel, G.S.; Young, R.F.; Baldwin, T.O. Use of regulated cell lysis in a lethal genetic selection in Escherichia coli: Identification of the autoinducer-binding region of the LuxR protein from Vibrio fischeri ATCC 7744. *J. Bacteriol.* **1990**, *172*, 3980–3987. [CrossRef] [PubMed]
16. Slock, J.; VanRiet, D.; Kolibachuk, D.; Greenberg, E.P. Critical regions of the Vibrio fischeri luxR protein defined by mutational analysis. *J. Bacteriol.* **1990**, *172*, 3974–3979. [CrossRef]
17. Zhang, R.-G.; Pappas, K.M.; Brace, J.L.; Miller, P.C.; Oulmassov, T.; Molyneaux, J.M.; Anderson, J.C.; Bashkin, J.K.; Winans, S.C.; Joachimiak, A. Structure of a bacterial quorum-sensing transcription factor complexed with pheromone and DNA. *Nature* **2002**, *417*, 971–974. [CrossRef]
18. Müh, U.; Hare, B.J.; Duerkop, B.A.; Schuster, M.; Hanzelka, B.L.; Heim, R.; Olson, E.R.; Greenberg, E.P. A structurally unrelated mimic of a Pseudomonas aeruginosa acyl-homoserine lactone quorum-sensing signal. *Proc. Natl. Acad. Sci. USA* **2006**, *103*, 16948–16952. [CrossRef]
19. Koch, B.; Liljefors, T.; Persson, T.; Nielsen, J.; Kjelleberg, S.; Givskov, M. The LuxR receptor: The sites of interaction with quorum-sensing signals and inhibitors. *Microbiology* **2005**, *151*, 3589–3602. [CrossRef]
20. Ding, X.; Yin, B.; Qian, L.; Zeng, Z.; Yang, Z.; Li, H.; Lu, Y.; Zhou, S. Screening for novel quorum-sensing inhibitors to interfere with the formation of Pseudomonas aeruginosa biofilm. *J. Med. Microbiol.* **2011**, *60*, 1827–1834. [CrossRef]
21. Grandclément, C.; Tannières, M.; Moréra, S.; Dessaux, Y.; Faure, D. Quorum quenching: Role in nature and applied developments. *FEMS Microbiol. Rev.* **2015**, *40*, 86–116. [CrossRef] [PubMed]

22. Martin, C.A.; Hoven, A.D.; Cook, A.M. Therapeutic frontiers: Preventing and treating infectious diseases by inhibiting bacterial quorum sensing. *Eur. J. Clin. Microbiol. Infect. Dis.* **2008**, *27*, 635–642. [CrossRef] [PubMed]

23. Kociolek, M. Quorum-Sensing Inhibitors and Biofilms. *Anti Infect. Agents Med. Chem.* **2009**, *8*, 315–326. [CrossRef]

24. Choudhary, S.; Schmidt-Dannert, C. Applications of quorum sensing in biotechnology. *Appl. Microbiol. Biotechnol.* **2010**, *86*, 1267–1279. [CrossRef]

25. Clatworthy, A.E.; Pierson, E.; Hung, D.T. Targeting virulence: A new paradigm for antimicrobial therapy. *Nat. Methods* **2007**, *3*, 541–548. [CrossRef]

26. Kalia, V.C. Quorum sensing inhibitors: An overview. *Biotechnol. Adv.* **2013**, *31*, 224–245. [CrossRef]

27. Chen, F.; Gao, Y.; Chen, X.; Yu, Z.; Li, X. Quorum Quenching Enzymes and Their Application in Degrading Signal Molecules to Block Quorum Sensing-Dependent Infection. *Int. J. Mol. Sci.* **2013**, *14*, 17477–17500. [CrossRef]

28. Wang, Z.; Yu, P.; Zhang, G.; Xu, L.; Wang, D.; Wang, L.; Zeng, X.; Wang, Y. Design, synthesis and antibacterial activity of novel andrographolide derivatives. *Bioorg. Med. Chem.* **2010**, *18*, 4269–4274. [CrossRef]

29. Qin, X.; Thota, G.K.; Singh, R.; Balamurugan, R.; Goycoolea, F.M. Synthetic homoserine lactone analogues as antagonists of bacterial quorum sensing. *Bioorg. Chem.* **2020**, *98*, 103698. [CrossRef]

30. Yang, L.; Rybtke, M.T.; Jakobsen, T.H.; Hentzer, M.; Bjarnsholt, T.; Givskov, M.; Tolker-Nielsen, T. Computer-Aided Identification of Recognised Drugs as Pseudomonas aeruginosa Quorum-Sensing Inhibitors. *Antimicrob. Agents Chemother.* **2009**, *53*, 2432–2443. [CrossRef]

31. Zeng, Z.; Qian, L.; Cao, L.; Tan, H.; Huang, Y.; Xue, X.; Shen, Y.; Zhou, S. Virtual screening for novel quorum sensing inhibitors to eradicate biofilm formation of Pseudomonas aeruginosa. *Appl. Microbiol. Biotechnol.* **2008**, *79*, 119–126. [CrossRef] [PubMed]

32. Annapoorani, A.; Umamageswaran, V.; Parameswari, R.; Pandian, S.K.; Ravi, A.V. Computational discovery of putative quorum sensing inhibitors against LasR and RhlR receptor proteins of Pseudomonas aeruginosa. *J. Comput. Mol. Des.* **2012**, *26*, 1067–1077. [CrossRef] [PubMed]

33. Tan, S.Y.-Y.; Chua, S.L.; Chen, Y.; Rice, S.A.; Kjelleberg, S.; Nielsen, T.E.; Yang, L.; Givskov, M. Identification of Five Structurally Unrelated Quorum-Sensing Inhibitors of Pseudomonas aeruginosa from a Natural-Derivative Database. *Antimicrob. Agents Chemother.* **2013**, *57*, 5629–5641. [CrossRef] [PubMed]

34. Goodford, P.J. A Computational procedure for determining energetically favorable binding sites on biologically important macromolecules. *J. Med. Chem.* **1985**, *28*, 849–857. [CrossRef] [PubMed]

35. Carosati, E.; Sciabola, S.; Cruciani, G. Hydrogen Bonding Interactions of Covalently Bonded Fluorine Atoms: From Crystallographic Data to a New Angular Function in the GRID Force Field. *J. Med. Chem.* **2004**, *47*, 5114–5125. [CrossRef] [PubMed]

36. Ahlström, M.M.; Ridderström, M.; Luthman, A.K.; Zamora, I. Virtual Screening and Scaffold Hopping Based on GRID Molecular Interaction Fields. *J. Chem. Inf. Model.* **2005**, *45*, 1313–1323. [CrossRef]

37. Sciabola, S.; Stanton, R.V.; Mills, J.E.; Flocco, M.M.; Baroni, M.; Cruciani, G.; Perruccio, F.; Mason, J.S. High-Throughput Virtual Screening of Proteins Using GRID Molecular Interaction Fields. *J. Chem. Inf. Model.* **2009**, *50*, 155–169. [CrossRef]

38. Sanjurjo, C.V.; Engwer, C.; Qin, X.; Hembach, L.; Verdía-Cotelo, T.; Remuñán-López, C.; Vila-Sanjurjo, A.; Goycoolea, F.M. A single intracellular protein governs the critical transition from an individual to a coordinated population response during quorum sensing: Origins of primordial language. *bioRxiv* **2016**, 074369. [CrossRef]

39. Skandamis, P.N.; Nychas, G.-J. Quorum Sensing in the Context of Food Microbiology. *Appl. Environ. Microbiol.* **2012**, *78*, 5473–5482. [CrossRef]

40. Galloway, W.R.; Hodgkinson, J.T.; Bowden, S.; Welch, M.; Spring, D.R. Applications of small molecule activators and inhibitors of quorum sensing in Gram-negative bacteria. *Trends Microbiol.* **2012**, *20*, 449–458. [CrossRef]

41. Takano, E. γ-Butyrolactones: Streptomyces signalling molecules regulating antibiotic production and differentiation. *Curr. Opin. Microbiol.* **2006**, *9*, 287–294. [CrossRef] [PubMed]

42. Gram, L.; De Nys, R.; Maximilien, R.; Givskov, M.; Steinberg, P.; Kjelleberg, S. Inhibitory Effects of Secondary Metabolites from the Red Alga Delisea pulchra on Swarming Motility of Proteus mirabilis. *Appl. Environ.*

Microbiol. **1996**, *62*, 4284–4287. [CrossRef] [PubMed]

43. Givskov, M.; De Nys, R.; Manefield, M.; Gram, L.; Maximilien, R.; Eberl, L.; Molin, S.; Steinberg, P.; Kjelleberg, S. Eukaryotic interference with homoserine lactone-mediated prokaryotuc signalling. *J. Bacteriol.* **1996**, *178*, 6618–6622. [CrossRef] [PubMed]

44. Manefield, M.; De Nys, R.; Naresh, K.; Roger, R.; Givskov, M.; Peter, S.; Kjelleberg, S. Evidence that halogenated furanones from Delisea pulchra inhibit acylated homoserine lactone (AHL)-mediated gene expression by displacing the AHL signal from its receptor protein. *Microbiology* **1999**, *145*, 283–291. [CrossRef] [PubMed]

45. Ren, D.; Sims, J.J.; Wood, T.K. Inhibition of biofilm formation and swarming of Escherichia coli by (5Z)-4-bromo-5-(bromomethylene)-3-butyl-2(5H)-furanone. *Environ. Microbiol.* **2001**, *3*, 731–736. [CrossRef]

46. Defoirdt, T.; Miyamoto, C.M.; Wood, T.K.; Meighen, E.A.; Sorgeloos, P.; Verstraete, W.; Bossier, P. The natural furanone (5Z)-4-bromo-5-(bromomethylene)-3-butyl-2(5H)-furanone disrupts quorum sensing-regulated gene expression in Vibrio harveyi by decreasing the DNA-binding activity of the transcriptional regulator protein luxR. *Environ. Microbiol.* **2007**, *9*, 2486–2495. [CrossRef]

47. Lönn-Stensrud, J.; Landin, M.A.; Benneche, T.; Petersen, F.C.; Scheie, A.A. Furanones, potential agents for preventing Staphylococcus epidermidis biofilm infections? *J. Antimicrob. Chemother.* **2009**, *63*, 309–316. [CrossRef]

48. Hentzer, M.; Wu, H.; Andersen, J.B.; Riedel, K.; Rasmussen, T.B.; Bagge, N.; Kumar, N.; Schembri, M.A.; Song, Z.; Kristoffersen, P.; et al. Attenuation of Pseudomonas aeruginosa virulence by quorum sensing inhibitors. *EMBO J.* **2003**, *22*, 3803–3815. [CrossRef]

49. Manefield, M.; Rasmussen, T.B.; Henzter, M.; Andersen, J.B.; Steinberg, P.; Kjelleberg, S.; Givskov, M. Halogenated furanones inhibit quorum sensing through accelerated LuxR turnover. *Microbiology* **2002**, *148*, 1119–1127. [CrossRef]

50. Steenackers, H.P.; Levin, J.; Janssens, J.C.; De Weerdt, A.; Balzarini, J.; Vanderleyden, J.; De Vos, D.E.; De Keersmaecker, S.C.J. Structure–activity relationship of brominated 3-alkyl-5-methylene-2(5H)-furanones and alkylmaleic anhydrides as inhibitors of Salmonella biofilm formation and quorum sensing regulated bioluminescence in Vibrio harveyi. *Bioorganic Med. Chem.* **2010**, *18*, 5224–5233. [CrossRef]

51. Janssens, J.C.A.; Steenackers, H.; Robijns, S.; Gellens, E.; Levin, J.; Zhao, H.; Hermans, K.; De Coster, D.; Verhoeven, T.L.; Marchal, K.; et al. Brominated Furanones Inhibit Biofilm Formation by Salmonella enterica Serovar Typhimurium. *Appl. Environ. Microbiol.* **2008**, *74*, 6639–6648. [CrossRef] [PubMed]

52. Ponnusamy, K.; Paul, D.; Kweon, J.H. Inhibition of Quorum Sensing Mechanism andAeromonas hydrophilaBiofilm Formation by Vanillin. *Environ. Eng. Sci.* **2009**, *26*, 1359–1363. [CrossRef]

53. Niu, C.; Afre, S.; Gilbert, E.S. Subinhibitory concentrations of cinnamaldehyde interfere with quorum sensing. *Lett. Appl. Microbiol.* **2006**, *43*, 489–494. [CrossRef] [PubMed]

54. Brackman, G.; Defoirdt, T.; Miyamoto, C.; Bossier, P.; Van Calenbergh, S.; Nelis, H.J.; Coenye, T. Cinnamaldehyde and cinnamaldehyde derivatives reduce virulence in Vibrio spp. by decreasing the DNA-binding activity of the quorum sensing response regulator LuxR. *BMC Microbiol.* **2008**, *8*, 149. [CrossRef] [PubMed]

55. Chang, C.-Y.; Krishnan, T.; Wang, H.; Chen, Y.; Yin, W.-F.; Chong, Y.-M.; Tan, L.Y.; Chong, T.M.; Chan, K.-G. Non-antibiotic quorum sensing inhibitors acting against N-acyl homoserine lactone synthase as druggable target. *Sci. Rep.* **2014**, *4*, 7245. [CrossRef] [PubMed]

56. Furuya, T.; Arai, Y.; Kino, K. Biotechnological Production of Caffeic Acid by Bacterial Cytochrome P450 CYP199A2. *Appl. Environ. Microbiol.* **2012**, *78*, 6087–6094. [CrossRef]

57. Hayman, M.; Kam, P.C. Capsaicin: A review of its pharmacology and clinical applications. *Curr. Anaesth. Crit. Care* **2008**, *19*, 338–343. [CrossRef]

58. Jones, N.L.; Shabib, S.; Sherman, P.M. Capsaicin as an inhibitor of the growth of the gastric pathogen Helicobacter pylori. *FEMS Microbiol. Lett.* **1997**, *146*, 223–227. [CrossRef]

59. Zeyrek, F.Y.; Oguz, E. In vitro activity of capsaicin against Helicobacter pylori. *Ann. Microbiol.* **2005**, *55*, 125–127.

60. Lee, H.S.; Lee, S.Y.; Park, S.H.; Lee, J.H.; Ahn, S.K.; Choi, Y.M.; Choi, D.J.; Chang, J.-H. Antimicrobial medical sutures with caffeic acid phenethyl ester and their in vitro/in vivo biological assessment. *MedChemComm* **2013**, *4*, 777. [CrossRef]

61. Murtaza, G.; Karim, S.; Akram, M.R.; Khan, S.A.; Azhar, S.; Mumtaz, A.; Bin Asad, M.H.H. Caffeic Acid

Phenethyl Ester and Therapeutic Potentials. *BioMed Res. Int.* **2014**, *2014*, 1–9. [CrossRef] [PubMed]

62. Norizan, S.N.M.; Yin, W.-F.; Chan, K.-G. Caffeine as a Potential Quorum Sensing Inhibitor. *Sensors* **2013**, *13*, 5117–5129. [CrossRef]

63. Koo, H.-J.; Song, Y.S.; Kim, H.-J.; Lee, Y.-H.; Hong, S.-M.; Lim, S.-J.; Kim, B.-C.; Jin, C.; Lim, C.-J.; Park, E.-H. Anti-inflammatory effects of genipin, an active principle of gardenia. *Eur. J. Pharmacol.* **2004**, *495*, 201–208. [CrossRef] [PubMed]

64. Kim, B.-C.; Kim, H.-G.; Lee, S.-A.; Lim, S.; Park, E.-H.; Kim, S.-J.; Lim, C.-J. Genipin-induced apoptosis in hepatoma cells is mediated by reactive oxygen species/c-Jun NH2-terminal kinase-dependent activation of mitochondrial pathway. *Biochem. Pharmacol.* **2005**, *70*, 1398–1407. [CrossRef] [PubMed]

65. Sanjurjo, C.V.; David, L.; Remuñán-López, C.; Goycoolea, F.M.; Vila-Sanjurjo, A. Effect of the ultrastructure of chitosan nanoparticles in colloidal stability, quorum quenching and antibacterial activities. *J. Colloid Interface Sci.* **2019**, *556*, 592–605. [CrossRef] [PubMed]

66. Lin, Y.-H.; Tsai, S.-C.; Lai, C.-H.; Lee, C.-H.; He, Z.S.; Tseng, G.-C. Genipin-cross-linked fucose–chitosan/heparin nanoparticles for the eradication of Helicobacter pylori. *Biomaterials* **2013**, *34*, 4466–4479. [CrossRef]

67. Hwang, Y.-J.; Larsen, J.; Krasieva, T.B.; Lyubovitsky, J.G. Effect of Genipin Crosslinking on the Optical Spectral Properties and Structures of Collagen Hydrogels. *ACS Appl. Mater. Interfaces* **2011**, *3*, 2579–2584. [CrossRef]

68. Canton, B.; Labno, A.; Endy, D. Refinement and standardisation of synthetic biological parts and devices. *Nat. Biotechnol.* **2008**, *26*, 787–793. [CrossRef]

69. Pe'delacq, J.-D.; Cabantous, S.; Tran, T.; Terwilliger, T.C.; Waldo, G.S. Corrigendum: Engineering and characterisation of a superfolder green fluorescent protein. *Nat. Biotechnol.* **2006**, *24*, 1170. [CrossRef]

70. Lin, J.-S.; Cheng, J.; Wang, Y.; Shen, X. The Pseudomonas Quinolone Signal (PQS): Not Just for Quorum Sensing Anymore. *Front. Microbiol.* **2018**, *8*. [CrossRef]

71. Price-Whelan, A.; Dietrich, L.E.; Newman, D.K. Rethinking 'secondary' metabolism: Physiological roles for phenazine antibiotics. *Nat. Methods* **2006**, *2*, 71–78. [CrossRef] [PubMed]

72. Pesci, E.C.; Milbank, J.B.J.; Pearson, J.P.; McKnight, S.; Kende, A.S.; Greenberg, E.P.; Iglewski, B.H. Quinolone signaling in the cell-to-cell communication system of Pseudomonas aeruginosa. *Proc. Natl. Acad. Sci. USA* **1999**, *96*, 11229–11234. [CrossRef] [PubMed]

73. McKnight, S.L.; Iglewski, B.H.; Pesci, E.C. The Pseudomonas Quinolone Signal Regulates rhl Quorum Sensing in Pseudomonas aeruginosa. *J. Bacteriol.* **2000**, *182*, 2702–2708. [CrossRef] [PubMed]

74. Mukherjee, S.; Moustafa, D.A.; Stergioula, V.; Smith, C.D.; Goldberg, J.B.; Bassler, B. The PqsE and RhlR proteins are an autoinducer synthase–receptor pair that control virulence and biofilm development in Pseudomonas aeruginosa. *Proc. Natl. Acad. Sci. USA* **2018**, *115*, E9411–E9418. [CrossRef] [PubMed]

75. Mahajan-Miklos, S.; Tan, M.; Rahme, L.G.; Ausubel, F.M. Molecular Mechanisms of Bacterial Virulence Elucidated Using a Pseudomonas aeruginosa– Caenorhabditis elegans Pathogenesis Model. *Cell* **1999**, *96*, 47–56. [CrossRef]

76. Dietrich, L.E.; Price-Whelan, A.; Petersen, A.; Whiteley, M.; Newman, D.K. The phenazine pyocyanin is a terminal signalling factor in the quorum sensing network of Pseudomonas aeruginosa. *Mol. Microbiol.* **2006**, *61*, 1308–1321. [CrossRef]

77. Seo, S.; Gao, Y.; Kim, N.; Szubin, R.; Yang, J.; Cho, B.-K.; Palsson, B.O. Revealing genome-scale transcriptional regulatory landscape of OmpR highlights its expanded regulatory roles under osmotic stress in Escherichia coli K-12 MG1655. *Sci. Rep.* **2017**, *7*, 2181. [CrossRef]

78. Jagmann, N.; Brachvogel, H.-P.; Philipp, B. Parastic growth of Pseudomonas aeruginosa in co-culture with the chitinolytic bacterium Aeromonas hydrophila. *Environ. Microbiol.* **2010**, *12*, 1787–1802. [CrossRef]

79. Bou-Abdallah, F.; Chasteen, N.D.; Lesser, M.P. Quenching of superoxide radicals by green fluorecent protein. *Biochim. Biophys. Acta* **2006**, *1760*, 1960–1965.

80. Mavrodi, D.V.; Bonsall, R.F.; Delaney, S.M.; Soule, M.J.; Phillips, G.; Thomashow, L.S. Functional Analysis of Genes for Biosynthesis of Pyocyanin and Phenazine-1-Carboxamide from Pseudomonas aeruginosa PAO1. *J. Bacteriol.* **2001**, *183*, 6454–6465. [CrossRef]

81. Haynes, W.C.; Stodola, F.H.; Locke, J.M.; Pridham, T.G.; Conway, H.F.; Sohns, V.E.; Jackson, R.W. PSEUDOMONAS AUREOFACIENS KLUYVER AND PHENAZINE α-CARBOXYLIC ACID, ITS

CHARACTERISTIC PIGMENT. *J. Bacteriol.* **1956**, *72*, 412–417. [CrossRef] [PubMed]

82.   Mazzola, M.; Cook, R.J.; Thomashow, L.S.; Weller, D.M.; Pierson, L.S. Contribution of phenazine antibiotic biosynthesis to the ecological competence of fluorescent pseudomonads in soil habitats. *Appl. Environ. Microbiol.* **1992**, *58*, 2616–2624. [CrossRef]

83.   Wang, Y.; Wilks, J.C.; Danhorn, T.; Ramos, I.; Croal, L.; Newman, D.K. Phenazine-1-Carboxylic Acid Promotes Bacterial Biofilm Development via Ferrous Iron Acquisition. *J. Bacteriol.* **2011**, *193*, 3606–3617. [CrossRef]

84.   Pierson, L.S.; Pierson, E.A. Metabolism and function of phenazines in bacteria: Impacts on the behavior of bacteria in the environment and biotechnological processes. *Appl. Microbiol. Biotechnol.* **2010**, *86*, 1659–1670. [CrossRef] [PubMed]

85.   Hassett, D.J.; Ma, J.-F.; Elkins, J.G.; McDermott, T.R.; Ochsner, U.A.; West, S.E.H.; Huang, C.-T.; Fredericks, J.; Burnett, S.; Stewart, P.S.; et al. Quorum sensing in Pseudomonas aeruginosa controls expression of catalase and superoxide dismutase genes and mediates biofilm susceptibility to hydrogen peroxide. *Mol. Microbiol.* **1999**, *34*, 1082–1093. [CrossRef] [PubMed]

86.   Morales, D.K.; Grahl, N.; Okegbe, C.; Dietrich, L.E.; Jacobs, N.J.; Hogan, D.A. Control of Candida albicans Metabolism and Biofilm Formation by Pseudomonas aeruginosa Phenazines. *mBio* **2013**, *4*, 00526-12. [CrossRef] [PubMed]

87.   Skindersoe, M.E.; Alhede, M.; Phipps, R.; Yang, L.; Jensen, P.Ø.; Rasmussen, T.B.; Bjarnsholt, T.; Tolker-Nielsen, T.; Høiby, N.; Givskov, M. Effects of Antibiotics on Quorum Sensing in Pseudomonas aeruginosa. *Antimicrob. Agents Chemother.* **2008**, *52*, 3648–3663. [CrossRef] [PubMed]

88.   Schertzer, J.W.; Boulette, M.L.; Whiteley, M. More than a signal: Non-signaling properties of quorum sensing molecules. *Trends Microbiol.* **2009**, *17*, 189–195. [CrossRef]

89.   Kubo, I.; Fujita, K.-I.; Lee, S.H.; Ha, T.J. Antibacterial activity of polygodial. *Phytother. Res.* **2005**, *19*, 1013–1017. [CrossRef]

90.   Wang, X.; Yao, X.; Zhu, Z.-A.; Tang, T.; Dai, K.; Sadovskaya, I.; Flahaut, S.; Jabbouri, S. Effect of berberine on Staphylococcus epidermidis biofilm formation. *Int. J. Antimicrob. Agents* **2009**, *34*, 60–66. [CrossRef]

91.   Sun, T.; Li, X.-D.; Hong, J.; Liu, C.; Zhang, X.-L.; Zheng, J.-P.; Xu, Y.-J.; Ou, Z.-Y.; Zheng, J.-L.; Yu, D.-J. Inhibitory Effect of Two Traditional Chinese Medicine Monomers, Berberine and Matrine, on the Quorum Sensing System of Antimicrobial-Resistant Escherichia coli. *Front. Microbiol.* **2019**, *10*, 2584. [CrossRef] [PubMed]

92.   Aswathanarayan, J.B.; Vittal, R.R. Inhibition of biofilm formation and quorum sensing mediated phenotypes by berberine in Pseudomonas aeruginosa and Salmonella typhimurium. *RSC Adv.* **2018**, *8*, 36133–36141. [CrossRef]

93.   Eiden, F.; Wendt, R.; Fenner, H. ChemInform Abstract: PYRONES AND PYRIDONES, PART 74. QUINOLYLIDENE DERIVATIVES. *Chem. Informationsdienst* **1978**, *9*, 561–568. [CrossRef]

94.   Evans, D.; Eastwood, F. Synthesis of an arylhydroxytetronimide and of 3-Hydroxy-4(1H)-quinolone derivatives. *Aust. J. Chem.* **1974**, *27*, 537. [CrossRef]

95.   Cornforth, J.W.; James, A.T. Structure of a naturally occurring antagonist of dihydrostreptomycin. *Biochem. J.* **1956**, *63*, 124–130. [CrossRef] [PubMed]

Permissions

List of Contributors

Pál Herczegh and Anikó Borbás
Department of Pharmaceutical Chemistry, University of Debrecen, Egyetem tér 1, H-4032 Debrecen, Hungary

Zsolt Szűcs
Department of Pharmaceutical Chemistry, University of Debrecen, Egyetem tér 1, H-4032 Debrecen, Hungary
Doctoral School of Pharmaceutical Sciences, University of Debrecen, Egyetem tér 1, H-4032 Debrecen, Hungary

Lieve Naesens and Annelies Stevaert
Rega Institute for Medical Research, KU Leuven, B-3000 Leuven, Belgium

Eszter Ostorházi
Department of Medical Microbiology, Semmelweis University, Nagyvárad tér 4, H-1089 Budapest, Hungary

Gyula Batta
Department of Organic Chemistry, University of Debrecen, H-4032 Debrecen, Hungary

Surendra Babu Lagu and Rajendra Prasad Yejella
Department of Pharmaceutical Sciences, Pharmaceutical Chemistry Division, A.U. College of Pharmaceutical Sciences, Andhra University, Visakhapatnam 530003, Andhra Pradesh, India

Richie R. Bhandare
Department of Pharmaceutical Sciences, College of Pharmacy & Health Sciences, Ajman University, UAE

Afzal B. Shaik
Department of Pharmaceutical Chemistry, Vignan Pharmacy College, Vadlamudi 522213, Andhra Pradesh, India

Kyriaki Marina Lyra, Katerina N. Panagiotaki, Aggeliki Papavasiliou, Elias Sakellis, Sergios Papageorgiou, Fotios K. Katsaros and Zili Sideratou
Institute of Nanoscience and Nanotechnology, National Centre of Scientific Research "Demokritos", 15310 Aghia Paraskevi, Greece

Nikolaos S. Heliopoulos
Institute of Nanoscience and Nanotechnology, National Centre of Scientific Research "Demokritos", 15310 Aghia Paraskevi, Greece
Department of Industrial Design & Production Engineering, University of West Attica, 12241 Egaleo, Attiki, Greece

Kostas Stamatakis
Institute of Biosciences and Applications, National Centre of Scientific Research "Demokritos", 15310 Aghia Paraskevi, Greece

Georgia Kythreoti
Institute of Nanoscience and Nanotechnology, National Centre of Scientific Research "Demokritos", 15310 Aghia Paraskevi, Greece
Institute of Biosciences and Applications, National Centre of Scientific Research "Demokritos", 15310 Aghia Paraskevi, Greece

Antonios Kouloumpis and Dimitrios Gournis
Department of Material Science & Engineering, University of Ioannina, 45110 Ioannina, Greece

Hang Yeon Jeong, Tae Ho Lee, Ju Gyeong Kim and Jae-Hak Moon
Department of Food Science and Technology, Chonnam National University, 77 Yongbongro, Gwangju 61186, Korea

Sueun Lee and Changjong Moon
Department of Veterinary Anatomy, College of Veterinary Medicine and BK21 FOUR Program, Chonnam National University, Gwangju 61186, Korea

Xuan Trong Truong and Tae-Il Jeon
Department of Animal Science, Chonnam National University, Gwangju 61186, Korea

Adriana Valls, Jose J. Andreu, Eva Falomir, Santiago V. Luis and Belén Altava
Departamento de Química Inorgánica y Orgánica, Universitat Jaume I, Av. Sos Baynat s/n, 12071 Castellón, Spain

Elena Atrián-Blasco and Scott G. Mitchell
Instituto de Nanociencia y Materiales de Aragón (INMA), Consejo Superior de Investigaciones Científicas-Universidad de Zaragoza, 50009 Zaragoza, Spain
CIBER de Bioingeniería, Biomateriales y Nanomedicina, Instituto de Salud Carlos III, 28029 Madrid, Spain

Luís M. T. Frija and Armando J. L. Pombeiro
Centro de Química Estrutural (CQE), Instituto Superior Técnico, Universidade de Lisboa, Av. Rovisco Pais, 1049-001 Lisboa, Portugal

Epole Ntungwe and Joana M. Andrade
CBIOS—Research Center for Health Sciences & Technologies, ULusófona de Humanidades e Tecnologias, Campo Grande 376, 1749-024 Lisboa, Portugal

Przemysław Sitarek
Department of Biology and Pharmaceutical Botany, Medical University of Lodz, Muszy´nskiego Street 1, 90-151 Łód´z, Poland

Monika Toma and Tomasz Śliwiński
Laboratory of Medical Genetics, Faculty of Biology and Environmental Protection, University of Lodz, 90-151 Lodz, Poland

Lília Cabral and M. Lurdes S. Cristiano
Department of Chemistry and Pharmacy (FCT) and Center of Marine Sciences (CCMar), Universidade do Algarve, P-8005-039 Faro, Portugal

Patrícia Rijo
CBIOS—Research Center for Health Sciences & Technologies, ULusófona de Humanidades e Tecnologias, Campo Grande 376, 1749-024 Lisboa, Portugal
iMed.ULisboa - Research Institute for Medicines, Faculdade de Farmácia, Universidade de Lisboa, Av. Prof. Gama Pinto, 1649-003 Lisboa, Portugal

Irene Magnifico, Giulio Petronio Petronio, Noemi Venditti, Marco Alfio Cutuli, Laura Pietrangelo and Roberto Di Marco
Department of Health and Medical Sciences "V. Tiberio" Università degli Studi del Molise, 8600 Campobasso, Italy

Franca Vergalito
Department of Agricultural, Environmental and Food Sciences (DiAAA), Università degli Studi del Molise, 86100 Campobasso, Italy

Katia Mangano
Department of Biomedical and Biotechnological Sciences, Universitá degli Studi di Catania, 95123 Catania, Italy

Davide Zella
Department of Biochemistry and Molecular Biology, School of Medicine, Institute of Human Virology, University of Maryland, Baltimore, MD 21201, USA

Volodymyr Horishny
Department of Chemistry, Danylo Halytsky Lviv National Medical University, Pekarska 69, 79010 Lviv, Ukraine

Victor Kartsev
InterBioScreen, 142432 Chernogolovka, Moscow Region, Russia

Vasyl Matiychuk
Department of Chemistry, Ivan Franko National University of Lviv, Kyryla i Mefodia 6, 79005 Lviv, Ukraine

Athina Geronikaki and Petrou Anthi
School of Pharmacy, Aristotle University of Thessaloniki, 54124 Thessaloniki, Greece

Pavel Pogodin and Vladimir Poroikov
Institute of Biomedical Chemistry, Pogodinskaya Street 10 Bldg.8, 119121 Moscow, Russia

Marija Ivanov, Marina Kostic and Marina D. Soković
Mycological Laboratory, Department of Plant Physiology, Institute for Biological Research, Siniša, Stanković-National Institute of Republic of Serbia, University of Belgrade, Bulevar Despota Stefana 142, 11000 Belgrade, Serbia

Phaedra Eleftheriou
Department of Biomedical Sciences, School of Health Sciences, International Hellenic University, Sindos, 57400 Thessaloniki, Greece

Sam Woong Kim, Song I. Kang, Da Hye Shin and Se Yun Oh
Gene Analysis Center, Gyeongnam National University of Science & Technology, Jinju 52725, Korea

Chae Won Lee, Yoonyong Yang, Youn Kyoung Son, Hee-Sun Yang, Byoung-Hee Lee and Woo Young Bang
National Institute of Biological Resources (NIBR), Environmental Research Complex, Incheon 22689, Korea

Hee-Jung An
Department of Pathology, CHA Bundang Medical Center, CHA University, Seongnam 13496, Korea

In Sil Jeong
Center for Immune Cell Research, CHA Advanced Research Institute, Seongnam 13488, Korea

Maikel Wijtmans and Iwan J. P. de Esch
Division of Medicinal Chemistry, Amsterdam Institute of Molecular and Life Sciences (AIMMS), Faculty of Science, Vrije Universiteit Amsterdam, De Boelelaan 1108, 1081 HZ Amsterdam, The Netherlands

Péter Ábrányi-Balogh, Aaron Keeley, László Petri and György Miklós Keserű
Medicinal Chemistry Research Group, Research Centre for Natural Sciences, Magyar tudósok krt 2, H-1117 Budapest, Hungary

David J. Hamilton
Division of Medicinal Chemistry, Amsterdam Institute of Molecular and Life Sciences (AIMMS), Faculty of Science, Vrije Universiteit Amsterdam, De Boelelaan 1108, 1081 HZ Amsterdam, The Netherlands
Medicinal Chemistry Research Group, Research Centre for Natural Sciences, Magyar tudósok krt 2, H-1117 Budapest, Hungary

Martina Hrast and Stanislav Gobec
Faculty of Pharmacy, University of Ljubljana, Ašker̆ceva 7, SI-1000 Ljubljana, Slovenia

Tímea Imre
MS Metabolomics Research Group, Research Centre for Natural Sciences, Magyar tudósok krt 2, H-1117 Budapest, Hungary

Munirah A. Almessiere
Department of Biophysics, Institute for Research & Medical Consultations (IRMC), Imam Abdulrahman Bin Faisal University, Dammam 31441, Saudi Arabia

Reem K. Aldakheel
Department of Biophysics, Institute for Research & Medical Consultations (IRMC), Imam Abdulrahman Bin Faisal University, Dammam 31441, Saudi Arabia
Department of Physics, College of Science, Imam Abdulrahman Bin Faisal University, Dammam 31441, Saudi Arabia

Suriya Rehman
Department of Epidemic Diseases Research, Institute for Research & Medical Consultations (IRMC), Imam Abdulrahman Bin Faisal University, Dammam 31441, Saudi Arabia

Firdos A. Khan
Department of Stem Cell Research, Institute for Research & Medical Consultations (IRMC), Imam Abdulrahman Bin Faisal University, Dammam 31441, Saudi Arabia

Mohammed A. Gondal
Department of Physics, Laser Research Group, King Fahd University of Petroleum & Minerals, Box 372, Dhahran 31261, Saudi Arabia

Ahmed Mostafa
Department of Pharmaceutical Chemistry, College of Clinical Pharmacy, Imam Abdulrahman Bin Faisal University, Dammam 31441, Saudi Arabia

Abdulhadi Baykal
Department of Nanomedicine Research, Institute for Research & Medical Consultations (IRMC), Imam Abdulrahman Bin Faisal University, Dammam 31441, Saudi Arabia

Ana Clara Lopes, Filipa Vaz and Melanie Filipe
School of Health Sciences, Polytechnic Institute of Guarda, Rua da Cadeia, 6300-035 Guarda, Portugal

Márcio Rodrigues, Maximiano P. Ribeiro and Paula Coutinho
School of Health Sciences, Polytechnic Institute of Guarda, Rua da Cadeia, 6300-035 Guarda, Portugal
Research Unit for Inland Development (UDI), Polytechnic Institute of Guarda, Av. Dr. Francisco Sá Carneiro, 50, 6300-559 Guarda, Portugal
CICS-UBI—Health Sciences Research Centre, University of Beira Interior, Av. Infante D. Henrique, 6200-506 Covilhã, Portugal

Gilberto Alves
CICS-UBI—Health Sciences Research Centre, University of Beira Interior, Av. Infante D. Henrique, 6200-506 Covilhã, Portugal

André R. T. S. Araujo
School of Health Sciences, Polytechnic Institute of Guarda, Rua da Cadeia, 6300-035 Guarda, Portugal
Research Unit for Inland Development (UDI), Polytechnic Institute of Guarda, Av. Dr. Francisco Sá Carneiro, 50, 6300-559 Guarda, Portugal
LAQV/REQUIMTE, Department of Chemical Sciences, Faculty of Pharmacy, University of Porto, Rua Jorge Viterbo Ferreira, 228, 4050-313 Porto, Portugal

Xiaofei Qin
Department of Bioengineering, Zhuhai Campus of Zunyi Medical University, Zhuhai 519041, China
Laboratory of Nanobiotechnology, Institute of Plant Biology and Biotechnology, University of Münster, Schlossplatz 8, D-48143 Münster, Germany

Celina Vila-Sanjurjo
Laboratory of Nanobiotechnology, Institute of Plant Biology and Biotechnology, University of Münster, Schlossplatz 8, D-48143 Münster, Germany
Department of Pharmacology, Pharmacy and Pharmaceutical Technology, University of Santiago de Compostela, Campus Vida, s/n, 15782 Santiago de Compostela, Spain

Ratna Singh
Laboratory of Molecular Phytopathology and
Renewable Resources, Institute of Plant Biology and
Biotechnology, University of Münster, Schlossplatz 8,
D-48143 Münster, Germany

Bodo Philipp
Institute of Molecular Microbiology and Biotechnology,
University of Münster, Corrensstraße 3, D-48149
Münster, Germany

Francisco M. Goycoolea
Laboratory of Nanobiotechnology, Institute of Plant
Biology and Biotechnology, University of Münster,
Schlossplatz 8, D-48143 Münster, Germany
School of Food Science and Nutrition, University of
Leeds, Leeds LS2 9JT, UK

Index

Printed in the USA
CPSIA information can be obtained
at www.ICGtesting.com
JSHW051408091023
49903JS00006B/331